616.028

is                                    re

OXFORD MEDICAL PUBLICATIONS

# Emergencies in Critical care

# Emergencies in Critical Care

Edited by

**Martin Beed**
Consultant in Critical Care and Anaesthesia
Nottingham University Hospitals
City Hospital Campus

**Richard Sherman**
Consultant in Critical Care and Anaesthesia
Nottingham University Hospitals
City Hospital Campus

**Ravi Mahajan**
Professor and Honorary Consultant in
Anaesthesia and Intensive Care Medicine
University of Nottingham &
Nottingham University Hospitals
City Hospital Campus

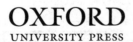

OXFORD
UNIVERSITY PRESS

# OXFORD
UNIVERSITY PRESS

Great Clarendon Street, Oxford OX2 6DP

Oxford University Press is a department of the University of Oxford.
It furthers the University's objective of excellence in research, scholarship,
and education by publishing worldwide in

Oxford New York

Auckland Cape Town Dar es Salaam Hong Kong Karachi
Kuala Lumpur Madrid Melbourne Mexico City Nairobi
New Delhi Shanghai Taipei Toronto

With offices in

Argentina Austria Brazil Chile Czech Republic France Greece
Guatemala Hungary Italy Japan Poland Portugal Singapore
South Korea Switzerland Thailand Turkey Ukraine Vietnam

Oxford is a registered trademark of Oxford University Press
in the UK and in certain other countries.

Published in the United States
by Oxford University Press Inc., New York

British Library Cataloguing in Publication Data
Data available

Library of Congress Cataloging in Publication Data
Data available

Typeset by Newgen Imaging Systems (P) Ltd., Chennai, India
Printed in Italy
on acid-free paper by
Legoprint

ISBN 978–0–19–856824–7 (flexicover: alk.paper)

10 9 8 7 6 5 4 3 2 1

# Preface

This book is intended to aid critical care staff during the management of emergencies in ICU/HDU, from an inexperienced junior doctor to the experienced staff nurse and consultant. Emergencies in critical care are often surprisingly predictable, and the knowledge of who is likely to be at risk, and how they may best be managed within a critical care environment, will provide those involved with the groundwork for a calm rational approach in otherwise stressful situations.

Many common conditions are managed in subtly different ways within a critical care environment, and some are peculiar to ICU (e.g. air-trapping in mechanically ventilated patients). We have tried to include a broad spectrum of diseases and emergencies, and where possible we have summarized those hard-to-remember facts in tables.

Mostly we have tried to keep an 'ABC' theme going through this book. This is not only the standard approach to emergency management, but also a widely used scheme for documenting daily reviews on ICU and for documenting trauma management.

The first half of the book describes the management of emergencies affecting various systems, whilst the second half concentrates on various groups of patients or conditions.

Most chapters begin with a generic description of how to manage emergencies affecting that system or patient group. This is followed by details of specific diagnoses and how they should be managed.

Where possible we have included references to our sister publications, the *Oxford Handbook of Emergencies in Anaesthesia* (OHEA), the *Oxford Handbook of Critical Care* (OHCC), and the *Oxford Handbook of Emergencies in Cardiology* (OHEC).

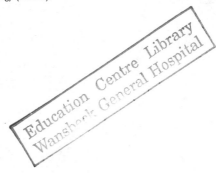

# Contents

# Contributors

**Myles Dowling**
Specialist Registrar in
Anaesthesia and
Intensive Care
Nottingham University
Hospitals

**Dan Harvey**
Specialist Registrar in
Anaesthesia and
Intensive Care
Nottingham University
Hospitals

**Gareth Moncaster**
Specialist Registrar in
Anaesthesia and
Intensive Care
Nottingham University
Hospitals

**Raj Rajendram**
Specialist Registrar in General
Medicine & Intensive Care,
Oxford Deanery

**Andrew Sharman**
Specialist Registrar in
Anaesthesia and
Intensive Care
Nottingham University
Hospitals

**Jonny Wilkinson**
Specialist Registrar in
Anaesthesia and
Intensive Care
Nottingham University
Hospitals

Additional help and advice was
also received from

**Dr Martin Levitt**
Consultant in Anaesthesia and
Intensive Care
City Campus, Nottingham
University Hospitals

**Dr Lina Hijazi**
Consultant in Genito-urinary
and HIV medicine
Whipps Cross Hospital

**Mandy Haughton**
Senior Staff Nurse
specialising in
Critical Care Medicine

**Sandy Whitehead**
Senior Staff Nurse
specialising in
Critical Care Medicine

**Miss Suzanne Wallace**
Specialist Registrar in
Obstetrics and Gynaecology

**Mr Steve Beed**
School Teacher and Artist

# Symbols and abbreviations

| | |
|---|---|
| 2,3 DPG | 2,3-diphosphoglycerate |
| 5HIAA | hydroxy-indole acetic acid |
| βHCG | human chorionic gonadotropin beta-subunit |
| A&E | accident and emergency |
| A-a | alveolar/arterial [oxygen gradient] |
| AAA | abdominal aortic aneurysm |
| ABC | airway, breathing, circulation |
| ABGs | arterial blood gases |
| AC | alternating current |
| ACA | anterior cerebral artery |
| Ach | acetylcholine |
| ACEi | angiotensin converting enzyme inhibitors |
| ACS | abdominal compartment syndrome |
| ACT | activated clotting time |
| ACTH | adrenocorticotropic hormone |
| ADH | anti-diuretic hormone |
| AF | atrial fibrillation |
| AFB | acid fast bacilli |
| AFE | amniotic fluid embolism |
| AIDS | acquired immune deficiency syndrome |
| ALI | acute lung injury |
| ALP | alkaline phosphatase |
| ALS | advanced life support |
| ALT | alanine aminotransferase |
| AMPLE history | allergies, medication, past medical history, last meal, environment |
| ANA | anti-nuclear antibodies |
| ANCA | anti-nuclear cytoplasmic antibodies |
| AP | antero-posterior [X-rays] |
| APACHE (II) | acute physiology and chronic health evaluation [score, version II] |
| APH | ante-partum haemorrhage |
| APP | abdominal perfusion pressure |
| APTT | activated partial thromboplastin time |
| ARDS | acute respiratory distress syndrome |
| ARF | acute renal failure |

| ASB | assisted spontaneous breathing |
| ASD | atrial septal defect |
| AST | aspartate aminotransferase |
| ATLS | advanced trauma life support |
| ATN | acute tubular necrosis |
| AVM | arterio-venous malformation |
| AVPU | **A**lert, responds to **V**oice, responds to **P**ain, **U**nresponsive, consciousness assessment |
| AXR | abdominal X-ray |
| BAL | broncho-alveolar lavage |
| BBB | blood brain barrier |
| BE | base excess |
| BIPAP | biphasic positive airways pressure |
| BIS | bispectral index |
| BLS | basic life support |
| BM | bone marrow |
| BM | blood monitoring [glucose] |
| BMI | body mass index |
| BNF | British national formulary |
| BOS | base of skull [fracture] |
| BP | blood pressure |
| BSA | body surface area |
| $Ca^{2+}$ | calcium |
| cAMP | cyclic adenosine monophosphate |
| CAP | community acquired pneumonia |
| CAPD | continuous ambulatory peritoneal dialysis |
| CAVH | continuous arterio-venous haemofiltration |
| CCF | congestive cardiac failure |
| CCHF | Crimean-Congo haemorrhagic fever |
| CCU | coronary care unit |
| CFI | cardiac function index |
| CF (A) M | cerebral function (analysing) monitor |
| CHF | congestive heart failure |
| CI | cardiac index |
| CIN | contrast induced nephropathy |
| CJD | Creutzfeld-Jacob disease |
| CK | creatinine kinase |
| CKMB | CK myocardial bound [portion] |
| CMV | cytomegalovirus |
| CMV | continuous mandatory ventilation |
| CNS | central nervous system |

| CO | cardiac output |
| CO | carbon monoxide |
| $CO_2$ | carbon dioxide |
| COHb | carboxyhaemoglobin |
| COPD | chronic obstructive pulmonary disease |
| CPAP | continuous positive airways pressure |
| CPIS | clinical pulmonary infection scores |
| CPP | cerebral perfusion pressure |
| CPR | cardio-pulmonary resuscitation |
| CPT | cryoprecipitate |
| CRBSI | catheter-related blood stream infection |
| CRP | C reactive protein |
| CRT | capillary refill time |
| CSL | compound sodium lactate [fluid] |
| C-spine | cervical spine |
| CSF | cerebrospinal fluid |
| CSM | committee for safety in medicine |
| CSU | catheter specimen urine |
| $C_T$ | lung compliance |
| CT | computed tomography |
| CTG | cardiotocograph |
| CTPA | CT pulmonary angiogram |
| CURB-65 | [a pneumonia scoring system] |
| CVA | cerebrovascular accident |
| CVP | central venous pressure |
| CVC | central venous catheter |
| CVS | cardiovascular system |
| CVVH | continuous veno-venous haemofiltration |
| CXR | chest X-ray |
| DC | direct current |
| DDT | dichloro diphenyl tricholoethane |
| DHI | dynamic hyperinflation |
| DI | diabetes insipidus |
| DIC | disseminated intravascular coagulopathy |
| DKA | diabetic ketoacidosis |
| DLT | double lumen [ET] tube |
| DM | diabetes mellitus |
| DMPS | sodium 2,3-dimercapto-1-propane sulphonate |
| DMSA | dimercaptosuccinic acid |
| DNAR | do not attempt resuscitation |
| $DO_2$ | oxygen delivery |

| DOB | date of birth |
| DOH | department of health |
| DNA | deoxyribonucleic acid |
| DPL | diagnostic peritoneal lavage |
| DRESS | drug rash with eosinophilia and systemic symptoms |
| ds-DNA | double stranded DNA |
| DTs | delirium tremens |
| DVT | deep vein thrombosis |
| EBV | Epstein-Barr virus |
| ECCO$_2$R | extra-corporeal carbon dioxide removal |
| ECG | electrocardiogram |
| ECHO | echocardiogram (TOE or TTE) |
| ECMO | extra-corporeal membrane oxygenation |
| EDTA | ethylene diamine tetraacetic acid |
| EEG | electroencephalogram |
| EF | ejection fraction |
| eGFR | estimated glomerular filtration rate |
| EMG | electromyograph |
| ENT | ear, nose and throat |
| ERCP | endoscopic retrograde cholangeopancreatography |
| ESR | erythrocyte sedimentation rate |
| ETCO$_2$ | end tidal $CO_2$ |
| ET(T) | endotracheal (tube) |
| EVLWI | extravascular lung water index |
| EWS | early warning score |
| FBC | full blood count |
| FDPs | fibrinogen degradation products |
| Fe | iron |
| FES | fat embolism syndrome |
| FEV$_1$ | forced expiratory volume in 1 second |
| FiO$_2$ | fraction of inspired $O_2$ |
| FFP | fresh frozen plasma |
| FOB | faecal occult blood |
| Fr | French gauge |
| FRC | functional residual capacity |
| FTc | corrected flow time |
| FVC | forced vital capacity |
| G | gauge |
| G&S | group and save |
| GBM | glomerular basement membrane |
| GBS | Guillain-Barré syndrome |

| | |
|---|---|
| GCS | Glasgow coma score |
| GEDVI | global end diastolic volume index |
| GFR | glomerular filtration rate |
| GGT | gamma-glutamyl transpeptidase |
| GHB | gammahydroxybutyric acid |
| GI (T) | gastro-intestinal (tract) |
| GP | general practitioner |
| GP2b3a | glycoprotein 2b3a receptor Inhibitor |
| GTN | glyceryl trinitrate |
| GU | genito-urinary |
| HAART | highly active anti-retroviral therapy |
| HAI | hospital acquired infection |
| HAP | hospital acquired pneumonia |
| HAS | human albumin solution |
| HAV | hepatitis A virus |
| HAV-IgM | hepatitis A antibody |
| Hb | haemoglobin |
| $HbA_{1C}$ | glycosylated haemoglobin |
| HBcore-IgM | hepatitis B core antibody |
| HbsAg | hepatitis B surface antigen |
| HBV | hepatitis B virus |
| HCAP | health-care associated pneumonia |
| Hct | haematocrit |
| HCV | hepatitis C virus |
| HD | haemodialysis |
| HELLP syndrome | **h**aemolysis, **e**levated **l**iver enzymes, **l**ow **p**latelets |
| HEPA [mask] | high-efficiency particulate air |
| HiB | *haemophilus influenzae* type b |
| HIT (S) | heparin induced thrombocytopaenia (syndrome) |
| HIV | human immunodeficiency virus |
| HMMA | hydroymethylmandelic acid |
| HONK | hyperosmolar non-ketotic [coma] |
| HPA (CFI) | health protection agency (centre for infections) |
| HR | heart rate |
| HRS | hepatorenal syndrome |
| HSP | Henoch-Schonlein purpura |
| HSV | herpes simplex virus |
| HUS | haemolytic uraemic syndrome |
| IABP | intra-aortic balloon pump |
| IAH | intra-abdominal hypertension |
| IAP | intra-abdominal pressure |

| | |
|---|---|
| IBC | iron binding capacity |
| IBW | ideal body weight |
| ICP | intra-cranial pressure |
| ICU | intensive care unit |
| ID card | identification card |
| IDDM | insulin dependent diabetes mellitus |
| I:E ratio | inspired:expired [air] ratio |
| IgE | immunoglobulin E |
| IHD | ischaemic heart disease |
| IJ | internal jugular |
| IM | intra-muscular |
| INR | international normalized ratio |
| IOP | intra-ocular pressure |
| IPPV | intermittent positive pressure ventilation |
| ITBVI | intrathoracic blood volume index |
| ITP | idiopathic thrombocytopaenia purpura |
| ITU | intensive therapy unit |
| IUFD | intra-uterine fetal death |
| IV | intra-venous |
| IVC | inferior vena cava |
| IVIG | intravenous immunoglobulin |
| IVU | intravenous urogram |
| IVF | in-vitro fertilization |
| JVP | jugular venous pressure |
| $K^+$ | potassium |
| $K_{CO}$ | transfer coefficient |
| LACS | lacunar syndrome |
| LAP | left atrial pressure |
| LBBB | left bundle branch block |
| LDH | lactate dehydrogenase |
| LFTs | liver function tests |
| LiDCO™ | lithium dilution cardiac output [monitor] |
| LMA | laryngeal mask airway |
| LMWH | low molecular weight heparin |
| LP | lumbar puncture |
| LRTI | lower respiratory tract infection |
| LSD | lysergic acid diethylamide |
| LV | left ventricle |
| LVAD | left ventricular assist device |
| LVEDP | left ventricular end-diastolic pressure |
| LVF | left ventricular failure |

| LVSWI | left ventricular stroke work index |
| MAOI | mono-amine oxidase inhibitor |
| MAP | mean arterial pressure |
| MARS | molecular adsorbent recirculating system |
| MBA | motor bike accident |
| MCA | middle cerebral artery |
| MCH | mean cell haematocrit |
| MCV | mean cell volume |
| MDMA | methylenedioxymethamfetamine (ecstasy) |
| MDR | multiple drug resistance |
| MEN | multiple endocrine neoplasia |
| MH | malignant hyperpyrexia |
| MI | myocardial infarction |
| MIBG | metaidobenzoguanidine [scan] |
| MODS | multiple organ dysfunction syndrome |
| MOF | multiple organ failure |
| MPAP | mean pulmonary artery pressure |
| MR | mitral regurgitation |
| MRI | magnetic resonance imaging |
| MRSA | methicillin-resistant *staphylococcus aureus* |
| MSSA | methicillin-sensitive *staphylococcus aureus* |
| MSU | mid-stream urine |
| $Na^+$ | sodium |
| $NaHCO_3$ | sodium bicarbonate |
| NBM | nil by mouth |
| NG / NGT | naso-gastric (tube) |
| NIBP | non-invasive blood pressure |
| NIV | non-invasive ventilation |
| NJ | naso-jejunal |
| nNRTI | non-nucleotide reverse transcriptase inhibitors |
| NPAs | naso-pharyngeal airways |
| NPIS | national poisons information service |
| NRTI | nucleotide reverse transcriptase inhibitors |
| NSAIDs | non-steroidal anti-inflammatory drugs |
| NSTEMI | non-ST elevation myocardial infarction |
| $O_2$ | oxygen |
| OCP | oral contraceptive pill |
| OD | overdose |
| ODC | oxygen dissociation curve |
| OGT | oro-gastric tube |
| OHCC | Oxford Handbook of Critical Care |

| OHEA | Oxford Handbook of Emergencies in Anaesthesia |
| OHEC | Oxford Handbook of Emergencies in Cardiology |
| OHSS | ovarian hyperstimulation syndrome |
| OPAs | oro-pharyngeal airways |
| $P_{0.1}$ | airway occlusion pressure at 0.1 sec |
| PA | pulmonary artery |
| $PaCO_2$ | partial pressure of arterial $CO_2$ |
| PACS | partial anterior circulation syndrome |
| PAFC | pulmonary artery flotation catheter |
| PAN | polyarteritis nodosa |
| $PaO_2$ | partial pressure of arterial $O_2$ |
| PAOP/PAWP | pulmonary artery occlusion [wedge] pressure |
| PAP | pulmonary artery pressure |
| PC | platelet concentrate |
| PCA | posterior cerebral artery |
| PCA(S) | patient controlled analgesia (system) |
| PCC | *pneumocystis carinii* |
| PCP | *pneumocystis carinii* pneumonia |
| PCR | polymerase chain reaction |
| PCT | Procalcitonin |
| PCWP | pulmonary capillary wedge pressure |
| PE | pulmonary embolus |
| PE | phenytoin equivalents |
| PEA | pulseless electrical activity |
| PEEP | positive end-expiratory pressure |
| PEEPi | intrinsic PEEP |
| PEFR | peak expiratory flow rate |
| PEG | percutaneous endoscopic gastrostomy |
| PET | pre-eclamptic toxaemia |
| PFTs | pulmonary function tests |
| PI | protease inhibitor |
| PICC | peripherally inserted central catheter |
| PICH | primary intracerebral haemorrhage |
| PIH | pregnancy induced hypertension |
| PMH | past medical history |
| PMR | polymyalgia rheumatica |
| PO/O | per oral/oral |
| POCS | posterior circulation syndrome |
| PPH | post-partum haemorrhage |
| PR | per rectum |
| PRN | pro re nata (as required) |

| PSV | pressure support ventilation |
| PT | prothrombin time |
| PTH | parathyroid hormone |
| PUO | pyrexia of unknown origin |
| PV | per vagina |
| PVL | Panton-Valentine leukocidin |
| PVR | pulmonary vascular resistance |
| PVRI | pulmonary vascular resistance index |
| QTc | corrected QT |
| RA | rheumatoid arthritis |
| RA | right atrium |
| RAP | right atrial pressure |
| RBBB | right bundle branch block |
| RBC | red blood cell |
| REJ | right external jugular |
| RIJ | right internal jugular |
| ROSC | return of spontaneous circulation |
| RPP | rate pressure product |
| RR | respiratory rate |
| RRT | renal replacement therapy |
| RS | respiratory system |
| RSI | rapid sequence intubation |
| RSV | respiratory syncytial virus |
| RTA | road traffic accident |
| RTA | renal tubular acidosis |
| Rt-PA | recombinant tissue plasminogen activator |
| RUQ | right upper quadrant |
| RV | right ventricle |
| RVEDP | right ventricle end-diastolic pressure |
| SA | *staphylococcus aureus* |
| SAFE | **s**hout for help, **a**pproach with caution, **f**ree from danger, **e**valuate ABC |
| SAH | subarachnoid haemorrhage |
| $SaO_2$ | arterial $O_2$ saturation |
| SARS (-CoV) | severe acute respiratory syndrome (corona virus) |
| SBP | spontaneous bacterial peritonitis |
| SC | subcutaneous |
| $ScvO_2$ | central venous $O_2$ saturation |
| SGC | Swan-Ganz catheter |
| SIADH | syndrome of inappropriate ADH |
| SICH | spontaneous intracerebral haemorrhage |

| | |
|---|---|
| SIRS | systemic inflammatory response syndrome |
| $SjO_2$ | jugular venous bulb $O_2$ saturations |
| SJS | Stevens-Johnson syndrome |
| SK | Streptokinase |
| SL | sublingual |
| SLE | systemic lupus erythematosus |
| SNP | sodium nitroprusside |
| SOB | shortness-of-breath |
| $SpO_2$ | plethysmographic [skin] $O_2$ saturation |
| SSB | Sengstaken-Blakemore tube |
| SSRI | selective serotonin reuptake inhibitor |
| STD | sexually transmitted disease |
| STEMI | ST elevation myocardial infarction |
| SV | stroke volume |
| SVC | superior vena cava |
| SVI | stroke volume index |
| $SvO_2$ | venous $O_2$ saturation |
| $S\bar{v}O_2$ | mixed venous $O_2$ saturation |
| SVR | systemic vascular resistance |
| SVRI | systemic vascular resistance index |
| SVT | supraventricular tachycardia |
| SVV | stroke volume variation |
| $T_3$ | tri-iodothyronine |
| $T_4$ | thyroxine |
| TACS | total anterior circulation syndrome |
| TB | tuberculosis |
| TBV | total blood volume |
| TCA | tricyclic antidepressants |
| TCD | trans-cranial Doppler |
| TEN | toxic epidermal necrolysis |
| TFTs | thyroid function tests |
| TGI | tracheal gas insufflation |
| TIA | transient ischaemic attack |
| TICA | terminal internal carotid artery |
| TICTAC | a tablet identification database |
| TIPSS | transjugular intrahepatic porto-systemic shunting |
| TLC | total lung capacity |
| TOD | trans-oesophageal Doppler |
| TOE | trans-oesophageal echocardiogram |
| Toxbase | a toxicology database |
| t-PA | tissue plasminogen activator |

| TPN | total parenteral nutrition |
| TR | tricuspid regurgitation |
| TRALI | transfusion related acute lung injury |
| TSH | thyroid-stimulating hormone |
| T-spine | thoracic spine |
| TT | thrombin time |
| TTE | trans-thoracic echocardiogram |
| TTP | thrombotic thrombocytopaenic purpura |
| TUR(P) | trans-urethral resection (of the prostate) |
| $T_V$ | tidal volume |
| U&Es | urea and electrolytes |
| UOP | urine output |
| URTI | upper respiratory tract infection |
| US | ultrasound |
| UTI | urinary tract infection |
| VAP | ventilator associated pneumonia |
| VC | vital capacity |
| $V_E$ | minute volume |
| VEs | ventricular ectopics |
| VF | ventricular fibrillation |
| VHF | viral haemorrhagic fever |
| VMA | vanillylmandelic acid |
| $VO_2$ | systemic oxygen consumption |
| V-P shunt | ventriculo-peritoneals shunt |
| VQ mismatch | ventilation perfusion mismatch |
| VRSS | vasopressor resistant septic shock |
| VSD | ventricular septal defect |
| VT | ventricular tachycardia |
| WBC | white blood cell |
| WCC | white cell count |
| WFNS | World Federation of Neurological Surgeons |
| WPW | Wolff-Parkinson-White syndrome |

# Emergency drug doses

**Adenosine**

| | |
|---|---|
| Narrow complex tachycardia | 6 mg IV (rapid bolus), repeat if required after 3 mins with 12 mg (up to 3 times), *caution with WPW syndrome* |

**Adrenaline/epinephrine**

| | |
|---|---|
| Cardiac arrest | 1 mg (10 ml 1in10,000, or 1 ml 1in1000) IV every 3–5 mins |
| Cardiac arrest & no IV access | 2–3 mg diluted in >10 mls sterile water via ET tube |
| Anaphylaxis/angiooedema | 500 µg (0.5 ml 1in1000) IM |
| Stridor or severe bronchospasm | 1–3 mg nebulised |
| Emergency infusions for bradycardia or bronchospasm | 0.04–0.4 µg/kg/min |
| Emergency infusions for hypotension | 0.04–0.4 µg/kg/min |

**Aminophylline**

| | |
|---|---|
| Bronchospasm | 250 mg IV slow (if not already on theophyllines), then 0.5 mg/kg/hr |

**Amiodarone**

| | |
|---|---|
| Cardiac arrest refractory & VF/VT | 300 mg (in 20 mls dextrose 5%) IV |
| Broad complex tachycardia | 150 mg (in 20 mls dextrose 5%) IV over 10 mins |
| Narrow complex tachycardia | 150 mg (in 20 mls dextrose 5%) IV over 10 mins, or 300 mg IV (in 100 mls dextrose 5% over 1 hour) according to severity of symptoms |
| Fast AF | 300 mg IV (in 100 mls dextrose 5% over 1 hour) |

**Atracurium**

| | |
|---|---|
| Difficulty ventilating/raised intracranial pressure (ONLY if intubated) | 50 mg IV (give anaesthetic agents as well to prevent awareness) |

**Atropine**

| | |
|---|---|
| Cardiac arrest | 3 mg IV *once* |
| Cardiac arrest & no IV access | 6 mg diluted in >10 mls sterile water via ET tube *once* |
| Severe or symptomatic bradycardia | 600 µg IV |

| Organophosphate/nerve agent poisoning | 2 mg IV should be given every 20 mins until pupils dilate, skin is dry and tachycardia occurs |
|---|---|
| **Benzylpenicillin** | |
| Meningitis/meningococcal septicaemia | 1.2 g IV |
| **Calcium chloride** | |
| Hyperkalaemic cardiac arrest | 10 ml 10% (6.8 mmol) IV |
| **Ceftriaxone** | |
| Meningitis/meningococcal septicaemia | 2 g IV |
| **Chlorphenamine** | |
| Anaphylaxis/angiooedema (*after* adrenaline) | 20 mg IV (slow) |
| **Dantrolene** | |
| Malignant hyperpyrexia | 1 mg/kg IV and repeat as needed up to 10 mg/kg |
| **Diamorphine** | |
| Pulmonary oedema | 2.5–5 mg IV |
| Severe pain | 2.5–5 mg IV/IM/SC |
| **Digoxin** | |
| Fast AF | 500 µg IV (over 30 mins) |
| **Dobutamine** | |
| Hypotension/heart failure | 2.5–10 µg/kg/min |
| **Ephedrine** | |
| Hypotension | 3–6 mg IV repeat every 3–4 mins as required |
| **Esmolol** | |
| Narrow complex tachycardia | 4–12 mg/min IV infusion |
| **Etomidate** | |
| Induction of anaesthesia | 0.1–0.4 mg/kg |
| **Flumazenil** | |
| Benzodiazepine overdose | 200 µg IV (repeat every minute as required up to 1 mg) |
| **Furosemide** | |
| Pulmonary oedema | 20–40 mg IV |
| **Glycopyrronium bromide** | |
| Severe or symptomatic bradycardia | 200–400 µg IV |
| **Glucagon** | |
| Hypoglycaemia | 1 mg IV/IM/SC |

**Glucose**

Hypoglycaemia | 25–50 mls of 25–50% Iv (via a large cannula/vein if possible)

**Haloperidol**

Severe agitation | 2.5–5 mg IV (always consider other causes, repeat up to 15 mg, continually review sedation/airway)

**Hydrocortisone**

Anaphylaxis | 200 mg IV (slow)
Severe bronchospasm | 200 mg IV (slow)
Addisons/hypoadrenalism | 200 mg IV (slow)

**Insulin and dextrose**

Severe hyperkalaemia | 15–20 U soluble insulin in 50 ml 50% dextrose IV over 30–60 mins

**Ipratropium bromide**

Bronchospasm | 500 µg nebulised

**Lidocaine**

Broad complex tachycardia | 50 mg IV (over 2 mins) repeat as required up to 200 mg

**Lorazepam**

Status epilepticus | 4 mg IV (slow)

**Magnesium sulphate**

Cardiac arrest & refractory VF/VT with possible hypomagnesaemia | 8 mmol (2 g or 4 ml $MgSO_4$ 50%) IV

Eclampsia | loading dose: 16 mmol (4 g) IV over 3–5 mins, followed by maintenance infusion of 5–10 mmol/hr

**Mannitol**

Raised ICP/intracranial mass effect | 0.5–1 g/kg (approx. 200–400 mls 20% solution)

**Metaraminol**

Hypotension requiring vasoconstriction | 0.5 mg IV

**Morphine**

Pulmonary oedema | 2.5–10 mg IV
Severe pain | 2.5–10 mg IV/IM/SC
Sedative infusion (combined with propofol, midazolam or equivalent) | 0–3 µg/kg/min

**Naloxone**

Opioid overdose | 200mcg IV followed by 100mcg every 2 minutes up to 2 mg; SC or IM routes can be used *in extremis)*

**Noradrenaline/norepinephrine**

| | |
|---|---|
| Hypotension requiring vasoconstriction | 0.04–0.4 µg/kg/min |

**Phenylephrine**

| | |
|---|---|
| Hypotension requiring vasoconstriction | 50 µg IV, or 30–60 µg/min |

**Phenytoin**

| | |
|---|---|
| Status epilepticus | loading dose 15 mg/kg (in 0.9% saline) IV infusion at a rate not exceeding 50 mg/min (ECG monitoring required) |

**Procyclidine**

| | |
|---|---|
| Oculogyric crisis/acute dystonia | 5–10 mg IV/IM |

**Propofol**

| | |
|---|---|
| Induction of anaesthesia | 1.5–2.5 mg/kg IV |
| Sedative infusion | 0–300 mg/hr |

**Salbutamol**

| | |
|---|---|
| Bronchospasm | 5 mg nebulised |
| Bronchospasm IV infusion | 250 mcg IV over 10 minutes, then 5–30 µg/min |

**Sodium bicarbonate**

| | |
|---|---|
| Cardiac arrest & tricyclic overdose or hyperkalaemia | 50 ml 8.4% IV |

**Suxamethonium**

| | |
|---|---|
| Rapid sequence intubation | 1–2 mg/kg IV |

**Terlipressin**

| | |
|---|---|
| Severe refractory septic shock | 1 mg IV 8 hourly |

**Thiopental**

| | |
|---|---|
| Induction of anaesthesia | 3–5 mg/kg |

**Vasopressin**

| | |
|---|---|
| Severe refractory septic shock | 0.01–0.04 units/min IV infusion |

# Assessment and stabilization

# ☠ /✛ /⚠ Assessment and immediate management of an emergency

The assessment and immediate management of critically ill patients follows the well-established ABC (**A**pproach/**A**irway, **B**reathing, **C**irculation) approach. What follows is a brief summary of the ABC approach adapted for patients within a critical care environment. Further details for each system are considered in individual chapters. Any deterioration during assessment and resuscitation should prompt a return to A.

Some interventions may need to be performed *whilst continuing assessment and emergency treatment*, particularly when emergencies are acute and life-threatening (e.g. BLS/ALS, see pp. 104–105, or needle thoracocentesis of a tension pneumothorax, see p. 78).

## Approach

- In all cases it is essential to ensure that those treating the patient are safe to carry out their work
- Consider C-spine immobilization where trauma is involved
- Give 100% oxygen in acute emergencies; in less acute scenarios titrate the oxygen required to keep $SaO_2$ >95%
- Connect any monitoring available: aim to have $SaO_2$, continuous ECG, and non-invasive BP monitoring as a minimum
  - Review any information from the monitoring devices (e.g. $SaO_2$, ventilatory parameters, heart rate and rhythm, blood pressure) alongside physical findings when examining the patient
  - Be alert for equipment malfunction (e.g. airway occlusion, ventilator failure, or infusion pump failure); and/or alarms from the monitoring systems which may indicate the cause or extent of problem
- Obtain a history and detailed information about the patient
  - From the patient where possible: the minimum history should include the AMPLE template advocated in trauma resuscitation
  - From attending staff or from any associated documentation
  - Review notes, observation charts, and blood results (fluid balance, blood gases, electrolytes)
  - Physiological scoring systems (e.g. early warning scores, EWS, or 'track and trigger' systems) may be used to 'flag up' patients at high risk of deterioration (see p. 9)
  - Assess the existing level of support required by the patient (e.g. requirement for inotropes or haemofiltration)

---

**The AMPLE history:**

- **A** Allergies
- **M** Medication
- **P** Past medical history
- **L** Last meal
- **E** Event (and environment)

## Airway

The most common cause for emergency related to airway is **airway obstruction**. It may be partial or complete

*In the intubated patient*
Work methodically from the ventilator to the patient
- Check the ventilator is working (with adequate pressures, tidal volumes and minute volumes) and that $O_2$ is connected; check that ventilator tubing is still connected and not obstructed
- High airway pressure (in mechanically ventilated patients) may cause ventilator alarms
- Listen for any air leaks from ventilator tubing or endotracheal cuff
- Check the endotracheal tube
  - Endotracheal tube position is normally 20–22 cm at lips; compare with any previously noted length)
  - Review CXR films for confirming correct placement of tube
  - Check tube patency (consider passing a suction catheter through the endotracheal tube to exclude obstruction)
  - Laryngoscopy may be required to confirm correct placement
  - Check end-tidal $CO_2$ to confirm endotracheal tube position (provided that there is also adequate cardiac output)
- Disconnect from ventilator and try ventilating with a self-inflating bag
  - Look for chest or other signs of airway obstruction (listed below)
  - Successful ventilation indicates obstruction at the level of ventilator tubing
  - If this is unsuccessful, then there is an obstruction within or beyond the endotracheal tube. Consider re-intubating with a fresh endotracheal tube and/or passing a fibre-optic scope. Also consider causes for failure to expand the lungs (e.g. tension pneumothorax or bronchospasm)

*In the unintubated patient*
- Assess the ability of the patient to breath, or in conscious patients the ability to speak, listening for:
  - Silence (caused by apnoea or complete obstruction); abnormally quiet or breath sounds
  - Stridor or wheeze
  - Gurgling
  - A hoarse voice
- In unconscious or uncooperative patients feel for breath with your hand or cheek; check for misting on an oxygen mask
- Look for evidence of airway obstruction
  - Bleeding, vomit, secretions, tissue swelling or foreign bodies
  - Obstruction of the pharynx by the tongue
  - Look for neck swelling or bruising, surgical/subcutaneous emphysema, or crepitus
- Look for chest and other signs of airway obstruction including:
  - Paradoxical chest and abdominal movements
  - Reduced chest exculsion

- Use of accessory muscles of respiration
- Hypoxia is a late sign and indicates extreme emergency
- Exclude obstruction of pharynx by the tongue
  - Chin lift: useful for infants, edentulous or unconscious patients
  - Jaw thrust: generally more effective than chin lift, and can be done one-handed (skilled) or two-handed (unskilled)
- Consider airway adjuncts
  - Oropharyngeal (Guedel) airways are only tolerated by unconscious patients
  - Nasopharyngeal airways are better tolerated by conscious patients but may cause nasal bleeding on insertion, worsening airway problems
  - Laryngeal mask airways (LMAs) are only tolerated by unconscious patients, do not protect from aspiration, and require basic training to insert
  - Orotracheal intubation is the gold standard for protecting and maintaining the airway, but is only tolerated by anaesthetized or unconscious patients and requires a skilled operator to insert (the nasotracheal route is rarely required outside operating theatres)
- Consider using a self-inflating bag and mask if possible, whilst continuing to look for causes of obstruction and how can it be relieved
- Consider endotracheal intubation or an emergency needle cricothyroidotomy/tracheostomy (see pp. 482 and 488)
  - Specialist anaesthetic and/or ENT airway skills will also be required at this point
- In patients who are unconscious, but maintaining an airway, patient positioning, or endotracheal intubation should be considered
  - The recovery position should be employed for unconscious patients, or 'head-down, left lateral' if they are lying on a trolley

## Breathing

The common causes for breathing difficulties include pleural diseases (pneumothorax, haemothorax, or pleural effusion), airway diseases (asthma, secretions, acute exacerbation of COPD), parenchymal disease (collapse, consolidation, ARDS) and cardiogenic disease (cardiogenic pulmonary oedema). Evidence of inadequate breathing should be looked for and corrected, including the following:

- Hypoxia: reduced $PaO_2$ or $SaO_2$
- Dyspnoea and/or tachypnoea (bradypnoea or Cheyne–Stokes breathing are late/severe signs)
- Obvious evidence of problem, e.g. pulmonary aspiration, massive bleeding
- Absent or abnormal chest movement
  - Unilateral movements may indicate pneumothorax, pleural effusion, collapse

- - Paradoxical chest-abdominal movement may indicate airway obstruction (asthma) or flail chest
  - Use of accessory muscles of respiration
- Raised JVP may be visible
- Apex beat or tracheal shift may be seen towards areas of collapse or away from pneumothoraces or pleural effusions
- Percussion may reveal effusions or pneumothoraces
- Abnormal breath sounds may be heard on auscultation
  - Silent chest or wheeze may be due to acute severe asthma/bronchospasm
  - Rattling noise suggests secretions
  - Absent unilateral sounds may be due to pleural effusion
  - Bronchial breathing suggests underlying consolidation
- Patients should be asked to cough to assess their ability to clear secretions, which may be limited by neuromuscular problems or pain
- Secretions themselves should be examined where possible, and patients encouraged to 'cough up' samples
- Check any intercostal drains, check if drains are still swinging or bubbling, and check the volume of blood or serous discharge
- Emergency management should be aimed at:
  - Excluding/treating life-threatening conditions (e.g. acute severe asthma, tension pneumothorax, pulmonary oedema, massive haemothorax)
  - Keeping $PaO_2$ >9 kPa, $PaCO_2$ within the normal limits for the patient with respiratory rate <35 breaths/min
- Consider:
  - A trial of bronchodilators if bronchospasm is suspected
  - Chest physiotherapy to clear secretions
  - CPAP/BIPAP in conscious and cooperative patients who do not respond to the above
  - Endotracheal intubation and mechanical ventilation if the above fail

*In the mechanically ventilated patient*
- Check the degree of any respiratory support:
  - Oxygen, peak pressures, PEEP, and minute volume requirements
  - Increased airway pressures or decreased tidal volumes may be due to increased airway resistance or reduced lung compliance.
  - If bronchospasm is present check the length of the expiratory-wheeze (in order to set I:E ratios), and check intrinsic PEEP
- Tracheal suction may reveal the amount and quality of secretions, and clear mucus plugs (critical care charts also often record the amount and character of secretions)
- Consider alveolar recruitment manoeuvres; these are often helpful in ARDS, atelectasis, or pulmonary oedema
- Consider ventilating with a self-inflating bag in order to assess compliance manually
- Consider urgent bronchoscopy
- Check any recent ABGs and CXR and repeat as required
- Chest US may help diagnose effusions or occult pneumothoraces

## Circulation

Cardiovascular emergencies often present as severe hypotension and shock, heart failure with pulmonary oedema, or cardiac arrest. Occasionally, the crisis may be due to uncontrolled hypertension. The causes for inadequate circulation include low-output states such as hypovolaemia or cardiogenic shock, and high-output states due to peripheral vasodilatation (e.g. sepsis).

Non-cardiovascular causes (e.g. endocrine disorders, electrolytes, pneumothorax) should also be considered. In addition, it should be remembered that certain interventions such as positive pressure ventilation or epidural analgesia can lead to relative hypovolaemia.

In critical care, a number of monitoring devices (e.g. ECG, arterial blood pressure, cardiac output monitor) may already be connected to the patient and may give important clues to the nature of emergency. Signs of cardiovascular compromise may include the following.

- Cardiovascular signs
  - Thready pulse, tachycardia, and hypotension
  - Cold peripheries, prolonged capillary refill (>2 seconds)
  - Alternatively, a bounding pulse may occur with hypotension in individuals capable of compensating
  - Bradycardia is a pre-terminal sign, or a sign of vagal stimulation (e.g. from intra-peritoneal blood)
  - JVP may be raised
- Other signs
  - Tachypnoea, reduced urine output, altered mental state
  - Decreased urine output (<0.5 ml/kg/hour)
  - Peripheral oedema
- Look for obvious or concealed blood/fluid loss
- Check any abdominal or wound drains; check they are still *in situ* and measure the volume of any blood loss
- Check Hb and haematocrit
- Check the status of any inotropic infusions
- Other signs of circulatory insufficiency may include lactataemia or metabolic acidosis
- Measured variables may also include:
  - CVP, pulmonary artery occlusion pressure (via SGC)
  - Stroke volume and cardiac output estimation (via echocardiography, PAFC, TOD, pulse contour analysis); these will also allow an estimation of systemic vascular resistance
  - TOD may give an estimation of cardiac filling and/or afterload changes by measuring the corrected flowtime (FTc)
  - Stroke volume variation may give an indication of assessing cardiac filling in ventilated patients
- Non-specific signs may be present in ventilated patients, including chest pulsation (indicating a hyperdynamic state), the presence of $ETCO_2$ (indicating both patent endotracheal access and that cardiac output is present), a swinging arterial line trace (a non-specific indicator of hypovolaemia)

- Venous blood saturations (either from the pulmonary artery ($S\bar{v}O_2$) or from a central line ($ScvO_2$)) which give a measure of oxygen extraction: too low a value indicates a low arterial oxygen supply or tissues which have poor perfusion and are extracting more oxygen than usual; a high value may be indicative of a shunt
- Immediate management should consist of:
  - Exclude life-threatening conditions such as cardiac tamponade (raised CVP/JVP, pulsus paradoxus, diminished heart sounds, low-voltage ECG, globular heart on CXR), haemorrhage, or arrhythmia that compromises circulation
  - Adequate fluid/blood replacement and treatment of hypovolaemic shock: give 500 ml of colloids within 5–10 minutes and reassess
  - For severe hypotension along with a low output state, consider starting an infusion of adrenaline until the cause is established
  - For severe hypotension along with high output state, start with IV fluids and vasoconstrictive agents such as noradrenaline
  - Cardiogenic shock should be treated with appropriate inotropes (e.g. dobutamine or adrenaline), and the management of any associated condition such as acute coronary syndrome, arrhythmias, or pulmonary oedema
  - Exclude and treat acid–base and electrolyte abnormalities, in particular severe metabolic acidosis, hypo-/hyperkalaemia, hypomagnesaemia, and hypocalcaemia
- In patients with sepsis and hypotension, or elevated serum lactate, suggested resuscitation goals include:
  - Central venous pressure of 8–12 mmHg
  - Mean arterial pressure ≥ 65 mmHg
  - Urine output ≥ 0.5 ml/kg/hour
  - $S\bar{v}O_2$ or $ScvO_2$ ≥ 70%

## Disability/neurology

Changes in neurological state may be related to neurological disease (head injury, space occupying lesion, subarachnoid haemorrhage), or worsening respiratory, circulatory, or metabolic disorders.

Exclude and treat hypoglycaemia, hypoxia, hypotension, or hypercapnia. Tracheal intubation may be necessary in unconscious patients (GCS <8) and/or if the gag reflex is absent. The immediate management aims for intracranial pathology should be to protect airway, ensure adequate breathing and gas exchange, and prevent blood pressure fluctuations.

- A rapid assessment of the patient's neurological status should be made by assessing whether or not the patient is **A**lert, responds to **V**oice, responds to **P**ain, or is **U**nresponsive (AVPU Scale). GCS will provide a more comprehensive scoring system
- Signs of altered neurological state may include:
  - Drowsiness, agitation, incoherence, or incontinence

- • Lack of response to verbal command and/or pain
- Other neurological signs may include:
  - • Focal neurological signs
  - • Pupil signs
  - • Lack of gag/cough reflex
- Check ICP if being monitored: raised ICP is >25 cmH$_2$O
- Jugular bulb saturation and/or transcranial Doppler measurements may be available
- Exclude blockage of V–P shunt (if *in situ*)
- Raised ICP may be treated with hypertonic saline or mannitol until more definitive measures are employed
- Urgent CT scan may be required for diagnosis and management

### Exposure/general

Other areas to assess or examine include:

- Temperature
- Rashes and stigmata
- Evidence of DVT
- Abdominal examination
- Trauma survey

Further emergency investigations should be guided by the general condition of the patient. If sepsis is suspected, two or more blood cultures should be obtained. Other cultures may be indicated (including cerebrospinal fluid, respiratory secretions, urine, wounds, and other body fluids). IV antibiotics should then be started as soon as possible.

### Pitfalls/difficult situations

- Certain groups of patients will be sicker than others with the same acute problem, including those patients who:
  - • Are at the extremes of age
  - • Have multi-system disease (e.g. diabetes or rheumatoid arthritis)
  - • Have chronic organ failure (e.g. heart, lung, kidney, or liver)
  - • Are immunosuppressed (e.g. those on steroids or chemotherapy, or those with liver disease or cancer)
  - • Are malnourished
- Others may compensate for longer despite being sicker
  - • Children, young adults, athletes, and pregnant women

**Early warning scores** (Table 1.1)

These score basic physiological variables (heart rate, blood pressure, respiratory rate, temperature, urine output, neurological status) in patients with the potential to deteriorate as a means of identifying developing critical illness earlier. Most patients identified by EWS systems need only basic management such as fluids, analgesia, or physiotherapy

### Further reading

Smith G, Nielsen M. ABC of intensive care: criteria for admission. *BMJ*, **318**, 1544–7.

Riley B, Faleiro R Critical care outreach: rationale and development. *Br J Anaesth CEPD Rev*, **1**, 146–9.

📖 OHCC p. 270.

**Table 1.1** Early Warning Score details

| | Score | | | | | |
|---|---|---|---|---|---|---|
| | 3 | 2 | 1 | 0 | 1 | 2 | 3 |
| Heart rate (bpm) | – | <40 | 40–50 | 51–100 | 101–110 | 111–130 | >130 |
| Respiration rate (breaths/min) | – | <8 | – | 9–14 | 15–20 | 21–30 | ≥30 |
| Temperature (°C) | – | <35 | – | 35–38.4 | – | ≥38.5 | – |
| Neurological status | – | – | – | Alert & orientated | Responds only to voice and/or confused | Responds only to pain | Unconscious |
| Urine output (ml/kg/hour) | Anuric | <0.5 | 0.5–1 | >1 and ≤1.5 | >1.5 | – | – |
| Systolic blood pressure (mmHg) | >70 below normal | >50 below normal | >20 below normal | Normal +30 or –20 | >30 above normal | >50 above normal | >80 above normal |

+1 if systolic is >150 mmHg below normal
Score 5 if systolic is ≤50 mmHg regardless of normal
Score 6 if systolic is ≤40 mmHg regardless of normal

+1 if systolic is ≥100 mmHg above normal
+2 if systolic is ≥110 mmHg above normal

If score is **≥4** request medical or outreach review.

If the patient has renal failure and is **normally anuric** do not score for urine output, but initiate medical review if score is **≥3**

Adapted from Nottingham University Hospitals Early Warning Score template

# ⑦ **Further management**

After the initial assessment and management of any emergency there may be further aspects of patient care to consider or plan for. Details of the further management of specific emergencies are considered in individual chapters; more generic areas of further management can be found below.

## General

- Following resuscitation patients should be nursed in an appropriate environment according to the level of care required: level 2 patients require a minimum of HDU care, whilst level 3 patients require ICU care. Other areas of care may be required for some specialist diseases (e.g. coronary care, cardiothoracic intensive care, neurosurgical, burns, spinal injury, or liver units)

---

**Levels of care**

Level 0   Normal ward-care patients
Level 1   Patients who can remain on a normal ward but who are at risk of acute deterioration (additional monitoring or out reach care may be required)
Level 2   Patients with, or at immediate risk of, single-organ failure. This may include the postoperative care of selected patients (continuous observation and/or single-organ support may be require, and there should be a 2:1 nurse to-patient ratio)
Level 3   Patients requiring support of two or more failing organs alongside basic respiratory support, or those who require advanced respiratory support alone

Levels 2 and 1 may be used to provide stepdown care to those recently discharged from a higher level of care

Adapted from *Levels of Critical Care for Adult Patients: Standards and Guidelines*, Intensive Care Society, 2002

---

- Continuous respiratory and cardiovascular monitoring combined with regular observations of physiological variables such as temperature and urine output should be carried out
- Pressure area care, oral toilet, and eye care should be attended to
- Contact lenses should be removed and corneas should be kept moist

## Airway

- Review CXR to confirm correct positioning of endotracheal tube
- The tube position at the teeth should be regularly checked/recorded
- In patients who are expected to require prolonged endotracheal intubation, the insertion of a tracheostomy should be considered

## Breathing

- Mechanical ventilation
  - CMV/IPPV, SIMV, and BIPAP/BiLevel, or their equivalent, are all available; there is no definitive evidence as to which is best

- Ventilator modes which allow patients to breath alongside the ventilator (e.g. SIMV or BIPAP) have advantages; using ASB or PSV may allow respiratory support to be titrated to a patient's needs
  - Moderate hypercapnia should be tolerated
- Initial ventilator settings
  - Start with a high $FiO_2$ (0.9–1) and titrate according to $SaO_2/PaO_2$
  - PEEP should be titrated to thoraco-pulmonary compliance and oxygen requirements; 5–10 $cmH_2O$ is appropriate initially (bronchospastic patients may require less/none at all, see p. 75)
  - Ventilator setting should be adjusted to achieve a minute volume which allows adequate oxygenation and moderate hypercapnia, a reasonable initial minute volume would be ~80 ml/kg (a tidal volume of 4–6 ml/kg × respiratory rate, i.e. in an 80 kg patient settings of 400 ml TV with a rate of 16 breaths/minute); where pressure-controlled ventilation is used, an initial inspiratory pressure of 20 $cmH_2O$ can be used and then adjusted to achieve acceptable tidal volume
  - Initial I:E ratios should be of the order of 1:2–1:1.5 (except in bronchospasm, see p. 75)
  - Volume, pressure, apnoea, low minute volume, and oxygen failure alarms should all be activated; a maximum upper pressure limit of 40 $cmH_2O$ should be set initially for all modes of ventilation
- Initial ventilator settings should be adjusted to ensure that a lung-protective ventilation strategy is maintained (ARDSnet guidelines, see p. 50)
- The bed head should be raised to 30°–45° (semi-recumbent) if possible in mechanically ventilated patients to prevent ventilator-associated pneumonia
- Regular chest physiotherapy should be attempted unless it is likely to worsen cardiovascular instability
- A weaning protocol should be initiated as soon as practicable

## Circulation
- Consider inserting an arterial line and central line for invasive cardiovascular monitoring
- Review CXR to confirm correct positioning of any thoracic CVCs
- Haemodynamic compromise may respond to bicarbonate therapy, but this should not used if pH ≥ 7.15

## Neurology
- Avoid muscle relaxants/neuromuscular blockade (NMBs) if possible (especially is there seizure activity); where a continuous infusion is required monitor train-of-four count
- Neurological status should be regularly assessed and recorded
- Sedation protocols should be used and the level of sedation measured against a recognized scoring system
- Where continuous infusions of sedation are used, daily interruptions of sedation 'holds' should be undertaken whenever possible

- Patients at risk of spinal trauma should be nursed supine with a whole bed tilt and assessed and stabilized as soon as possible; hard collars should be removed according to protocol (see p. 189)
- Patients at risk of raised ICP should be positioned 30°–45° head up to improve venous drainage

### Endocrine/metabolism
- Managing blood glucose
  - There are many available insulin regimens: glycaemic control should keep blood glucose <8.3 mmol/L, whilst avoiding episodes of hypoglycaemia
  - Regularly check blood glucose at least every 4 hours
- Adrenal support
  - Continue steroid support in patients who take long-term steroids
  - In shocked patients at risk of adrenal suppression (e.g. those with sepsis, or following induction with etomidate) commence steroid support and consider performing an ACTH stimulation test

### Renal
- Catheterization of critically ill or immobile patients will allow accurate monitoring of hourly urine output
- Strict measurement of fluid balance should be maintained
- Where renal replacement therapy is required (see p. 277) intermittent haemodialysis or continuous veno-venous haemo-filtration (CVVH) may be used; haemodynamic stability may be better using CVVH

### Gastrointestinal and hepatic
- Inserting a nasogastric tube will facilitate enteral feeding; in cases of base of skull fractures or nasal trauma consider an orogastric tube
- Review CXR to confirm correct positioning of NGT
- Provide stress ulcer prophylaxis
  - Institute enteral feeding where possible
  - Consider $H_2$ receptor inhibitors (e.g. ranitidine 50 mg IV 8-hourly, reduced to 12-hourly in the presence of significant renal failure; oral dose 150 mg 12-hourly
  - IV proton pump inhibitors (e.g. omeprazole 40 mg IV/oral 24-hourly): alternative to $H_2$ antagonists with no proven superiority in prophylaxis; dose reduction not required in renal failure
  - Alternatively sucralfate 2 g NG 8-hourly may be used but provides less protection against clinically significant GI haemorrhage. It may also block NG tubes or result in bezoars, and care is required in renal failure

### Haematology
- Consider DVT prophylaxis in all patients who are immobile or otherwise at high risk of developing DVT
  - Subcutaneous low molecular weight heparin (e.g. enoxaparin 40 mg SC 24-hourly, or dalteparin 5000 units SC 24-hourly)
  - Subcutaneous heparin 5000–10000 units SC 12-hourly: alternative to low molecular weight heparin, may be easier to reverse if the patient develops active bleeding

- Prophylaxis may be withheld in coagulopathic, anti-coagulated, or actively bleeding patients or in patients at high risk of catastrophic bleeding (e.g. following neurosurgery)
- Consider compression stockings or an intermittent pneumatic compression device alongside pharmacological prophylaxis, or where heparins are contraindicated
- Treatment of anaemia and clotting abnormalities
  - In the absence of coronary artery disease, significant tissue hypoperfusion, or ongoing haemorrhage, haemoglobin may safely be allowed to fall to 7.0 g/dl
  - If transfusing red blood cells aim for a haemoglobin of 7.0–9.0 g/dl
  - Where coronary artery disease or active bleeding is present a suggested alternative transfusion 'trigger' is ≤10 g/dl
  - Avoid correcting clotting if possible unless there is bleeding or invasive procedures are planned
  - Platelets should be transfused if counts are $<50 \times 10^9/L$ and surgery or invasive procedures are planned, or counts are $<30 \times 10^9/L$ and there is a significant bleeding risk; or whenever counts are $<5 \times 10^9/L$

## Microbiology
- Antimicrobial therapy should initially be based on the broad-spectrum coverage for the most likely local pathogens
- After 48 hours therapy should be adjusted, guided by culture results, to a narrow spectrum regimen if possible. Some antimicrobials require regular serum concentration measurement
- Asepsis and strict handwashing protocols should be adopted, and where necessary patients infected with multiply resistant organisms should be isolated. Routine surveillance swabs may be needed

## Analgesia
- Analgesia should be used when required. As a bare minimum patients should be able to cough and deep breathe with no pain or minor pain only
- Epidurals should be examined daily for any complications (see p. 395)

## Surgical patients
- Wound drain/stoma output and stoma perfusion should be monitored
- In cases where abdominal compartment syndrome is possible (see p. 294), intra-abdominal pressures should be measured
- In vascular patients, regular monitoring of the appropriate peripheral pulses may be required

## Trauma patients
- Trauma patients admitted to ICU/HDU should undergo tertiary surveys to identify any injuries missed during the initial resuscitation

## Obstetric patients
- Obstetric patients require intermittent or continuous fetal monitoring

## Discussion of care

- Discussions with the patient and/or their family covering the likely progression of the illness should take place as soon as is practicable
- Where appropriate the resuscitation status of the patient should be discussed with the patient

## Further reading

Intensive Care Society (2002). *Levels of Critical Care for Adult Patients: Standards and Guidelines.* Intensive Care Society, London.

Dellinger RP, Carlet JM, Masur H, *et al.* (2004) Surviving Sepsis Campaign: guidelines for management of severe sepsis and septic shock. *Crit Care Med* **32**, 858–73.

# Chapter 2

# Airway

# ☠ Airway obstruction

An obstructed airway is a medical emergency requiring immediate treatment. Where possible, patients at risk should be identified early so that airway obstruction can be prevented. Although upper airway obstruction may be gradual in onset, it more commonly progresses very rapidly. Medical personnel should be present near the patient constantly, continuously assessing whether or not there are signs of impending total obstruction. Total obstruction should be relieved within 1–2 min.

Whilst the eventual aim when managing airway disorders is to obtain a definitive airway, patients die because of failed oxygenation and ventilation—not failed intubation. Basic airway management skills (e.g. bag and mask ventilation) are crucial.

## Causes

*Internal obstruction*
- Foreign body or tumour
- Airway bleeding
- Upper airway infection (e.g. epiglottitis or diphtheria)
- Swelling/oedema
  - Angio-oedema (ACE inhibitors, aspirin, hereditary)
  - Anaphylaxis
  - Following upper airway interventions or surgery (including post-extubation laryngeal oedema)
  - Airways burns or inhalation of smoke/toxic fumes

*External compression*
- Swelling/oedema: neck trauma, external mass, or tumour
- Haematoma (especially in coagulopathic or anti-coagulated patients)
  - Neck trauma
  - Following thyroid or carotid surgery
  - Following internal jugular line insertion

*Neurological causes*
- Diminished level of consciousness
- Laryngospasm (vocal cords closed against respiration in semi-conscious patient)
- Paralysis of vocal cords
  - Neurological disease (e.g myasthenia gravis, Guillain–Barré syndrome, polyneuritis, or recurrent laryngeal nerve damage)
  - Inadequate reversal of muscle relaxants

## Presentation and assessment

May present as a cardiac arrest (see p. 105) or as an unconscious patient where bag and mask ventilation is impossible

*Partial obstruction*
- Anxiety
- Patient prefers sitting, standing, or leaning forward
- Inability to speak or vocal changes (muffled or hoarse voice)
- Stridor (inspiratory noise accompanying breathing) or noisy breathing

- Obvious neck swelling
- Lump in throat, difficulty in swallowing
- Choking
- Coughing
- Drooling
- Respiratory distress
  - Tachypnoea and dyspnoea
  - Use of accessory muscles of respiration
  - Paradoxical breathing: indrawn chest and suprasternal recession
  - Tracheal tug
  - 'Hunched' posture

*Total or near-total obstruction*
- Anxiety
- Hypoxaemia, cyanosis
- Altered consciousness
- Diminished or absent air entry
- Minimal respiratory excursions
- Tachypnoea and respiratory distress
- Bradycardia

**Investigations**
Diagnosis is mainly clinical and some investigations may have to wait until the patient is stabilized with a secure airway
- ABGs
- FBC, cross-match, clotting screen, U&Es
- Blood cultures and swabs where appropriate
- Neck X-ray, CXR
- CT scan may be required
- Endoscopy or direct laryngoscopy will aid diagnosis and allow interventions to restore airway patency, but both require ENT or anaesthetic experience in order to be performed safely

**Airway interventions in a patient with a partially obstructed airway can provoking complete airway obstruction**

**Differential diagnoses**
- Equipment failure (e.g. incorrectly assembled self-inflating Ambu-bag)
- ETT or tracheostomy obstruction (see pp. 38, 41)
- Conditions which result in noisy breathing:
  - Bronchospasm
  - Hysterical stridor
- Conditions which result in difficulty breathing spontaneously or high airway pressures when ventilating patient
  - Bronchospasm
  - Tension pneumothorax
- Conditions which result in patients adopting a sitting or leaning forward position
  - SVC obstruction
  - Cardiac tamponade

## Immediate management

- 100% $O_2$, pulse oximetry
- Assess condition of patient and likely cause of airway obstruction

**If patient is peri-arrest**
  - Call for skilled help: anaesthetist, ENT surgeon
  - Total obstruction requires immediate laryngoscopy and tracheal intubation
  - Surgical airway, i.e. cricothyroidotomy or tracheostomy, for total obstruction if the above fails

**If patient has suffered cardiac arrest**
  - Follow BLS guidelines (see p. 104): remove obvious obstruction, give two rescue breaths, and commence CPR

**If airway obstruction is due to diminished level of consciousness**
  - Call for skilled anaesthetic assistance
  - If traumatic: simultaneously assess C-spine and other injuries
  - Consider replacing hard collar with manual in-line stabilization: often helpful when supporting airway; always advisable prior to attempting intubation
  - **Ensuring an adequate airway always overrides concerns about potential C-spine injuries**
  - Support/open airway: use adjuncts (oropharyngeal or naso-pharyngeal airways)
  - Support ventilation with bag and mask if required
  - Proceed to definitive airway: most commonly rapid-sequence intubation (see p. 482)
  - Cricothyroidotomy or tracheostomy is indicated in the event of failed intubation

**If airway obstruction is due to airway swelling, infection, or physical obstruction:**
  - Call for senior help (anaesthetic and ENT)
  - Consider humidified oxygen or heliox whilst waiting
  - Consider nebulized adrenaline (5 mg/5 ml 1:1000 in a nebulizer)
  - Elective intubation: prior to complete airway obstruction
  - Equipment for inhalational induction (anaesthetic machine with anaesthetic gas (sevoflurane or halothane))
  - Prepare difficult airway equipment (see p. 23)
  - Consider transferring patient to operating theatre or critical care area where above equipment is present if this is quicker
  - Cricothyroidotomy or tracheostomy is indicated in the event of failed intubation

**Early intubation should be considered to reduce the risk of sudden deterioration and airway obstruction**

**Other considerations requiring simultaneous treatment**
- Anaphylaxis/angio-oedema (see p. 112): IV or IM adrenaline, steroids, anti-histamines
- Haematoma after neck surgery: remove dressings, cut open sutures
- Airway bleeding (see p. 36): correct any clotting abnormalities
- Facial trauma (see p. 26): simultaneous assessment of C-spine and other associated trauma, as with diminished level of consciousness caused by trauma
- Laryngospasm: support ventilation with bag and mask ventilation; if possible apply PEEP (easier if using a Water's or C-circuit). Often laryngospasm will resolve, but re-intubation may be required (low-dose propofol 10–20 mg IV and low-dose suxamethonium 10–15 mg IV have successfully been used)
- Inadequate reversal of muscle relaxants: treat for laryngospasm as above, but also consider treating with IV neostigmine 2.5 mg mixed with glycopyrronium bromide 0.5 mg (only works if reversing a non-depolarizing muscle relaxant that is already beginning to wear off)
- In stable patients where diagnosis/degree of obstruction is in doubt nasal endoscopy performed by an experienced ENT surgeon may help. Be prepared to intubate or perform cricothyroidotomy/tracheostomy if total airway obstruction is provoked
- Once **A**irway is secure continue **ABC** approach
- Assess breathing and oxygenation
- Assess circulation
- Establish IV access
- Fluid/colloid to restore circulatory volume as appropriate
- Transfer to critical care environment for close observation

**Further management**
Only if condition is stable and the airway obstruction has been relieved
- Consider dexamethasone to reduce any further airway swelling
- Ventilation and sedation for a number of days on ICU may be required for intubated patients until the cause of obstruction has been resolved
- Adopt a lung-protective ventilation strategy (see p. 50)
- Surgical or microbiology opinions may be required
- Supportive measures on the ICU for septic patients (see pp. 120–122)
- Assessment of airway swelling (laryngoscopy and/or cuff-leak test) prior to extubation
- Where intubation is likely to be prolonged, or airway obstruction may recur after extubation, consider electively performing a tracheostomy

**Pitfalls/difficult situations**
- Delaying intubation may make a difficult intubation impossible
- Deterioration may be rapid, progressing from normal to complete airway obstruction in only a few hours
- Cardiovascular collapse may be severe, masking airway signs

- Airway interventions in a patient with a partially obstructed airway can provoke complete airway obstruction
- Insertion of oropharyngeal or nasopharyngeal airway in patients with retropharyngeal abscess may burst the abscess and soil the airway
- Other, non-airway, indications for intubation also exist (see p. 22)
- It is important to recognize patients in whom endotracheal intubation is likely to be difficult (see p. 22)
- Obtaining a definitive airway via endotracheal intubation or surgical tracheostomy can be challenging in the face of airway obstruction. The priority is always to maintain oxygenation, and intubation or cricothyroidotomy (see p. 488) should only be attempted by inexperienced operators in circumstances where the patient is otherwise likely to die (the most common technique of intubation, rapid-sequence intubation, is described on p. 482 only so that non-anaesthetic trained critical care practitioners are familiar with a technique with which they may be required to assist)
- Anyone who may be required to manage an airway or intubate patients in elective or emergency settings must be able to recognize a misplaced endotracheal tube (see p. 25) and be aware of what to do in the event of a failure to intubate (see p. 24)

**Further reading**

📖 OHCC p. 280, OHEA pp. 80, 124, 194, 434, 439.

# Complications at intubation

**Indications for endotracheal intubation**

*To protect the airway*
- From risk of aspiration: blood/vomit
- From risk of obstruction (see preceding pages)
- Because sedation/anaesthesia is required to allow assessment or treatment, particularly in agitated or combative patients

*To permit mechanical ventilation*
- Apnoea, bradypnoea
- Hypoxaemia or inadequate respiratory effort
- Hypercarbia or requirement for hyperventilation
- Cardiovascular instability—to maximize oxygenation

**Features predictive of difficult endotracheal intubation**
- Previous difficult intubation
- Current airway obstruction, inflammation, or haemorrhage
- Previous neck/jaw surgery or previous tracheostomy
- Receding jaw, or cannot protrude bottom incisors in front of top incisors
- Limited mouth opening (≤3 cm or two finger breadths)
- Prominent front teeth
- Unable to extend neck
- Morbid obesity, bull neck, large breasts
- Mallampati class III or IV: with mouth fully open and tongue protruding, the back of the mouth, uvula, and faucal pillars cannot be seen

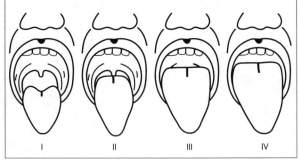

| I | II | III | IV |

**Equipment for intubation**

- A range of facemasks and a means of ventilating (i.e. self-inflating bag)
- Airway adjuncts (OPAs, NPAs)
- Range of cuffed endotracheal tubes (size 6.5–10)
- Lubricant
- 10 cm syringe (for inflating ETT cuff)
- Laryngoscope with Mackintosh blades size 3 and 4
- Tape or ties
- Stethoscope
- End-tidal $CO_2$ monitoring
- Suction apparatus, tubing; Yankauer suckers and suction catheters
- Magill forceps

**Equipment for difficult intubation**

- Microlaryngeal tubes (size 5–6)
- Bougies and stylets
- Special laryngoscopes (McCoy, short-handled, polio blade)
- LMAs (sizes 3, 4, 5) (intubating LMA if available)
- Airway exchange catheters
- Intubating fibrescope
- Berman airways
- Emergency cricothyroidotomy kit
  - Needle cricothyroidotomy kits
  - Surgical cricothyroidotomy equipment

## :ʘ: Failed intubation drill

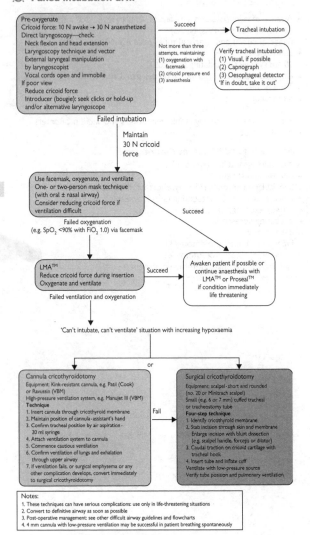

Notes:
1. These techniques can have serious complications: use only in life-threatening situations
2. Convert to definitive airway as soon as possible
3. Post-operative management: see other difficult airway guidelines and flowcharts
4. 4 mm cannula with low-pressure ventilation may be successful in patient breathing spontaneously

Adapted with permission from Difficult Airway Society Guidelines Flowchart, 2004. (Reproduced with kind permission of the Difficult Airway Society.)

### Recognizing a misplaced endotracheal tube

*Oesophageal intubation*
- Vocal cords not visualized
- No air entry into either side of chest
- No chest movement
- No misting of ETT
- 'Gurgling' on epigastric auscultation
- $CO_2$ trace on capnograph absent or only lasts for 1–2 breaths

*Bronchial intubation*
- Unilateral air entry (listen with stethoscope in both axillae)
- Hypoxaemia (may be gradual onset)
- High airway pressures
- Position of ETT at lips too far (*average* position at the lips is 20–22 cm for females, and 22–24 cm for males)

Auscultation may be unreliable, particularly in the obese

### Further reading

Vaughan RS (2001). Predicting difficult airways. *Br J Anaesth CEPD Rev* **1**, 44–7.
Difficult Airway Society. http://www.das.uk.com/
📖 OHEA pp. 68, 70, 76, 94.

# :✪: Airway and facial trauma

Trauma to the face and neck can directly damage airway structures or result in swelling/haematoma formation which may compress the airway. Trauma is also a major cause of airway haemorrhage (see p. 36).

## Causes
- Blunt force trauma: commonly car crash or assault
- Penetrating trauma: commonly stabbing or shooting
- All can affect
  - Midface: LeFort fractures, associated with base-of-skull fractures
  - Mandible or zygoma: both may occasionally disrupt the tempero-mandibular joint, limiting mouth opening
  - Larynx: severe injury rapidly leads to asphyxiation
  - Trachea: associated with severe thoracic or great vessel damage
- Associated with severe head injury and/or intoxication (factors associated with life-threatening injury from trauma, see p. 398)

## Presentation and assessment
- History of trauma or attempted hanging
- Obvious facial disruption, airway haemorrhage, spitting blood, epistaxis
- Altered consciousness
- Respiratory distress
  - Tachypnoea, dyspnoea, hypoxaemia, cyanosis
  - Use of accessory muscles of respiration
  - Paradoxical breathing: indrawing chest and suprasternal recession
  - Tracheal tug
  - Diminished or absent air entry, minimal respiratory excursions
- Patient prefers sitting, standing, or leaning forward

Laryngeal/tracheal trauma
- Surgical emphysema, neck swelling or bruising
- Palpable fracture
- Inability to speak or vocal changes (muffled or hoarse voice)
- Stridor (inspiratory noise accompanying breathing) or noisy breathing

## Investigations
Diagnosis is mainly clinical and some investigations may have to wait until the patient is stabilized with a secure airway
- ABGs
- FBC, cross-match, coagulation screen, U&Es, LFTs
- CXR
- CT scan may be required to evaluate head or facial injuries
- C-spine and trauma X-rays

## Differential diagnoses
- Epistaxis
- Airway tumour
- Tension pneumothorax

## Immediate management

- 100% $O_2$, pulse oximetry
- Assess degree of airway disruption, obstruction, bleeding
- Simultaneously assess C-spine and any other associated injuries
- If the patient is *in extremis* or injury is severe
  - Call for senior help (anaesthetic and surgical)
  - Assist ventilation via bag and mask if required. Care with airway adjuncts; oropharyngeal airways may provoke bleeding and nasal airways must be used only as a last resort in facial injuries because of the risk of disrupting the dura in base-of-skull fractures
  - Total obstruction requires immediate laryngoscopy and tracheal intubation. Uncut endotracheal tubes should be used in case of later facial swelling
  - Two suction devices may be needed if bleeding is rapid
  - Surgical airway, i.e. cricothyroidotomy or tracheostomy, for total obstruction if the above fails
- If airway bleeding or disruption makes difficult intubation likely
  - Prepare equipment for inhalational induction (anaesthetic machine with anaesthetic gas (sevoflurane or halothane))
  - Prepare difficult airway equipment (see p. 23)
  - Surgical tracheostomy by a skilled surgeon is indicated in the event of a 'failed intubation', or as the first-line technique
- Once **A**irway is secure continue **ABC** approach
- Assess breathing and oxygenation
- Establish IV access
- Fluid/colloid to restore circulatory volume
- Blood and blood product transfusion if required
- Obtain AMPLE history (see p. 2)

## Further management

- Complete secondary surveys
- Trauma screen X-rays
- Assess and treat other traumatic injuries
- Once stabilized, ventilation and sedation on ICU will be required for intubated patients and will be required until inflammation has resolved
- Consider antibiotics and check tetanus status
- Carry out full tertiary survey after suitable delay
- Consider delaying extubation until after any surgical repairs
- Assess airway swelling (laryngoscopy and/or cuff-leak test) prior to extubation

## Pitfalls/difficult situations

- Associated head, chest and cervical spine injuries are common

## Further reading

Chesshire NJ, Knight DJW (2001). The anaesthetic management of facial trauma and fractures. *Br J Anaesth CEPD Rev.* **1**, 108–12.

American College of Surgeons Committee on Trauma, ATLS Guidelines.

📖 OHEA p.198.

# :⚙: Airway and facial burns

Airway burns can cause airway obstruction within hours. Corrosive/toxic gases may also cause impaired gas exchange or oxygenation.

## Causes
- Direct-contact thermal burns to the face or airway
  - Airway fires (rare outside operating theatres)
  - Self-immolation
  - Trapped/unconscious near a heat source
- Inhalation of hot or corrosive gas
  - Entrapment near a burning substance (house fire, car fire)
  - 'Flashbacks' of hot gases (foundry accidents, aerosol can fires)
- Inhalation of steam or drinking hot fluids
  - Drinking corrosive fluids (e.g. bleach)

Airway and facial burns are associated with alcoholism, chronic ill health, psychiatric illness, trauma, and extremes of age

## Presentation and assessment
There is a high risk of airway oedema leading to obstruction if there is:
- On examining the face
  - Facial oedema already present
  - Marked facial burns (blistering, peeling skin)
- On examining the inside of the mouth and nose
  - Airway oedema present, blistering/peeling of mucosal membranes
  - There is loss of nasal hair
- On examining the neck
  - Circumferential or marked anterior neck burns are present
  - Laryngeal structures are no longer palpable
- Difficulty swallowing, drooling
- Carbonaceous sputum
- Inability to speak or vocal changes (muffled or hoarse voice)
- Stridor (inspiratory noise accompanying breathing) or noisy breathing
- Respiratory distress
  - Tachypnoea, dyspnoea, and/or wheeze/bronchospasm
  - Use of accessory muscles of respiration, tracheal tug
  - Paradoxical breathing (indrawing chest and suprasternal recession)
  - Patient prefers sitting, standing, or leaning forward

## Investigations
The diagnosis is mainly clinical and some investigations may have to wait until the patient is stabilized with a secure airway
- ABGs
- Carboxyhaemaglobin (using co-oximetry)
- FBC, cross-match, U&Es
- CXR
- C-spine and trauma series X-rays if appropriate

## Differential diagnoses
- Facial swelling secondary to anaphylaxis or angio-oedema

## Immediate management

- 100% $O_2$, pulse oximetry
- Assess degree of burn and airway obstruction
- Anaesthetic assessment of airway may be required
- If there is associated trauma simultaneously assess C-spine and other injuries
- If the patient is *in extremis* or the injury is severe:
  - Call for senior help (anaesthetic and ENT)
  - Consider humidified oxygen or heliox whilst waiting
  - Consider nebulized adrenaline (5 mg/5 ml 1:1000 in a nebulizer)
  - Elective intubation: prior to complete airway obstruction (uncut tubes should be used in case of facial swelling)
  - Prepare equipment for inhalational induction (anaesthetic machine with anaesthetic gas (sevoflurane or halothane))
  - Prepare difficult airway equipment (see p. 23)
  - Cricothyroidotomy or tracheostomy is indicated in the event of failed intubation, or as the first-line technique

**Early intubation should be considered to reduce the risk of sudden deterioration and airway obstruction**

Once **A**irway is secure continue **ABC** approach

- Assess breathing and oxygenation
- Ventilation may be required in the event of lung damage
- Assess any associated chest injuries
- In the case of circumferential chest injuries consider escharotomies
- Establish IV access and fluid resuscitate using a burns protocol (see p. 405)
- Obtain an 'AMPLE' history (see p. 2)

## Further management

- Assess and treat other traumatic injuries
- Once stabilized, ventilation and sedation on ICU will be required for intubated patients for a number of days until inflammation has resolved
- Consider transfer to burns unit (see p. 407). Anaesthetic assessment of airway risk may be required in unintubated patients
- Treat any inhalational injury (see p. 66)
- Consider antibiotics and check tetanus status
- Assess of airway swelling (laryngoscopy and/or cuff-leak test) prior to extubation

## Pitfalls/difficult situations

- If in doubt intubate as delay may make a difficult intubation impossible
- Failure to appreciate how rapidly these conditions can progress: normal to complete airway obstruction in only a few hours
- Hoarse voice is an early sign of laryngeal oedema
- Trauma, including chest, head, and neck injuries, is common

## Further reading

Papini RPG, Wood FM (1999). Current concepts in the management of burns with inhalation injury. *Care Crit. Ill* **15**, 61–5.

Hettiaratchy S, Papini R (2004). Initial management of a major burn. I: Overview. *BMJ*, **328**, 1555–7.

# ☼ **Airway infections** (See also p. 330)

Airway infections are associated inflammation and/or obstruction (partial or complete) which may be extrinsic or intrinsic to the upper airway.

## Causes

*Extrinsic*
- Pharyngeal, retropharyngeal, or peri-tonsillar abscess
- Ludwig's angina (soft tissue infection of the floor of the mouth)
- Deep-neck infections

All are mostly polymicrobial infections (aerobes include β-haemolytic streptococci and *Staphylococcus aureus*; anaerobes include bacteroides, and Gram-negatives include *Haemophilus parainfluenzae*)

*Intrinsic*
- Diphtheria: airway inflammation and a greyish pseudo-membrane in the respiratory tract (caused by *Corynebacterium diphtheriae*)
- Epiglottitis: inflammation of epiglottis vallecula, aryepiglottic folds, and arytenoids (commonly *Haemophilus influenzae*, also *H.parainfluenzae*, *Streptococcus pneumoniae* and *Staph.aureus*)

*Risk factors for airway infections include*
- Poor dental hygiene
- Recent sore throat
- Recent oral/pharyngeal surgery

## Presentation and assessment

Depending on cause, may include
- Tachypnoea, dyspnoea, hypoxaemia, and cyanosis
- Stridor
- 'Hunched' posture: sitting forward, mouth open, tongue protruding
- 'Muffled' or hoarse voice, sore throat, painful swallowing, drooling
- Neck swelling
- Trismus
- Fever and signs of systemic sepsis (see p. 322)
- Diphtheria exotoxin may cause CNS symptoms or cardiac failure

## Investigations
- FBC, U&Es
- Blood cultures and throat swabs
- CXR for all intubated patients
- Lateral soft tissue neck X-ray may demonstrate swelling and loss of airway cross-section ('thumb print' and 'vallecula' signs)
- Laryngoscopy (indirect or fibreoptic) performed by a skilled operator
- CT or MRI of head and neck may assist with diagnosis

**Airway interventions in a patient with a partially obstructed airway can provoke complete airway obstruction**

## Differential diagnoses
- Trauma
- Airway foreign body or tumour

Immediate management

- Humidified 100% $O_2$, pulse oximetry
- Rapid assessment, although manipulating airway or patient position may completely obstruct airway, particularly in children
- If the patient is *in extremis* or obstruction is severe:
  - Call for senior help (anaesthetic and ENT)
  - Elective intubation prior to complete airway obstruction
  - Equipment for inhalational induction (anaesthetic machine with anaesthetic gas (sevoflurane or halothane))
  - Prepare difficult airway equipment (see p. 23)
  - Consider transferring patient to an operating theatre or critical care area where equipment is present if this is quicker
  - Surgical tracheostomy by a skilled surgeon is indicated in the event of a 'failed intubation', or as the first-line technique
- If there is a need to 'buy' time waiting for senior help consider
  - Heliox
  - Nebulized adrenaline (5 mg/5 ml 1:1000 in a nebulizer)

**For those patients in-extremis, blood cultures and epiglottic swabs should not be obtained until the airway has been secured.**

- In more stable patients
  - Transfer to critical care environment for close observation
  - Early intubation should still be considered to reduce the risk of sudden airway obstruction
- Once Airway is secure continue **ABC** approach
- Blood cultures and pharyngeal/epiglottic swabs
- Obtain IV access and consider
  - Hydrocortisone 100–200 mg IV
- Suggested antibiotics: cefuroxime 1.5 g IV 8-hourly with metronidazole 500 mg IV 8-hourly
  - In severe infections consider adding chloramphenicol
- For diphtheria consider erythromycin 0.5–1 g IV 6-hourly

Further management

- Ventilation and sedation on ICU is obligatory for intubated patients and may be required for a number of days until inflammation has resolved
- Surgical drainage of abscesses and collections may be required
- Supportive measures on the ICU for septic patients (see p. 322)
- Assess of airway swelling (laryngoscopy and/or cuff-leak test) prior to extubation

Pitfalls/difficult situations

- Delaying intubation may make a difficult intubation impossible
- Failure to appreciate how rapidly these conditions can progress: normal to complete airway obstruction in only a few hours

Further reading

Ames WA, Ward VMM, Tranter RMD, *et al.* (2001). Adult epiglottitis: an under-recognized, life-threatening condition. *Br J Anaesth* **85**, 795–7.
  OHEA p. 426.

## ☠ **Airway foreign bodies**

The most common causes are food boluses (including sweets and nuts), dentures, toys (in children), chewed items (e.g. pen tops), blood clots, and vomit.

### Causes
Foreign bodies are commonly associated with
- Decreased consciousness from alcohol or CVA
- Dementia
- Children

### Presentation and assessment
- May be witnessed
- May present as a cardiac arrest (see p. 105) or as an unconscious patient where bag and mask ventilation is impossible
- May present as sudden total or near-total airway obstruction

*Total or near-total obstruction*
- Anxiety or altered consciousness
- Hypoxaemia, cyanosis
- Diminished or absent air entry
- Minimal respiratory excursions
- Tachypnoea and respiratory distress
- Bradycardia

*Partial obstruction*
- Anxiety
- Patient prefers sitting, standing, or leaning forward
- Inability to speak, lump in throat, difficulty in swallowing
- Stridor (inspiratory noise accompanying breathing) or noisy breathing
- Choking, coughing or drooling
- Respiratory distress
  - Tachypnoea and dyspnoea
  - Use of accessory muscles of respiration
  - Paradoxical breathing: indrawing chest and suprasternal recession

*Late presentation*
- Monophonic wheeze or lobar pneumonia which does not respond to treatment

### Investigations
- CXR or neck X-ray (although many foreign bodies are radiolucent, partial collapse and/or volume loss may be seen in the lung fields)
- Endoscopy or direct laryngoscopy will aid diagnosis and allow intervention to restore airway patency, but both require ENT or anaesthetic experience in order to be performed safely
- Consider chest CT

### Differential diagnoses
- Bronchospasm
- Pneumonia

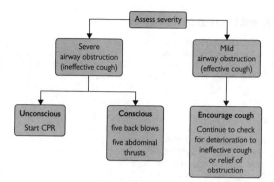

**Fig. 2.1** Adult choking algorithm (UK Resuscitation Council Guidelines 2005) (Reproduced with kind permission of the RCUK.)

## Immediate management

- If patient is choking, follow choking algorithm (see Fig. 2.1), otherwise:
- 100% $O_2$, pulse oximetry
- If patient has suffered cardiac arrest
  - Follow BLS guidelines (see p. 104). Remove obvious obstruction, give two rescue breaths, and commence CPR
- If the patient is *in extremis* or obstruction is severe
  - Call for senior help (anaesthetic and ENT)
  - Consider heliox whilst waiting
  - Elective intubation, prior to complete airway obstruction
  - Equipment for inhalational induction (anaesthetic machine with anaesthetic gas (sevoflurane or halothane))
  - Prepare difficult airway equipment (see p. 23)
  - Consider transferring patient to an operating theatre or critical care area where above equipment is present if this is quicker
  - Surgical tracheostomy is indicated in the event of failed intubation
  - Foreign body may be removed at laryngoscopy or bronchoscopy
- In more stable patients awake flexible bronchoscopy may be possible
- Once **A**irway is secure continue **ABC** approach
- Consider transfer to critical care environment for close observation

## Further management

- Consider antibiotics and dexamethasone

## Pitfalls/difficult situations

- Some foreign bodies (nuts) can cause secondary airway inflammation
- There may be more than one foreign body

## Further reading

📖 OHEA p. 196.

# :Ö: **Airway tumours**

Airway obstruction can develop in patients with primary malignant or metastatic tumours of the head, neck, respiratory tract, or mediastinum. Obstruction may be caused by extrinsic or intrinsic compression due to the tumour itself, or any associated lymphadenopathy.

## Causes
- Smoker
- Previous history of cancer

## Presentation and assessment
- Airway haemorrhage or haemoptysis
- Recurrent or persistent pneumonia
- Persistent cough and/or hoarse voice
- Cervical, supraclavicular, or axillary lymphadenopathy
- Obstruction or respiratory distress of gradual onset

*Total or near-total obstruction*
- Anxiety or altered consciousness
- Hypoxaemia, cyanosis
- Diminished or absent air entry
- Minimal respiratory excursions
- Tachypnoea and respiratory distress
- Bradycardia

*Partial obstruction*
- Anxiety
- Patient prefers sitting, standing, or leaning forward
- Inability to speak, lump in throat, difficulty in swallowing
- Stridor (inspiratory noise accompanying breathing) or noisy breathing
- Respiratory distress
  - Tachypnoea and dyspnoea
  - Use of accessory muscles of respiration
  - Paradoxical breathing: indrawing chest and suprasternal recession

## Investigations
Some investigations may have to wait until the patient is stabilized
- ABGs
- FBC, group and save, U&Es, LFTs, coagulation screen
- Blood and sputum cultures if evidence of coexisting infection
- CXR
- CT scan may be required
- When possible, endoscopy, bronchoscopy, or direct laryngoscopy will aid diagnosis and allow interventions to restore airway patency

## Differential diagnoses
- Upper airway infection
- Foreign body
- Asthma, COPD
- Pulmonary oedema

**Immediate management**

- 100% $O_2$, pulse oximetry
- Make as full assessment as possible, including CT scanning if the clinical situation allows
- Primary aim is to establish a patent airway and palliate symptoms; senior anaesthetic and surgical assistance likely to be required
- If upper airway obstruction suspected and the patient is *in extremis* or obstruction is severe
  - Call for senior help (anaesthetic and ENT)
  - Consider heliox whilst waiting
  - Elective intubation prior to complete airway obstruction
  - Equipment for inhalational induction (anaesthetic machine with anaesthetic gas (sevoflurane or halothane))

Prepare difficult airway equipment (see p. 23)
  - Surgical tracheostomy is indicated in the event of failed intubation
- If lower airway obstruction suspected and the patient is *in extremis* or obstruction is severe
  - Call for senior help (anaesthetic and ENT or thoracic)
  - Consider heliox whilst waiting
  - Equipment for inhalational induction (anaesthetic machine with anaesthetic gas (sevoflurane or halothane)) may be needed
- Consider transferring patient to operating theatre or critical care area where above equipment is present if this is quicker or more appropriate
- Avoid IPPV until obstruction bypassed—risk of barotrauma
- Airway manipulation may provoke complete obstruction
- Assess degree of bleeding and extent of lung soiling, if severe
- Once **A**irway is secure continue **ABC** approach

**Further management**

Only if condition is stable and airway obstruction has been relieved
- Ventilation and sedation on ICU may be required for intubated patients for a number of days until inflammation has resolved
- Antibiotics for prophylaxis or treatment of concurrent infection may be required
- Supportive measures on the ICU for septic patients (see p. 322)
- Assess of airway swelling (laryngoscopy and/or cuff-leak test) prior to extubation

**Pitfalls/difficult situations**

- Do not use sedatives before securing an airway
- Do not induce general anaesthesia without senior assistance present
- Do not use positive pressure ventilation until obstruction is relieved

**Further reading**

Mason RA, Fielder CP (1999). The obstructed airway in head and neck surgery. *Anaesthesia* **54**, 625–8.

# ☹ Airway haemorrhage

This is an emergency that can cause airway obstruction, deterioration in gas exchange (due to flooding of alveoli with blood), or circulatory collapse.

## Causes
- Following airway surgery
- Following upper airway interventions, especially tracheostomy
- Upper airway infection
- Airway or neck trauma
- Coagulopathic or anti-coagulated patients
- Epistaxis may occasionally be so severe as to compromise the airway

## Presentation and assessment
- Anxiety
- Haemoptysis
- Persistent cough
- Airway obstruction: stridor, use of accessory muscles, paradoxical breathing
- Alveolar soiling: widespread crepitations, diminished air entry
- Respiratory distress: tachypnoea, dyspnoea, decreased $SpO_2$, cyanosis, altered consciousness
- Signs of blood loss: pallor, tachycardia, hypotension

## Investigations
Diagnosis is mainly clinical and some investigations may have to wait until the patient is stabilized
- ABGs
- FBC, cross-match
- Coagulation screen
- Neck X-ray
- When possible, endoscopy or direct laryngoscopy will aid diagnosis and allow interventions to restore airway patency

## Differential diagnoses
- Haemoptysis due to pulmonary haemorrhage
- Pulmonary oedema

## Immediate management

- 100% $O_2$, pulse oximetry
- For trauma patients: simultaneous assessment of C-spine and other associated trauma
- Assess degree of bleeding and extent of lung soiling, if severe:
  - Call for senior help (anaesthetic and surgical)
  - first line of management should be to secure patency of airway
  - Airway obstruction will require immediate laryngoscopy, suction of upper airway and tracheal intubation
  - Two suction devices may be needed if bleeding is rapid
  - Surgical airway (cricothyroidotomy or tracheostomy) may be needed if intubation fails
  - Aim is to place cuff of ETT beyond site of haemorrhage in the first instance
  - Surgical control of bleeding should then be attempted
- Once **A**irway is secure continue **ABC** approach
- Urgent bronchoscopy may be required to remove clots from lower airways if the patient has inhaled large amounts of blood
- Establish IV access
- Fluid/colloid may be needed to restore circulatory volume
- Blood and blood product transfusion may be required

## Further management

Only if condition is stable and airway obstruction has been relieved or is not deteriorating
- Fibreoptic laryngoscopy or bronchoscopy to assess the source of haemorrhage
- Assessment by ENT surgeon and/or thoracic surgeon for more definitive management of bleeding
- Sedate and ventilate in intensive care until haemorrhage is controlled or if oxygenation is poor despite a patent airway
- Circulatory support including inotropes may be required

## Pitfalls/difficult situations

- Deterioration may be rapid
- In extensive lung soiling hypoxia may not be relieved by securing airway and ventilation. Watch for development of pneumonia or ARDS

## Further reading

📖 OHEA pp. 212, 424.

# :⊙: **Endotracheal tube complications**

Indications for intubation can be found on p. 22; a description of how to perform rapid-sequence intubations can be found on p. 482, and what to do if unable to pass a endotracheal tube at the time of intubation (the failed intubation) can be found on p. 24. Other endotracheal tube complications include
- Tube obstruction (malposition, cuff herniation, mucous plugging)
- Cuff leak
- Aspiration of gastric contents
- Accidental extubation

## Causes

Complications are more likely
- In agitated or very mobile patients, or patients with abnormal anatomy
- During transfer
- If there are large amounts of airway secretions

Aspiration is more likely where patients have
- Been intubated as an emergency, or by inexperienced operator
- Had a full stomach at time of intubation, or intubation was delayed in a patient at risk of aspiration

## Presentation and assessment
- Occluded, semi-occluded, or malpositioned ETT:
  - Agitation
  - Hypoxia and cyanosis
  - Diminished or unilateral air entry
  - Difficulty ventilating with high airway pressures
  - ETT position at lips has changed
- Cuff leak:
  - Audible leak on inspiration if ventilated
  - Ventilator may alarm indicating a leak, low airway pressure, or low expiratory volumes
- Airway soiling with gastric contents:
  - Widespread crepitations, wheeze, or high airway pressures
  - Hypoxia

## Investigations

Diagnosis is mainly clinical and some investigations may have to wait until airway is secure and the patient is stabilized
- ABGs
- Endoscopy (may reveal malpositioning or airway soiling with gastric contents)
- CXR to check ETT position (above carina)

## Differential diagnoses
- Bronchospasm

## Immediate management

- 100% oxygen, pulse oximetry
- Assess degree of airway obstruction
- Check ETT position (*average* position at the lips is 20–22 cm for females, and 22–24cm for males; these distances may still be too far). If too far try withdrawing tube slowly, preferably under direct vision using laryngoscope to avoid accidental extubation
- Try manually ventilation, check ventilator tubing and connections
- Pass a suction catheter via ETT: removes secretions and checks patency of lumen
- If the patient is *in extremis* or obstruction is severe:
  - Try deflating the cuff; if it has herniated the obstruction should relieve quickly
  - If this fails, consider laryngoscopy to check tube position (cuff should be just below cords)
- Consider removing ETT and re-intubating. This will require
  - Sedation (if not already commenced; may have to be increased)
  - Muscle relaxants (suxamethonium, atracurium, or other)
  - Suction immediately available
  - Consider changing ETT over bougie or airway exchange catheter
- In the event of accidental decannulation
  - Assist ventilation via bag and mask with airway adjuncts (oropharyngeal/nasal airways) if required
  - Consider re-intubation (sometimes not required; patient may achieve adequate ventilation breathing spontaneously without support or with non-invasive ventilation)

If ever in doubt, oxygenate by any means possible. This may mean removing ETT and inserting an LMA or simply using bag and mask ventilation until help arrives

- Once **A**irway is secure continue **ABC** approach
- Check to ensure adequate ventilation. If poor, consider the possibility of pneumothorax
- In the event of airway soiling pass suction catheter
- In the event of a cuff leak try further inflating the cuff. If this fails or the cuff gradually deflates, consider electively changing tracheostomy when the patient is stable

## Further management

If condition is stable and any severe airway obstruction has been relieved or airway re-secured
- Continue ventilation in an ICU setting
- If the patient has airway soiling:
  - Send tracheal aspirate samples
  - Use appropriate antibiotics
  - Consider bronchodilators, chest physiotherapy, and regular suction

## Further reading
OHEA pp. 90, 92.

# :O: **Tracheostomy complications**

Complications can arise on first or subsequent insertions of tracheostomy tube and may obstruct or soil the airway or hamper ventilation. Complications include

- Aspiration of gastric contents
- Bleeding
- Malpositioning (including para-tracheal tracheostomy placement)
- Infection
- Tracheostomy occlusion (malposition, cuff herniation, mucous plugging)
- Cuff leak, or accidental decannulation (removal)

## Causes

Complications are more likely if

- The tracheostomy was performed as an emergency procedure, or by an inexperienced operator
- The tracheostomy was performed in a patient who had
  - A full stomach
  - Severe chest problems ($FiO_2$ >0.6 and/or PEEP >10 $cmH_2O$)
  - Coagulation abnormalities or platelet dysfunction
  - Large amounts of airway secretions
- Agitated or very mobile patients, or patients with abnormal anatomy

## Presentation and assessment

- Occluded/semi-occluded airway
  - Agitation
  - Hypoxia and cyanosis
  - Diminished air entry
  - Difficulty ventilating with high airway pressures
- Airway soiling with gastric contents
  - Widespread crepitations, wheeze, or high airway pressures
  - Hypoxia
- Bleeding
  - Obvious blood loss from or around the tracheostomy
  - Presence of blood in airway
  - Increased airway pressure
  - Hypoxia
- Malpositioning
  - Difficulty ventilating with increased airway pressures
  - Rapidly developing respiratory insufficiency and hypoxia
  - Pneumothorax or pneumomediastinum
  - Subcutaneous emphysema
- Cuff leak
  - Audible leak on inspiration if ventilated
  - Ventilator may alarm, indicating a leak, low airway pressure, or low expiratory volumes
  - Able to talk past cuffed tube
- Infection
  - Cellulitis, skin erosion, or frank pus

## Investigations
Diagnosis is mainly clinical and some investigations may have to wait until the airway is secure and the patient is stabilized.
- ABGs
- FBC, coagulation studies
- Endoscopy (may reveal malpositioning, or airway soiling with blood or gastric contents)
- CXR

## Differential diagnoses
- Bronchospasm

## Immediate management
- 100% oxygen, pulse oximetry
- Assess degree of airway obstruction
- Check tracheostomy position, try manually ventilating, check ventilator tubing and connections
- Pass suction catheter via tracheostomy: removes secretions and checks patency of lumen
- If the tracheostomy has an inner tube remove/replace
- If the patient is *in extremis* or obstruction is severe
  - Try deflating the cuff; if it has herniated the obstruction should relieve quickly
  - If this fails, stop ventilating through the tracheostomy tube and establish airway using endotracheal tube
- In the event of accidental decannulation
  - Attempt ventilation via a bag and mask using airway adjuncts (oropharyngeal/nasal airways) if required. If the tracheostomy was sited for upper respiratory tract obstruction attempt to resite the tracheostomy as soon as possible
  - Some tracheostomies will remain patent and ventilation may be assisted via the stoma
  - Consider endotracheal intubation
- In the event of airway bleeding
  - Assess degree of bleeding and extent of lung soiling
  - Call for skilled help (experienced anaesthetist)
  - Airway obstruction will require immediate laryngoscopy, suction of upper airway, and tracheal intubation
  - Urgent endoscopy may be required to remove clots from airway and lungs

**If ever in doubt, secure airway using endotracheal intubation**
- Once **A**irway is secure continue **ABC** approach
- Check to ensure adequate ventilation; if poor consider the possibility of pneumothorax
- In the event of airway soiling, pass suction catheter
- In the event of a cuff leak, try further inflating cuff; if this fails or the cuff gradually deflates, consider electively changing tracheostomy when patient stable
- Fluid/colloid to restore circulatory volume
- Correct any coagulopathy if there is airway bleeding

## Further management

If the condition is stable and any severe airway obstruction has been relieved
- Continue ventilation in an ICU setting
- If obstruction only mild or after the airway is re-established using ETT
  - Re-explore tracheostomy wound and re-insert tube. This can be difficult, particularly with recent (<7 days) percutaneous tracheostomy wounds. Senior anaesthetic or ENT help may be required
  - Re-siting over an endoscope may help to ensure correct positioning
- If the patient has airway soiling or cellulitis
  - Send wound or tracheal aspirate samples
  - Use appropriate antibiotics
  - Consider bronchodilators, chest physiotherapy, and regular suction
- If the patient has airway bleeding
  - Fibreoptic laryngoscopy or bronchoscopy to assess the source of haemorrhage
  - Assessment by ENT surgeon and/or thoracic surgeon for more definitive management of bleeding
  - Circulatory support including inotropes may be required

## Pitfalls/difficult situations

- Haemorrhage may appear after a few hours
- Malpositioning is obvious almost immediately

## Further reading

Quigley RL (1988). Tracheostomy: an overview. Management and complications. *Br J Clin Pract* **42**, 430–4.

Seay SJ, Gay SL, Strauss M (2002). Tracheostomy emergencies. *Am J Nurs* **102**, 59, 61, 63.

# Breathing

# ☼ Respiratory failure

Respiratory failure occurs when air transfer in and out of the lungs is reduced, or when gas exchange within the lungs fails (due to shunt, VQ mismatch, or poor gas diffusion), resulting in either
- Type 1 respiratory failure—causing hypoxia
- Type 2 respiratory failure—causing hypoxia and hypercapnia

Type 1 respiratory failure typically has parenchymal causes. Type 2 respiratory failure occurs with mechanical/obstructive causes or as a result of fatigue or decreased consciousness, especially when occurring with any causes of respiratory failure.

---

**Definitions:**

- Hypoxia: $PaO_2$ <8 kPa or $PaO_2$ <11 kPa on $FiO_2$ ≥40%
- Hypercapnia: $PaCO_2$ >6.3 kPa

Blood gas values must be interpreted flexibly with regard to
- Inspired oxygen concentration ($FiO_2$) required to avoid hypoxia
- Respiratory distress in the presence of normal blood gases
- Lack of symptoms of respiratory distress in patients with chronic lung conditions giving rise to abnormal blood gases
- Intracardiac shunt
- Pre-existing metabolic alkalosis leading to hypercapnia

---

## Causes
- Upper airway obstruction (see p. 16)
- Lower airway obstruction
  - Acute bronchoconstriction, asthma, anaphylaxis
  - Chronic obstructive pulmonary disease
  - Mucous plugging, atelectasis
  - Foreign body
- Lung tissue damage/gas exchange failure
  - Pneumonia
  - Lung contusion
  - ARDS
  - Pulmonary haemorrhage
  - Cardiogenic pulmonary oedema
  - Lung fibrosis
- Pulmonary circulatory compromise
  - Pulmonary embolus
  - Pulmonary vascular disease
  - Heart failure
  - Excessively raised cardiac output
- Neuromuscular damage
  - Decreased level of consciousness: intracranial catastrophe, sedative agents
  - Paralysis/weakness (e.g. spinal damage, tetanus, Guillain–Barré syndrome, myasthenia gravis)

- Mechanical compromise of lung tissue
  - Pneumothorax, haemothorax, pleural effusion
  - Skeletal deformation: flail chest, kyphopscoliosis, diaphragmatic rupture
  - Raised intra–abdominal pressure
  - Obesity or ascites
- Inadequate mechanical ventilation
- Hypercapnia may be caused by increased $CO_2$ production (see p. 52)

**Presentation and assessment**
Respiratory failure may present with respiratory or cardiac arrest (see p. 105).

**Evidence of respiratory distress which may precede or accompany respiratory failure includes**
- Agitation, sense of impending doom
- Sense of 'tight chest' or breathlessness in conscious patients
- Inability to talk normally or in full sentences
- Sweating, clamminess
- Tachypnoea >25 breaths/minute
- Dyspnoea, or laboured breathing, with use of accessory muscles
- Gasping or 'pursed-lip' breathing
- Sitting, or hunched posture
- Cyanosis
- Hypoxaemia, as evidenced by arterial blood gas or $SpO_2$ <92%
- Hypercapnia: flapping tremor, warm peripheries, and bounding pulse
- Tachycardia (>110 beats/minute)

**Pre-terminal signs include**
- Bradycardia, dysrhythmia, or hypotension
- Silent chest
- Bradypnoea or exhaustion
- Confusion or decreased level of consciousness

**In mechanically ventilated patients evidence of respiratory failure may also be accompanied by**
- High, or low, pressure ventilator alarms
- Evidence of low delivered tidal volume, or low minute-volume alarm
- Audible leak from ventilator circuit, or leak alarm
- Inability to ventilate using self-inflating bag
- Lack of chest movement
- Lack of respiratory sounds on auscultation

**Other features associated with respiratory failure depend upon the cause, but may include**
- Pleuritic chest pain; haemoptysis; evidence of sepsis (pyrexia, rigors, purulent sputum); reduced peak flow; cough or audible wheeze; wheeze, rub, or bronchial breathing on auscultation; reduced air entry or altered percussion note associated with pneumothorax,

consolidation or effusion; evidence of mediastinal deviation(tracheal deviation, altered apex); raised JVP; evidence of cardiac failure

## Investigations

In most cases clinical assessment will reveal evidence of respiratory distress. Investigations which may aid in assessing severity or establishing a diagnosis include
- ABGs
  - The $PaO_2/FiO_2$ ratio may be calculated to give a measure of the degree of respiratory failure (see back endpapers)
  - Alternatively, the alveolar arterial (A–a) $O_2$ gradient may be calculated: A–a difference = $(FiO_2 \times 94.8) - (PaCO_2 + PaO_2)$
- FBC
- U&Es, LFTs
- Peak flow measurements (where appropriate)
- ECG
- CXR
- Chest ultrasound

Further investigations may be required depending on cause or clinical progress:
- Coagulation studies
- CRP
- D-dimers (of limited use in the ICU)
- Culture (blood, sputum)
- Atypical serology
- Urine for Legionella and pneumococcal antigen
- Bronchoscopy or non-directed BAL
- Echocardiogram
- CT chest
- CT pulmonary angiogram

## Differential diagnoses

Patients may appear to be in respiratory distress despite having adequately saturated arterial blood. In these cases it is important to consider
- Anaemia
- Cytotoxic hypoxia, e.g. cyanide or carbon monoxide poisoning
- Metabolic acidosis
- Hyperventilation, either hysterical or associated with disease (e.g. thyrotoxicosis) or pain

Also consider
- Upper airway obstruction (see p. 16)
- Endotracheal tube/breathing system obstruction (see pp. 38 and 40)

**Immediate management**

- If the patient is spontaneously breathing without ventilatory support:
  - Ensure that the airway is secure and patent
  - Increase $FiO_2$ to near 100% (see p. 48)
  - Assist breathing with bag and mask if required
  - Consider escalating respiratory support in a stepwise progression (non-invasive CPAP or BIPAP may be indicated (see p. 50))
  - Endotracheal intubation and mechanical ventilation may be required
- If patient is already intubated and/or receiving ventilatory support (non-invasive or invasive) consider the following
  - Increase $FiO_2$ to 100%
  - Check that the airway is patent; in intubated patients check the patency and position of the endotracheal tube (check with suction catheter if in doubt (see p. 38))
  - If already on a ventilator, ensure ventilation is possible; check equipment is working and not disconnected
  - If in doubt switch to self-inflating Ambubag and ventilate manually

Establish a probable diagnosis as soon as possible and treat as appropriate, especially any reversible causes such as pneumothorax, pulmonary oedema, secretions and mucous plugs, bronchospasm, and pleural effusions

- Once **A**irway and **B**reathing are stabilized, continue **ABC** approach
  - Patients may require aggressive circulatory support

**Further management**

- Titrate oxygen therapy and respiratory support to keep $PaO_2$ >8 kPa and $PaCO_2$ <6.3 kPa (and respiratory rate <30 breaths/minute if spontaneously breathing) where possible
- If basic ventilatory support is not enough consider additional manoeuvres for hypoxaemia (see p. 56) or hypercapnia (see p. 52)
- Consider invasive monitoring with serial arterial blood gas analysis
- If mechanical ventilation is necessary, sedation (with or without muscle relaxation) will be required at least initially; attempt to follow a lung-protective ventilation strategy (see p. 50)
- If endotracheal intubation is likely to last for more than a few days consider early tracheostomy

**Pitfalls/difficult situations**

- Double-check equipment as it may be faulty or not be delivering sufficiently high $O_2$; switch to alternative equipment if in doubt
- Cold limbs or poor skin perfusion may make $SpO_2$ readings unreliable or difficult to maintain
- CXR interpretation can be difficult in supine patients; certain conditions such as anterior pneumothoraces or pleural effusions may require additional imaging (CT or US)
- The presence of a metabolic acidosis increases dyspnoea; do not ignore circulatory support and correction of acidosis

## Oxygen delivery devices

Devices which deliver variable concentrations (and *estimated* FiO$_2$):
- Nasal cannulae[*]
  - At 2 L/minute O$_2$ flow – maximum FiO$_2$ = 28%
  - At 4 L/minute O$_2$ flow – maximum FiO$_2$ = 35%
  - At 6 L/minute O$_2$ flow – maximum FiO$_2$ = 45%
- Non-Venturi masks (e.g. Hudson mask)
  - At 5 L/minute O$_2$ flow – maximum FiO$_2$ = 35%
  - At 8 L/minute O$_2$ flow – maximum FiO$_2$ = 55%
  - At 12 L/minute O$_2$ flow – maximum FiO$_2$ = 65%
- Reservoir bag masks (non-rebreathing masks, trauma masks)
  - At 15 L/minute O$_2$ flow – maximum FiO$_2$ = 80–90%

Devices which deliver fixed O$_2$ concentrations:
- All Venturi masks: 24–60% if O$_2$ flow rate is set according to instructions written on adapter (to change FiO$_2$, change adapter)
- Ventilator circuits: upto100% O$_2$ as set
- Oxylog portable ventilators: if set to 'Airmix', 50–60%; if set to 'No airmix', 100%

[*] High-flow O$_2$ (at rates of >20 L/minute) can be delivered by some delivery devices which obtain near 100% humidification (e.g. Vapotherm™)

**Indications for ventilatory support**

Invasive (and in some cases or non-invasive) ventilatory support should be considered where

Endotracheal intubation is required:
- Airway protection
- Secretion clearance

Respiratory failure is present or likely to occur:
- Respiratory rate >30 breaths/minute, or apnoea/bradypnoea
- Vital capacity <10–15 ml/minute
- Hypercapnia with pH <7.35
- $PaO_2$ <11 on $FiO_2$ <40%
- Fatigue, exhaustion, inadequate respiratory effort
- Decreased level of consciousness
- Acute pulmonary oedema

Cardiopulmonary support is required:
- Following cardiac arrest
- Post-operative support of certain high risk patients
- Severe shock or LVF

Sedation, anaesthesia, and/or paralysis is required to:
- Control intracranial pressure
- Transfer critically ill patients
- Control muscle spasms (e.g. tetanus)
- Allow assessment or treatment, particularly in agitated or combative patients

See also indications for endotracheal intubation (p. 22)

## Lung-protective mechanical ventilation

Lung-protective strategies help in avoiding barotrauma, volutrauma, and/ or the development of ARDS
- Use tidal volumes of approximately 6 ml/kg
- Keep maximum ventilatory pressure at <30 cmH$_2$O
- Keep I:E ratio >1:1 where possible
- Use assist-controlled ventilation where possible
- Use adequate level of PEEP
- Use the minimum required FiO$_2$ to keep SpO$_2$ above 90% (or PaO$_2$ above 8 kPa)
- Allow CO$_2$ to rise if necessary (permissive hypercapnia)

## Non-invasive ventilation

### Potential advantages
- Decreased incidence of ventilator-associated pneumonia
- No endotracheal intubation or tracheostomy required
  - No risk of failure to intubate,
  - No risk of long-term tracheal damage
- No sedation required
  - Patient can communicate
  - Patients can often eat and drink

### Indications
- Acute pulmonary oedema
  - (Use CPAP or BIPAP* with PEEP of 10–15 cmH$_2$O)
- Obstructive sleep apnoea
  - (Use CPAP or BIPAP with PEEP and inspiratory pressure adjusted to alleviate obstruction)
- COPD
  - (Use CPAP or BIPAP with inspiratory pressure adjusted to ease work of breathing or avoid hypercapnic acidosis and PEEP adjusted to approximately 80% of intrinsic PEEP)
- Weaning from mechanical ventilation
- Respiratory failure in immunocompromised patients at high risk of VAP (e.g. neutropaenic patients)
- Other causes of acute respiratory failure where there are no contraindications

### Contraindications[†]
- Risk of airway obstruction or inability to protect the airway
- Facial abnormalities, trauma or burns; or recent facial/airway surgery
- Upper airway obstruction
- Excessive secretions or vomiting; bowel obstruction
- Very high oxygen requirement/life-threatening hypoxaemia
- Severe acidaemia
- Haemodynamic instability, dysrhythmias, or severe comorbidity
- Confusion, agitation, or patient refusal

- Pneumothoraces (an intercostal drain should be inserted first)
- Upper GI surgery is a relative contraindication

**Complications**
- Intolerance of mask (up to 25%)
- Airway may still become obstructed, especially if patient becomes obtunded or if there is airway trauma
- Skin damage
- Gastric distension

\* Current evidence suggests that CPAP *may* be preferable to BIPAP

† NIV may be used in the presence of contraindications provided there is a contingency plan for intubation or the decision not to proceed to invasive ventilation has previously been made

**Further reading**

Levy MM (2005). Pathophysiology of oxygen delivery in respiratory failure. *Chest* **128**(Suppl 2), 547S–53S.

Malarkkan N, Snook NJ, Lumb AB (2003). New aspects of ventilation in acute lung injury. *Anaesthesia* **58**, 647–67.

Riley B (1999). Strategies for ventilatory support. *Br Med Bull* **55**, 806–20.

Baudouin S, Blumenthal S, Cooper B, *et al.* (2002). Non-invasive ventilation in acute respiratory failure. *Thorax* **57**, 192–211.

OHCC pp. 278, 282, OHEA pp. 48, 304, 306, OHEC p. 22.

# ⚠ **Hypercapnia**

Hypercapnia is defined as a $PaCO_2$ >6.3 kPa. It can occur as a result of decreased clearance of $CO_2$ or, less commonly, as a result of increased production.

## Causes

- Decreased ventilation
  - All causes of type 2 respiratory failure (see p. 44), including COPD or bronchospasm, airway obstruction, inadequate respiratory rate (e.g. head injury or overdose), inadequate ventilation (e.g. neuromuscular disease or traumatic damage), impaired gas exchange (e.g. acute lung injury, ARDS, or infection)
  - Inadequate mechanical ventilation
- Increased production
  - Sepsis and pyrexia (rarely causes very severe hypercapnia)
  - Thyroid storm
  - Reperfusion event (e.g. following release from crush injury)
  - Malignant hyperpyrexia
  - Neuroleptic malignant syndrome
  - Drug reaction: serotinin syndrome, ecstasy (MDMA) poisoning
- Equipment failure may lead to re-breathing of expired $CO_2$; this is more common with breathing circuits in anaesthetic rather than ICU practice.

## Presentation and assessment

- Most commonly revealed by arterial blood gas analysis
  - Hypercapnia results in a respiratory acidaemia, which may be compensated for metabolically by retention of bicarbonate ions in chronic conditions (e.g. COPD)
- Where end-tidal $CO_2$ measurements are available, these will be raised
- Symptoms of hypercapnia include
  - Agitation, sweating, flapping tremor
  - Respiratory distress: tachypnoea, dyspnoea
  - Tachycardia, hypertension, bounding pulse
  - Peripheral vasodilatation
  - Decreased consciousness level, narcosis

## Investigations

- ABGs
- FBC, coagulation studies
- U&Es, LFTs
- TFTs
- CK and urine myoglobin (where MH or reperfusion injury suspected)
- ECG

## Differential diagnoses

- Inaccurate ABG sample result

**Immediate management**

- Titrate $O_2$ to maintain $SpO_2$ oxygen ≥95% via reservoir mask, if spontaneously breathing, or ventilator if receiving respiratory support
- Secure airway if required
- Where hyperpyrexia is suspected (MH, neuroleptic malignant syndrome, serotinin syndrome, MDMA poisoning) treat accordingly (see p. 252)
- Where thyroid storm is suspected treat accordingly (see p. 246)
- Treat any underlying cause of type 2 respiratory failure
- Consider intubation and mechanical ventilation if the patient is tiring, hypercapnia or oxygenation are worsening, or if airway needs to be secured
- Tolerate moderate hypercapnia ($PaCO_2$ <8 kPa)
- Consider altering ventilation parameters*
  - Increase inspiratory pressure, inspiratory time, or tidal volume if ventilatory volumes are inadequate
  - Increase respiratory rate if minute volumes are inadequate despite good tidal volumes
  - Increase PEEP to maintain lung recruitment
- Consider increasing sedation or short-term muscle relaxation to allow greater tolerance of hypercapnia and to reduce $CO_2$ produced by the work of breathing
- Consider advanced airway manoeuvres or oxygenation techniques
  - Alveolar recruitment measures (see p. 63)
  - If lung pathology is unilateral try positioning bad lung uppermost
  - Consider prone position
- Once **A**irway and **B**reathing are stabilized, continue **ABC** approach

* Follow a lung-protective strategy where possible (see p. 50)

**Further management**
- If acidaemia is severe and has both mixed metabolic and respiratory components, consider commencing renal replacement therapy or using bicarbonate infusions
- Aggressively treating pyrexia with anti-pyretics and/or cooling
- High-frequency oscillatory ventilation may aid $CO_2$ clearance as may tracheal gas insufflation (TGI)
- Extra-corporeal $CO_2$ removal ($ECCO_2R$) may be possible

**Pitfalls/difficult situations**
- Avoid hypercapnia where possible in patients with head injuries or where ICP control is required
- Where hypercapnia has been tolerated for a prolonged period and metabolic compensation has occurred be careful not to correct it too rapidly as the relative hypocapnia may result in cerebral vasoconstriction

**Further reading**
📖 OHEA p. 44.

# ☼ Complications of mechanical ventilation

Complications of mechanical ventilation which may require emergency treatment include
- Failure to ventilate
- Failure to oxygenate
- Barotrauma
- Haemodynamic instability

*Other complications covered in more detail in other sections include*
- Hypercapnia (see p. 52)
- Air trapping (see p. 76)
- Ventilator associated pneumonia (see p. 58 and 332)
- Mucous plugging and atelectasis (see p. 62)

## Causes
Complications are more likely in
- Agitated, under-sedated, or very mobile patients
- Patients with abnormal anatomy
- Patients with severe respiratory diseases, especially severe pneumonia, ARDS, bronchospasm, trauma, and contusions
- Patients with underlying chronic chest conditions
- Patients with chest abnormalities or chest trauma
- Patients requiring airway pressures >35 cmH$_2$O or receiving high volumes via mechanical ventilation

Haemodynamic instability
- May result from decreased venous return or cardiac output
- Is made worse by coexisting dehydration, hypovolaemia, sepsis, cardiac ischaemia or failure

## Presentation and assessment
Difficulty in ventilating/oxygenating may present with
- Hypoxaemia (SpO$_2$ <92%, or PaO$_2$ <8kPa), cyanosis
- Increasing airway pressures[*]
- High, or low, pressure ventilator alarms
- Evidence of low delivered tidal volume, or low minute-volume alarm
- Audible leak from ventilator circuit, or leak alarm
- Inability to ventilate using self-inflating Ambubag
- Lack of chest movement or respiratory sounds on auscultation
- Hypercapnia
- Dynamic hyperinflation (next inspiratory cycle starts before last expiratory cycle finished)

Where the patient is conscious and/or spontaneously breathing alongside mechanical ventilatory support, complications of ventilation may result in
- Agitation, sweating, clamminess
- Increasing respiratory distress, tachypnoea, dyspnoea

[*] Increasing airway pressures will occur if using volume-controlled ventilation; decreasing tidal volumes will occur with pressure-controlled ventilation

Cardiovascular abnormalities may include
- Cardiac arrest
- Tachycardia, bradycardia, or dysrhythmia
- Hypotension

Evidence of barotrauma may also include
- Tracheal deviation away from affected side (pneumothorax)
- Absent/diminished breath sounds on affected side
- Hyper-resonant percussion note on affected side
- Subcutaneous emphysema
- Pneumothorax or pneumomediastinum on CXR

**Investigations**
- ABGs
- FBC, U&Es, LFTs
- Serum CRP
- D-dimers (of limited use in the ICU)
- ECG
- CXR
- Chest ultrasound
- Bronchoscopy
- Echocardiogram
- CT chest
- CT pulmonary angiogram

---

**Indications for fibreoptic bronchoscopy in ventilated patients**

- To obtain microbiological samples via suction or lavage, particularly if patients are immunocompromised or suspected to have atypical infections
- To localize and control haemoptysis
- Removal of secretions, blood clots, or foreign bodies allowing lung re-expansion
- To examine for strictures, tumours, or tracheobronchial trauma
- To assess patency or position of endotracheal tube
- To evaluate degree of tracheobronchial trauma following airway burns or smoke inhalation

*Relative contraindications include*
- Moderate/severe hypoxaemia or hypercapnia
- Coagulopathy, SVC obstruction, or other risk of bleeding
- Near-complete tracheal obstruction
- Myocardial ischaemia, dysrhythmias or hypotension

---

**Differential diagnoses**
- Where there is difficulty in ventilating always consider the possibility of an occluded or semi-occluded airway (see pp. 38 and 40)

## Immediate management

### If there is difficulty in ventilating the patient

- Increase $FiO_2$ to near 100%
- Airway: check patency and position of endotracheal tube or tracheostomy (see pp. 38 and 40)
- Check for equipment failure and disconnection; if in doubt switch to self-inflating Ambubag and ventilate manually
- Consider the possibility of the following; treat as appropriate
  - Endobronchial intubation (see p. 38)
  - Equipment failure or disconnection
  - Bronchospasm (see p. 68)
  - Breathing against ('fighting') the ventilator
  - Foreign body, mucous plugs, retained chest secretions, or major collapse of the lung tissue (see p. 62)
  - Tension pneumothorax, tension haemothorax, massive effusion (see pp. 78 and 80)
  - ARDS (see p. 90)
- Consider increasing sedation or short-term muscle relaxation
- Consider altering ventilation parameters*
  - Increase inspiratory pressure, inspiratory time, or tidal volume if ventilatory volumes are inadequate
  - Increase respiratory rate if minute volumes are inadequate despite good tidal volumes
  - Increase PEEP to maintain lung recruitment

### Where there is evidence of barotrauma

- Increase $FiO_2$ to maintain oxygenation
- Treat tension pneumothorax immediately (see p. 490)
- Treat non-tension pneumothoraces in mechanically ventilated patients by insertion of chest drains (see p. 492)
- Alter ventilation parameters where appropriate* following a lung-protective strategy where possible (see p. 50), or a strategy targeted at controlling the effects of bronchospasm (see p. 75)
- Where there is evidence of 'fighting the ventilator' consider increasing sedation/anxiolysis

### Treat any haemodynamic instability

- Aggressively treat hypotension using fluid to restore circulatory volume, and inotropes where required
- Consider the possibility of the following – treat as appropriate:
  - Cardiac tamponade (see p. 146)
  - Hypovolaemia (see p. 106)
  - Sepsis (see p. 118)
  - Tension pneumothorax (see p. 78)
  - Cardiac ischaemia, failure or dysrhythmia (see pp. 124, 128, 136 and 140)

**Where there is hypoxia despite adequate ventilation**
- Increase $FiO_2$ to 100%: double check this value and switch to alternative supply if concerned
- Consider the possibility of the following; treat as appropriate:
  - Endobronchial intubation (see p. 38)
  - Pneumothorax (see p. 492)
  - Pleural effusions (see p. 492)
  - Mucous plugs, retained chest secretions, or major collapse of the lung tissue (see p. 62)
  - Acute pulmonary oedema (see p. 84)
  - Pulmonary embolism (see p. 92)
  - ARDS (see p. 90)
  - Cardiac shunting/ASD
- Consider altering ventilation parameters as above*
  - Consider decreasing the I:E ratio to 1:1.5, 1:1, or even inverting the ratios in order to maximize inspiration and allow intra-pulmonary gas redistribution with airway lower pressures
  - Tolerate hypercapnia
- Consider advanced airway manoeuvres or oxygenation techniques:
  - Alveolar recruitment measures (see p. 62)
  - Bronchoscopy to aid diagnosis or remove secretions
  - If lung pathology is unilateral try positioning bad lung uppermost
  - Prone position
  - Inhaled nitric oxide or nebulized prostacyclin
  - High frequency oscillatory ventilation
  - ECMO

* Follow a lung-protective strategy where possible (see p. 50).

**Further management**
- Identify and treat any coexisting/exacerbating infections
- If endotracheal intubation is likely to be prolonged consider early tracheostomy
- Where possible use assist-controlled or pressure-support ventilation

**Pitfalls/difficult situations**
- Have a high index of suspicion for tension pneumothorax in patients with cardiovascular collapse.
- CXR interpretation can be difficult in supine patients; certain conditions such as anterior pneumothoraces or pleural effusions may require additional imaging (CT or US)
- Obese patients may require much higher inspiratory pressures and levels of PEEP than expected
- Consider inserting prophylactic chest drains in patients with severe chest trauma who require ventilation
- Minimize volume replacement in patients who have had lung surgery

**Further reading**

Bell D (2003). Avoiding adverse outcomes when faced with 'difficulty with ventilation'. *Anaesthesia* **58**, 945–50.
📖 OHEA pp. 62, 350, 354, 358.

## :💠: Severe pneumonia (see also p. 332)

Acute severe lower respiratory tract infection causing respiratory compromise or sepsis (see p. 332) is a common reason for, and complication of, admission to critical care.

### Causes

Advancing age and any coexisting medical conditions (particularly heart disease, lung disease, immunocompromised patients (e.g. HIV, haematological malignancy, hepatic failure, drug use)) increase the likelihood of severe pneumonia.

### Community-acquired pneumonia

- Common bacterial organisms include: *S.pneumoniae*, *H.influenzae*
- Common viruses: influenza A and B
- Less common organisms (often associated with COPD): *S.aureus*, *M.catarrhalis*, *K.pneumonia*, *Pseudomonas*
- Atypical organisms: *Legionella*, *Mycoplasma*, *Chlamydia psittaci*, *Coxiella burnetti*

### Hospital-acquired pneumonia

Aspiration (see also p. 64) is a common cause of hospital-acquired infection especially where aspiration is witnessed or where there is neurological injury. Other risk factors include prolonged hospital stay, supine position, severe illness, immune system compromise, and mechanical ventilation.

- Common organisms: *S.aureus*, *Pseudomonas*, *Bacteroides*, *Klebsiella*, and Gram-negative enterobacteria

### Where there is no response to treatment or the patient is immunocompromised consider less common causes of pneumonia

- Other: TB, *Pneumocystis carinii*, *Cryptococcus neoformans*
- Resistant species: especially *S.aureus* and *Pseudomonas*
- Viral: varicella, CMV
- Fungal: *Candida species*, *Aspergillus*

### Presentation and assessment

- Agitation or malaise
- Increasing respiratory distress, tachypnoea, dyspnoea
- Cough, purulent sputum, haemoptysis
- Pleuritic chest pain or abdominal pain
- Rigors, pyrexia, sweating, clamminess
- Hypoxia, hypercapnia
- Pleural effusion
- Tachycardia
- Hypotension, sepsis

*Where the patient is mechanically ventilated the only indications may be*

- Worsening oxygenation
- Increased sputum production
- Indices of infection (pyrexia, WCC, CRP, culture results)
- CXR changes on routine films

**Assessing the severity of pneumonia (CURB-65)**

- **C**onfusion: new mental confusion
- **U**rea: >7 mmol/L
- **R**espiratory rate: raised >30/minute
- **B**lood pressure: systolic <90 mmHg and/or diastolic blood pressure <60 mmHg

Severe pneumonia can be diagnosed if there are more than two criteria

*Adverse prognostic features*
- Age ≥65 years
- Presence of any coexisting disease
- Hypoxaemia ($SaO_2$ <92% or $PaO_2$ <8 kPa) regardless of $FiO_2$

**Investigations**
- ABGs
- FBC (WCC may be high, >12 × 10$^9$/L, or low <4 × 10$^9$/L)
- U&Es, LFTs, CRP
- CXR
- ECG, echocardiogram,
- Culture: blood, sputum
- Atypical serology
- Urine for pneumococcal and Legionella antigen
- Bronchoscopy or non-directed BAL
- CT chest

**Differential diagnoses**
- Acute myocardial infarction/pulmonary oedema
- Pulmonary embolism
- Pneumothorax
- Pneumonitis, vasculitis, sarcoidosis, or malignancy

**Immediate management**

- 100% $O_2$ initially, then titrate to blood gas result
- Consider urgent physiotherapy and/or tracheal suctioning
- Non-invasive ventilation may reduce the need for endotracheal intubation
- Consider intubation and mechanical ventilation* if patient tiring, oxygenation worsening, or if airway needs to be secured
- Antibiotics as soon as possible preferably after cultures
- Once **A**irway and **B**reathing are stabilized, continue **ABC** approach
- Support circulation with IV fluid/inotropes/vasopressors

* Follow a lung-protective strategy where possible (see p. 50)

**Further management**

- Antibiotic management should be guided by local protocols, culture results and sensitivity. Empirical treatment protocols may include:
  - Severe community-acquired pneumonia: co-amoxiclav 1.2 g 8-hourly, or cefuroxime 1.5 g 8-hourly IV AND erythromycin 500 mg 6-hourly IV
  - Severe hospital-acquired pneumonia: ceftazidime 2 g 8-hourly IV AND gentamicin (with dose monitoring)
  - *Legionella*: clarithromycin 500 mg 12-hourly IV ± rifampicin 600 mg 12-hourly
- Apply the general measures for sepsis management (see p. 322)
- Remember analgesia for chest pain where required
- Consider invasive monitoring and serial blood gas analysis

**Pitfalls/difficult situations**

- Pneumonia is more common in patients with chronic lung conditions which may require concurrent treatment
- Malignancies or foreign bodies may give rise to pneumonia
- Organisms found on tracheal aspirates may not be causative
- Pneumonia can be caused by mixed organisms
- Consider *Legionella* where there is evidence of other organ failure (especially renal) and/or a community outbreak

**Further reading**

BTS (2001). BTS Guidelines for the management of community acquired pneumonia in adults. *Thorax* **56**(Suppl 4), iv1–64.

Macfarlane JT, Boldy D, Boswell T, *et al.* (2004). Update of BTS pneumonia guidelines: what's new? *Thorax* **59**, 364–6.

OHCC p. 288.

# ① Mucous plugging and atelectasis

Excess mucus secretion or sputum production can lead to blockage within the bronchial tree.

## Causes
- Respiratory tract infection
- Asthma
- COPD
- Inhalational injury
- Aspiration pneumonitis

## Presentation and assessment

Features indicative of mucous plugging include:
- Excessive mucus/sputum production
- Episodes of desaturation and respiratory distress
  - Tachypnoea, dyspnoea
  - Hypoxaemia, cyanosis
- CXR changes: distal atelectasis, segmental/lobar collapse
- Increasing airway pressures in the ventilated patient*

Range of severity from
- Minor: area of atelectasis
- Moderate: segmental collapse
- Severe: lobar collapse
- Life-threatening: tracheal/ETT obstruction and failure to ventilate

## Investigations

In most cases the diagnosis will be clinical
- CXR
- ABGS
- FBC
- Blood and sputum cultures
- Bronchoscopy may be indicated (see p. 55 and 506)
- Broncho-alveolar lavage samples (if performing bronchoscopy)

## Differential diagnoses
- Pulmonary embolism
- Bronchospasm
- Airway or endotracheal tube obstruction from any cause including
  - Foreign body
  - Airway/bronchial tumour

---

* Increasing airway pressures will occur if using volume-controlled ventilation; decreasing tidal volumes will occur with pressure-controlled ventilation

## Immediate management

- If the patient is spontaneously breathing
  - Give 100% oxygen via reservoir mask
  - Consider urgent physiotherapy
  - Tracheal suction: awake patients may require insertion of a nasopharyngeal airway to facilitate suction catheters to be passed into the trachea
  - Nebulized therapy: $\beta_2$-agonists (salbutamol 5 mg) to bronchodilate, 0.9% saline (5–10 ml) to loosen secretions
  - Consider starting non-invasive ventilation (see p. 50) with a PEEP of 5–10 cmH$_2$O; make sure that this is not contraindicated (e.g. impaired swallowing or cough reflex)
  - *In extremis* consider assisting ventilation using bag and mask
  - Intubation and mechanical ventilation may be required
- In already intubated patients consider the following
  - Increase FiO$_2$ to maintain adequate O$_2$ saturation
  - Increase PEEP to improve lung recruitment
  - Chest physiotherapy, airway suctioning (± saline lavages)
  - Recruitment manoeuvres (various techniques described including: stepwise increase in PEEP and $V_t$ up to a maximum peak airway pressure of 35 cmH$_2$O which is maintained for ~5 minutes, then PEEP and $V_t$ returned to previous settings)
  - Nebulized therapy as above; *N*-acetylcysteine (5–10 mg in 3 ml 0.9% saline) may also be tried in patients with tenacious sputum
  - Fibreoptic bronchoscopy and bronchial toilet
- Once **A**irway and **B**reathing are stabilized, continue **ABC** approach

## Further management

- Consider regular physiotherapy and/or nebulizers
- Commence antibiotics as appropriate, guided by microbiology results
- Occasionally elective endotracheal or tracheostomy tube change may be required if secretions become encrusted and cause obstruction

## Pitfalls/difficult situations

- Failure to treat underlying cause or recognize areas of collapse which require aggressive physiotherapy, PEEP, or bronchoscopy
- Failure to try simple manoeuvres first with minor/moderate atelectasis

## Further reading

Stiller K (2000). Physiotherapy in intensive care: towards an evidence-based practice. *Chest* **118**, 1801–13.

Goodfellow LT, Jones M (2002). Bronchial hygiene therapy: from traditional hands-on techniques to modern technological approaches. *Am J Nurs* **102**, 37–43.

Mentzelopoulos SD, Tzoufi MJ (2002). Anesthesia for tracheal and endobronchial interventions. *Curr Opin Anaesthesiol* **15**, 85–94.

Mehrishi S (2002). Is bronchoscopy indicated in the management of atelectasis? Pro: bronchoscopy. *J Bronchol* **9**, 46–51.

📖 OHCC p. 284.

# :⚙: **Aspiration**

Aspiration presents either with acid inhalation leading to acid pneumonitis, or with the inhalation of particulate matter causing small airway obstruction and/or community- or hospital-acquired aspiration pneumonia.

## Causes
Risk factors include:
- Neurological injury or decreased consciousness level
- Difficulty swallowing (e.g. stroke and Parkinson's disease)
- Complicated endotracheal intubation, especially if the patient
  - was intubated as an emergency, or by an inexperienced operator
  - was at risk of aspiration: full stomach, hiatus hernia, delayed gastric emptying, incompetent lower oesophageal sphincter
- General anaesthesia: aspiration can occur as an occult event
- Mechanical ventilation

*Where there is pneumonia common bacterial organisms include*
- Community-acquired: anaerobes and streptococci
- Hospital-acquired: *S.aureus, E.coli, Klebsiella, Enterobacter, Pseudomonas*

## Presentation and assessment
- Both pneumonia and pneumonitis may coexist and presentation may be subacute/delayed
- Aspiration may be witnessed
- Increasing respiratory distress, tachypnoea, dyspnoea
- Cough and/or wheeze, particularly with acid pneumonitis
- Rigors, pyrexia, sweating, and purulent sputum production
- Tachycardia, hypotension, sepsis
- Indices of infection (pyrexia, WCC, CRP, culture results)

## Investigations
- ABGs
- FBC, U&Es, LFTs, CRP
- CXR
- Culture (blood and sputum)
- Bronchoscopy

## Differential diagnoses
- Bronchospasm
- Acute pulmonary oedema
- Endobronchial intubation
- Mucous plugging or foreign body inhalation
- Undiagnosed pre-operative chest infection

## Immediate management

- 100% $O_2$ initially (humidified if possible): titrate to blood gas result
- Consider intubation and mechanical ventilation* (with PEEP if required), especially if airway needs securing, patient is tiring, or oxygenation worsening
- Bronchodilators should be prescribed as appropriate
- If patients require further respiratory support, non-invasive techniques are usually contraindicated

*Acid pneumonitis treatment (mostly supportive in nature)*
- Patients with particulate aspirate matter may require rigid bronchoscopy to remove large obstructing pieces
- Evidence does not support the use of prophylactic antibiotics

*Aspiration pneumonia*
- Antibiotic therapy is the basis of management (see below)
- Consider fibreoptic bronchoscopy to collect lavage specimens for microbiological diagnosis and exclude obstructing neoplasms
- Once **A**irway and **B**reathing are stabilized, continue **ABC** approach

* Follow a lung-protective strategy where possible (see p. 50)

## Further management

- Where antibiotic therapy is indicated it should be guided by local protocols, culture results and sensitivity. Empirical treatment protocols may include co-amoxiclav 1.2 g 8-hourly IV and metronidazole 500 mg IV 8-hourly
- Apply the general measures for sepsis management (see p. 322)
- Consider invasive monitoring and serial blood gas analysis

## Pitfalls/difficult situations

- Complications of aspiration include lung abscess formation, empyema, lobar collapse, and ARDS
- A 45° head-up tilt in ventilated patients may reduce the likelihood of ventilator-acquired pneumonia

## Further reading

Englehart T, Webster NR (2000). Pulmonary aspiration of gastric contents in anaesthesia. *Br J Anaesth* **83**, 453–60.
📖 OHEA p. 96.

# :⚙: **Inhalational injury**

Inhalational injury occurs following burns where adherent soot particles cause tracheitis, bronchitis, bronchiolitis, and alveolitis. Systemic absorption of toxins also occurs, and both/either may lead to the severe systemic inflammatory response syndrome and subsequent infectious complications. Inhalational injury increases the mortality from burns.

## Causes
- Commonly occurs in burns victims trapped in an enclosed space
- Can also occur with self-immolation
- Inhalation of steam or hot/corrosive gas

Associated with alcoholism, chronic ill health, psychiatric illness, trauma, and extremes of age (young children and the elderly)

## Presentation and assessment
Significant inhalational injury is suggested by
- Compatible history
- Severe generalized burns, or burns associated with
  - The face: oedema, blistering, pealing skin
  - The neck: circumferential or anterior neck burns
  - The airway: airway oedema present or blistering/pealing of mucosal membranes
  - Airway injury requiring intubation (see p. 28)
- Loss of consciousness
- Carbonaceous sputum
- Respiratory distress
  - Tachypnoea, dyspnoea and/or wheeze/bronchospasm
  - Hypoxaemia (although $SpO_2$ may appear misleadingly normal in the presence of CO poisoning)
  - Cyanosis (although a pink flush may occur due to CO poisoning)

## Investigations
- ABGs
- COHb: elevated levels of carboxyhaemoglobin in the blood make inhalational injury more likely
- FBC
- U&Es, LFTs
- CXR
- ECG
- Consider bronchoscopy: the presence of soot within the bronchial tree confirms inhalational injury

## Differential diagnoses
- CO poisoning without inhalational injury
- Facial burns without inhalational injury
- Burns injury with associated COPD, ARDS, pneumonia, or PE

**Immediate management**

- Give 100% oxygen
- Consider intubation and mechanical ventilation* if patient is tiring, oxygenation is worsening, or airway needs to be secured
- Continue ventilation initially with 100% $O_2$ to minimize/reverse effects of carboxyhaemoglobin
- Once **A**irway and **B**reathing are stabilized, continue **ABC** approach
- Support circulation with IV fluid as guided by burns fluid regimes (see p. 405)
- Any associated skin and airway burns should be managed appropriately (see p. 28 and 404)

* Follow a lung-protective strategy where possible (see p. 50)

**Further management**
- Supportive medical treatment includes nebulized bronchodilators
- Bronchoscopic saline lavage and toilet of adherent soot should be performed on a daily basis until the trachea and bronchi are soot free
- Alternatively, it has been suggested that frequent blind lavages with weak bicarbonate solutions may diminish the direct epithelial injury (and possibly the degree of associated SIRS)
- High-dose steroids are contraindicated, and as yet there is no evidence for the use of low-dose steroids
- There is also no evidence to support the use of prophylactic antibiotics

**Pitfalls/difficult situations**
- Patients with inhalational injury are highly likely to require early intubation for airway protection
- The development of ARDS and pneumonia is common in burns patients

**Further reading**

Young CJ, Moss J (1989). Smoke inhalation: diagnosis and treatment. *J Clin Anesth* **1**, 377–86.
□ OHCC p. 306.

# :☻: Asthma/severe bronchospasm

Acute wheeze severe enough to cause respiratory and/or cardiovascular compromise.

## Causes
- Known asthma/COPD
- Eczema, hayfever, atopy
- Trigger agent exposure in susceptible individuals (e.g. cigarette smoke and ozone)

## Presentation and assessment
- Sense of 'tight chest' or 'can't breathe' in conscious patient
- Increasing respiratory distress associated with bilateral wheeze
Bronchospasm may vary in degree of severity:
- Evidence of severe bronchospasm:
  - Unable to talk in full sentences
  - Tachypnoea >25 breaths/minute
  - Tachycardia >110 beats/minute
  - Peak flow 33–50% of predicted or best
- Evidence of severe bronchospasm which is imminently **life-threatening**:
  - Silent chest
  - Bradycardia, dysrhythmia, or hypotension
  - Bradypnoea or exhaustion
  - Confusion or decreased level of consciousness
  - Peak flow <33% of predicted or best
  - Cyanosis, $SpO_2$ <92%, or $PaO_2$ <8 kPa
  - $PaCO_2$ normal or raised (>4.6 kPa), or acidaemia (pH <7.35)
- Evidence of severe bronchospasm in the mechanically ventilated patient:
  - Cyanosis, $SpO_2$ <92%, or $PaO_2$ <8 kPa
  - Increasing airway pressures[*]
  - Dynamic hyperinflation (next inspiratory cycle starts before last expiratory cycle finished): may present as hypotension

Where COPD is suspected from the patients history it may be appropriate to follow a slightly different treatment pathway (see p. 72), although if in doubt, or if the patient is *in extremis* and further history is unavailable, then **treat as for acute bronchospasm** and review once the patient is stable.

## Investigations
- Peak flow measurements
- ABGs
- FBC, U&Es
- Blood and sputum cultures
- CXR to check for pneumothorax, foreign body, pneumonia, or malpositioned ETT

---

[*] Increasing airway pressures will occur if using volume-controlled ventilation; decreasing tidal volumes will occur with pressure-controlled ventilation

**Differential diagnoses**

- Anaphylaxis causing bronchospasm
- Acute pulmonary oedema: 'cardiac wheeze'
- Endobronchial intubation
- Breathing against ('fighting') the ventilator
- Airway/ETT/breathing system obstruction or foreign body
- Pneumothorax/tension pneumothorax
- Pulmonary embolism

**Immediate management**

- Give 100% oxygen via reservoir mask if spontaneously breathing or ventilator if receiving respiratory support
- Secure airway if required
- Nebulized $\beta_2$-agonist (salbutamol 5 mg or terbutaline 10 mg) up to every 15 minutes
- Hydrocortisone 100–200 mg IV
- Consider aminophylline 250 mg IV (if not on regular theophyllines) and/or salbutamol 250 µg IV over 10 minutes
- Consider adrenaline 250–500 µg SC if *in extremis*
- Once **A**irway and **B**reathing are stabilized, continue **ABC** approach
- Patients are often dehydrated and may require aggressive fluid resuscitation, especially after induction of anaesthesia for intubation

**Further management**

- If bronchospasm persists consider
  - Repeated $\beta_2$-agonist nebulizers
  - Ipratropium bromide nebulizers 500 µg 6-hourly
  - Magnesium infusion 25–100 mg/kg over 20 minutes
  - Aminophylline infusion: 0.5 mg/kg/hour
  - $\beta_2$-agonist infusion: salbutamol 5 mg/0.9% saline 500 ml at 1–3 ml/minute (5–30 µg/minute)
- In patients who require endotracheal intubation, or are already intubated, sedation (with or without muscle relaxation) may be difficult and may require the combination of several agents including
  - Propofol (may obtund airway irritation)
  - Alfentanil, fentanyl or remifentanil (morphine may exacerbate bronchospasm)
  - Midazolam
  - Ketamine: has bronchodilator activity, but should not be used without benzodiazepine cover
  - The volatile agents isoflurane and sevoflurane (halothane may provoke cardiac arrhythmias) have sedative and bronchodilator properties but are difficult to manage on ICU if scavenging is not available
  - Neuromuscular blockade can be useful when trying to establish ventilatory support (vecuronium or rocuronium may be preferable to atracurium, as they cause less histamine release). It should be stopped as soon as is safe because combining steroids and neuro-muscular blockade increases the risk of critical illness myopathy

- In ventilated patients
  - Follow a lung-protective strategy aimed at avoiding lung damage or air trapping (see p. 75)
  - Establish normal levels of respiratory function if possible
- Identify and treat any coexisting/exacerbating infections; send appropriate blood and sputum cultures
- Monitor oxygenation and arterial $CO_2$ with serial arterial blood gas analyses
- Monitor serum potassium concentrations; many asthma treatments decrease serum potassium which may need supplementing
- Continue steroid therapy; convert to oral prednisolone when appropriate
- In patients where COPD is suspected rapidly decrease oxygen after the initial resuscitation (provided that the patient is stable) in order to avoid precipitating $CO_2$ retention (type 2 respiratory failure (p. 44))
- In patients where COPD is suspected or who are known to be $CO_2$ retainers titrate ventilation aiming for whatever the 'normal' levels of arterial $O_2$, $SpO_2$ and arterial $CO_2$ are for the patient (these may be recorded in the patient's notes or may have to be estimated according to the patient's exercise tolerance)

## Pitfalls/difficult situations
- Be aware that a silent chest or bradycardia are pre-terminal events
- It may be difficult to ventilate severe asthmatics adequately whilst avoiding using high inflation pressures
- It is important to allow a sufficiently long I:E ratio to prevent dynamic hyperinflation/air trapping
- As bronchospasm improves remember to alter ventilator settings so as to avoid barotrauma
- Tension pneumothorax is common in asthmatic patients

## Further reading

British Thoracic Society et al. (1997). British guidelines on asthma management. Thorax 52(Suppl), 51.

BTS/SIGN (2003). Update of British guidelines on the management of asthma. Thorax 58(Suppl I) pp. 1–83.

Papiris S, Kotanidou A, Malagari K, Roussos C (2002). Clinical review: severe asthma Crit Care 6, 30–44.

Jagoda A, Shepherd S, Spevitz A, Joseph MM (1997). Refractory asthma. Part 1: Epidemiology, pathophysiology, pharmacologic interventions. Ann Emerg Med 29, 262–74.

Jagoda A, Shepherd S, Spevitz A, Joseph MM (1997). Refractory asthma. Part 2: Airway interventions and management. Ann Emerg Med 29, 275–81.

📖 OHCC pp. 296–8, OHEA pp. 56, 122.

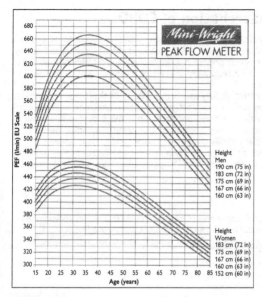

**Fig. 3.1** Peak expiratory flow rate – normal values. Adapted by Clement Clarke International Ltd. for use with EN13826/EU Scale peak flow meters from Nunn AJ, Gregg I (*BMJ* **298**: 1068–70).

---

### Indications for mechanical ventilation in acute asthma

#### Absolute
- Apnoea
- Decreased consciousness

#### Relative
- Increasing hypercapnia
- Exhaustion (normal or low respiratory rate)
- Drowsiness
- Haemodynamic instability
- Refractory hypoxaemia

Endotracheal intubation should be performed semi-electively before acute decompensation occurs

# ☼ Exacerbation of COPD

Chronic obstructive pulmonary disease (COPD) includes diseases causing chronic airflow limitation (CAL) such as chronic bronchitis and emphysema. Patients may present as a result of gradual deterioration leading to type 1 or type 2 respiratory failure (see p. 44), or may present with an exacerbation.

It is important to fully assess the severity of their underlying disease prior to any current exacerbation. It may be desirable to avoid endotracheal intubation, or inappropriate to treat the patient within a critical care environment. Any decision to limit treatment should be made by senior clinicians, ideally involving the patient and/or their relatives.

If in doubt, or if the patient is in extremis and further history is unavailable **treat as for acute bronchospasm** and review once the patient is stable.

## Causes
* Infection:
    * Bacterial (commonly *H.influenzae*, *H.parainfluenzae*, *S.pneumoniae*, *S.aureus*, *M.catarrhalis*, *K.pneumonia*, and *Pseudomonas*)
    * Viral (commonly influenza A and B, parainfluenza, rhinovirus, coronavirus)
* Trigger agent exposure (e.g. ozone)
* Following anaesthesia or major surgery
* Major systemic illness
* Pneumothorax
* Pulmonary embolism
* Cardiac failure

## Presentation and assessment
If possible assess the severity of the patient's airway disease when they are 'well', and the degree of reversibility of the current exacerbation:
* Exercise tolerance when well
* Any previous history and investigations
    * Pulmonary function tests
    * Normal $SpO_2$ on air
    * Previous CXRs and/or chest CT scans
* History and examination may reveal any of the causes listed above as triggers for an acute exacerbation

*Unlike acute bronchospasm indicators of hypoxia and respiratory distress may be chronic. Signs more likely to be associated with acute deterioration include:*
* New sensation of 'tight chest', breathlessness, or inability to talk
* Worsening respiratory distress with or without bilateral wheeze
* $SpO_2$ <90%, or $PaO_2$ <8 kPa
* Tachypnoea (>25 breaths/minute) or bradypnoea (<10 breaths/minute)
* Raised $PaCO_2$ (>6.3 kPa) with associated acidaemia (pH <7.35)

- Exhaustion, confusion, or decreased level of consciousness,
- Tachycardia (>110 beats/minute) or bradycardia (<50 beats/minute)
- Dysrhythmia or hypotension
- Pyrexia

## Investigations

- Peak flow measurements
- ABGs
- FBC, U&Es
- Theophylline concentration (in patients using theophyllines)
- Blood cultures, sputum cultures
- ECG
- CXR to check for pneumothorax, foreign body, pneumonia

## Differential diagnoses

- Bronchospasm due to acute asthma or anaphylaxis
- Pneumonia
- Acute pulmonary oedema: 'cardiac wheeze'
- Endobronchial intubation
- Breathing against ('fighting') the ventilator
- Airway/ETT/breathing system obstruction or foreign body
- Pneumothorax/tension pneumothorax
- Pulmonary embolism

## Immediate management

- 100% $O_2$ initially; then titrate to achieve $SpO_2$ >90%
  - Venturi masks allow good control of $FiO_2$ (see p. 48)
  - Monitor arterial blood gases to identify development or worsening of type 2 respiratory failure
- Nebulized $\beta_2$-agonist (salbutamol 5 mg or terbutaline 10 mg) up to every 15 minutes
- Consider ipratropium bromide nebulizers 500 µg 6-hourly
- Hydrocortisone 100–200mg IV or prednisolone PO 30–40 mg
- Consider aminophylline 250 mg IV (if not on regular theophyllines) and/or salbutamol 250 µg IV over 10 minutes
- Consider non-invasive ventilation (see p. 50), especially if $PaCO_2$ >6.3 kPa or pH 7.25–7.35
  - Start with CPAP or BIPAP titrate $O_2$ as above; titrate inspiratory pressure (10–20 cmH$_2$O), and titrate PEEP starting at 4 cmH$_2$O
  - CPAP/BIPAP may decrease work of breathing or acidaemia
  - CPAP/BIPAP may obviate the need for invasive ventilation; may be used as a trial before, or a bridge to, endotracheal intubation; or may be the 'ceiling' of intervention
- If the patient fails to respond and there is any doubt as to the reversibility of the patient's condition, proceed to endotracheal intubation/mechanical ventilation; **treat as for acute bronchospasm**
- Once **A**irway and **B**reathing are stabilized, continue **ABC** approach
- Patients are often dehydrated and may require aggressive fluid resuscitation – especially after induction of anaesthesia for intubation

**Further management**

- Consider the use of respiratory stimulants such as doxapram where there is an absolute contraindication to non-invasive ventilation
- Where there is evidence of infection treat accordingly (see pp. 58 and 332)
- Consider early tracheostomy in intubated patients as it may assist weaning by allowing less sedation and decreasing dead-space (hence less work of breathing)
- Increased sputum production is common; physiotherapy, suctioning, and tracheostomy insertion may help

**Pitfalls/difficult situations**

- Patients with COPD who require intubation often take a long weaning from mechanical ventilation
- Bullae may mimic the appearances of pneumothoraces
- Coexisting cardiac disease is common in patients with COPD
- Chronic infection is common and organisms cultured in tracheal aspirates may not represent the cause of an acute exacerbation
- Where mechanical ventilation is considered inappropriate, non-invasive ventilation may still be beneficial even in situations where it might normally be contraindicated (e.g. decreased level of consciousness)

**Further reading**

Currie GP, Wedzicha JA (2006). ABC of chronic obstructive pulmonary disease, acute exacerbations. *BMJ* **333**, 87–9.
📖 OHCC p. 286.

**Ventilator management of bronchospasm**

- Initially use manual ventilation with a Waters circuit or self-inflating bag until ventilator settings configured
- Aim for tidal volumes of approximately 4–8 ml/kg IBW
- Low respiratory rate (6–10 breaths/minute)
- Aim for a long I:E ratio (1:3–1:5)
- Aim for an inspiratory flow of approximately 100 L/minute
- Aim for 'permissive hypercapnia', allowing $PaCO_2$ to rise to as much as 10kPa; if pH falls too severely consider a bicarbonate infusion
- Where ventilation is difficult consider heavy sedation or short-term neuromuscular blockade
- Avoid PEEP if possible; if it is required to improve oxygenation, consider setting extrinsic PEEP to 80% of calculated PEEPi

## ☠ Air trapping

Air trapping occurs in ventilated patients when there is insufficient time for all the air to escape from the lungs during expirations. As a result extra air accumulates within the lungs with each breath until the lungs become hyperinflated and respiratory or cardiovascular collapse occurs. This phenomenon is also known as breath-stacking, increased auto-PEEP, intrinsic PEEP (PEEPi), or dynamic hyperinflation (DHI)

### Causes
- Only occurs in ventilated patients
- Severe bronchospasm: leads to very long expiratory times. Air trapping typically occurs when attempts are made to maintain normocapnia by hyperventilating
- Inverse ratio ventilation where the inspiratory time on the ventilator is longer than expiratory times (used in conditions such as ARDS)
- Possibly more likely to occur in patients who are under-sedated or breathing against ('fighting') the ventilator
- Can occur in chest trauma or mechanical obstruction ('ball-valving')

### Presentation and assessment
Not associated with spontaneous ventilation
- Gradually increasing airway pressures will occur if using volume-controlled ventilation and decreasing tidal volumes will occur with pressure-controlled ventilation
- Bilateral breath sounds with wheeze or a silent chest may be present
- High auto-PEEP (see below)
- Sudden cardiovascular collapse or inability to ventilate
- Can present as PEA arrest

### Investigations
In severe cases the diagnosis is one of exclusion
- Many ventilators have a facility for measuring PEEPi (auto-PEEP); a PEEPi >15 $cmH_2O$ should be considered high (temporary disconnection from ventilator will decrease PEEPi)
- CXR may show hyperinflation

### Differential diagnoses
- Tension pneumothorax
- ETT/airway obstruction, or ventilator failure

### Immediate management
- Check ETT, ventilator, and ventilator tubing to exclude blockage or malfunction
- *In extremis* or arrest: disconnect ventilator and allow chest to empty
- Once **A**irway and **B**reathing are stabilized, continue **ABC** approach

**Further management**
- Treat bronchospasm (see p. 68)
- Set ventilator settings as advised below
- If already on appropriate ventilator setting consider
  - Further decreasing minute ventilation (rate and/or tidal volume)
  - Increasing expiratory time further (IE ratio >1:5)
  - Tolerating greater levels of hypercapnia
  - Further sedation and paralysis

**Pitfalls/difficult situations**
- Tension pneumothorax can occur alongside air trapping

**Further reading**
Mehrishi S, George L, Awan A (2004). Intrinsic PEEP: an underrecognized cause of pulseless electrical activity. *Hosp Physician* **40**, 30–6.
📖 OHEA p. 208.

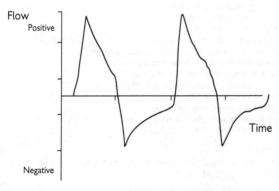

**Fig. 3.2** Ventilator flow–time display for a patient with air trapping.

## ☠ Tension pneumothorax

A tension pneumothorax (progressive accumulation of air in the pleural cavity) leads to over-expansion of one side of the thorax, which in turn compresses the contralateral side and the great vessels.

### Causes
- Chest trauma, especially where fractured ribs are present
- Subclavian or internal jugular central line insertion
- High ventilation pressures (especially severe asthma)
- Chronic lung disease
- Following chest or upper GI surgery

### Presentation and assessment
- Patient may have already suffered a PEA cardiac arrest (see p. 105)
- Sense of impending doom in conscious patient
- Increasing respiratory distress
  - Tachypnoea, dyspnoea
  - Hypoxaemia, cyanosis
- Cardiovascular compromise or complete cardiovascular collapse
- Increasing airway pressures in the ventilated patient[*]
- Tracheal deviation away from affected side
- Absent/diminished breath sounds on affected side
- Hyper-resonant percussion note on affected side
- Distended external jugular veins
- Surgical emphysema may be present

It is important to have a high index of suspicion for tension pneumothorax in patients with cardiovascular collapse.

### Investigations
In most cases the diagnosis of a tension pneumothorax should be clinical. It should not require a CXR.

Once treatment has been initiated consider
- ABGs
- FBC, U&Es
- CXR (to confirm lung re-expansion)

### Differential diagnoses
Other potential diagnoses to consider include
- Severe acute bronchospasm
- Pulmonary embolism
- Cardiac tamponade
- Massive haemothorax
- Endobronchial intubation
- ETT/breathing system obstruction
- Anaphylaxis

---

[*] Increasing airway pressures will occur if using volume-controlled ventilation; decreasing tidal volumes will occur with pressure-controlled ventilation

**Immediate management**

- Give 100% oxygen via reservoir mask if spontaneously breathing or ventilator if receiving respiratory support
- Secure airway if required
- Needle decompression: large-bore cannula (14G or larger) inserted through the anterior chest wall in the mid-clavicular line at the second intercostal space (at the level of the angle of Louis). Insert just above top of third rib to avoid neurovascular bundle along lower edge of second rib
- Once **A**irway and **B**reathing are stabilized, continue **ABC** approach

**Further management**

- Insertion of chest drain should follow rapidly after initial decompression to avoid re-tensioning (see p. 492)
- Where the patient is ventilated a lung-protective strategy should be adopted when possible (see p. 50)
- Check CXR for position of chest drain and to confirm re-expansion of lung (the diagnosis of a tension pneumothorax should be clinical and investigations should not delay immediate management)
- Consider arterial blood gas analysis to monitor changes in hypoxaemia

**Pitfalls/difficult situations**

- Tension pneumothorax may be spontaneous, without apparent cause
- Tension pneumothorax may be present without significant tracheal deviation
- The external jugular veins may not be distended if there is associated hypovolaemia (e.g. in trauma patients)
- May recur despite the presence of a functioning chest drain, especially with positive pressure ventilation
- Standard cannula may not be long enough to reach pleural cavity in obese or muscular patients
- Bilateral tension pneumothoraces may occur causing absent bilateral chest sounds with equal percussion notes
- Tension pneumothorax in an asthmatic patient may be difficult to diagnose, and treatment may not reduce airway pressures

**Further reading**

Laws D, Neville E, Duffy J (2003). BTS guidelines for the insertion of a chest drain. *Thorax* **58**(Suppl II), ii53–9.

American College of Surgeons Committee on Trauma. ATLS Guidelines. Available online at: www.facs.org/trauma/atls/index.html

Friend KD (2000). Prehospital recognition of tension pneumothorax. *Prehosp Emerg Care* **4**, 75–7.

Plewa MC, Ledrick D, Sferra JJ (1995). Delayed tension pneumothorax complicating central venous catheterization and positive pressure ventilation. *Am J Emerg Med* **13**, 532–5.

Campbell-Smith TA, Bendall SP, Davis J (1998). Tension pneumothorax in the presence of bilateral intercostal chest drains. *Injury* **29**, 556–7.

OHCC p. 300, OHEA pp. 50, 52.

## ☠ **Massive haemothorax**

Massive haemothorax is defined as more than 1500 ml of blood in the chest cavity. Haemothorax often results from vascular damage at the time of the original injury, although other causes including rib fractures and infection may cause vascular damage some time after injury and so delay presentation.

### Causes

- Penetrating chest injury
- Blunt chest trauma, especially where fractured ribs are present
- Subclavian or internal jugular central line insertion
- Following chest or upper GI surgery

### Presentation and assessment

- Anxiety
- Increasing respiratory distress
    - Tachypnoea, dyspnoea
    - Hypoxaemia, cyanosis
- Dull percussion note on the affected side (although may have an accompanying pneumothorax)
- May be associated with signs of tension (see p. 78)
    - Increasing airway pressures in the ventilated patient[*]
    - Trachea deviated to the opposite side
    - Absent or diminished breath sounds on the affected side
- Signs of associated hypovolaemia may predominate (see p. 114)
    - Tachycardia
    - Hypotension
    - Oliguria
    - Delayed capillary refill
    - Decreased level of consciousness

### Investigations

- ABGs
- Cross-match blood
- FBC, U&Es, coagulation screen,
- CXR (may show evidence of tension with mediastinal shift, or may not differentiate from pleural effusion)
- Ultrasound if available and time allows
- Echocardiography (to exclude tamponade)

In an emergency, strong clinical suspicion should guide first line treatment

### Differential diagnoses

- Pleural effusion:
- Chest consolidation
- Tension pneumothorax:
- Cardiac tamponade

---

[*] Increasing airway pressures will occur if using volume-controlled ventilation; decreasing tidal volumes will occur with pressure-controlled ventilation

## Immediate management

- Give 100% oxygen via reservoir mask if spontaneously breathing or ventilator if receiving respiratory support
- Secure airway: endotracheal intubation and ventilation are likely to be required in extreme situations
- Needle decompression may be required *in extremis* to treat any associated tension pneumothorax (see p. 490)
- Inser large-bore IV cannula for fluid resuscitation; blood cross-match
- Insert chest drain: this may precipitate rapid blood loss in extreme cases
- Restore circulatory volume/blood transfusion
- Once **A**irway and **B**reathing are stabilized, continue **ABC** approach

## Further management

- Emergency thoracotomy if blood loss persists at >200 ml/hour
- Check CXR for position of chest drain and to confirm re-expansion of lung
- Invasive monitoring

## Pitfalls/difficult situations

- May be bilateral
- Signs of tension not always present
- Cardiovascular collapse may be severe, masking chest signs
- Thoracocentesis cannula may not be long enough in obese patients
- A number of people may be required for successful resuscitation

## Further reading

American College of Surgeons Committee on Trauma. ATLS Guidelines. Available online at: www.facs.org/trauma/atls/index.html
📖 OHCC p. 302.

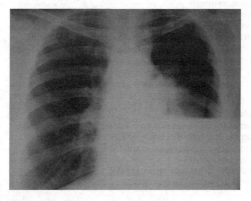

**Fig. 3.3** CXR of a haemopneumothorax.

# ⚙ Pulmonary haemorrhage

Haemoptysis most commonly presents as bloodstained sputum or small amounts of fresh blood. Occasionally bronchial artery or vein rupture can occur, or bleeding can be so widespread that haemorrhage is massive and life threatening by obstructing the airway and disrupting gas exchange, or by leading to hypovolaemia.

## Causes

Minor haemoptysis
- Pneumonia
- Pulmonary embolism
- Cancer
- Suction catheter trauma

Major haemoptysis
- TB or bronchiectasis
- Arterio-venous malformations
- Vasculitides: RA, Wegener's granulomatosis, microscopic polyangiitis, systemic lupus erythematosus (SLE), Goodpasture's syndrome, Henoch–Schönlein purpura (HSP), and idiopathic haemosiderosis
- Severe coagulopathy
- Pulmonary artery flow catheters can rupture a pulmonary artery

Trauma can cause pulmonary haemorrhage, but more often causes haemothorax.

## Presentation and assessment

- Frank blood or bloody sputum
- Anxiety
- Increasing respiratory distress
  - Tachypnoea, dyspnoea
  - Hypoxaemia, cyanosis
- Signs of associated hypovolaemia (see p. 114)
  - Tachycardia, hypotension, oliguria, delayed capillary refill

Signs of respiratory distress and hypoxaemia are likely to occur before signs of hypovolaemia

## Investigations

- ABGs
- CXR
- FBC, coagulation screen
- U&Es (rheumatological causes may have associated renal compromise)
- Vasculitis screen (e.g. auto-antibodies, ANCA, ANA, rheumatoid factor, immunoglobulins complement, anti-GBM antibodies)
- Blood and sputum cultures
- Urine microscopy (for red cell casts suggestive of glomerulonephritis)
- Bronchoscopy and washings if appropriate
- CT chest

**Differential diagnoses**
- Pulmonary oedema
- Oropharyngeal bleeding or epistaxis
- Airway infection
- Foreign body

**Immediate management**

- Give 100% oxygen via reservoir mask if spontaneously breathing or ventilator if receiving respiratory support
- Secure airway if required: intubation may be required in the event of massive haemoptysis
  - If bleeding source is one-sided rather than diffuse it may be possible to isolate that side using a double-lumen tube (DLT); as a temporary measure consider managing the patient with the bleeding side lowermost
- Once ventilated
  - Increasing PEEP (>10 cmH$_2$O if tolerated) may aid lung recruitment and decrease bleeding
  - Repeated recruitment manoeuvres may be required (see p. 63)
- Depending upon likely diagnosis
  - Urgent bronchoscopy may be required to identify and treat bleeding lesions
  - Urgent pulmonary angiography may be required to identify and treat bleeding lesions
- Once **A**irway and **B**reathing are stabilized, continue **ABC** approach
- If haemorrhage is severe, blood replacement may be required
- Replace clotting products/platelets where indicated

**Further management**
- Exclude oropharyngeal bleeding
- Blood clots can cause large casts to form obstructing the bronchial tree. These may require bronchoscopy to remove
- Once the diagnosis has been arrived at specific treatments may be available:
  - Immunomodulatory therapy for rheumatological conditions
  - Antibiotics for infections
  - Bronchial artery embolization

**Pitfalls/difficult situations**
- Conscious patients will often swallow blood; blood loss is often higher then can be seen by examining receivers
- Epistaxis and oropharyngeal trauma can cause copious bleeding to occur. Careful examination is required. In unconscious patients intubation and tracheal suction will confirm haemoptysis

**Further reading**
OHCC p. 304, OHEA p. 60.

# ⑦ Pulmonary oedema

Pulmonary oedema is characterized by accumulation of excessive fluid in the lung which leads to respiratory distress and impaired gas exchange. Causes of pulmonary oedema may be cardiogenic, resulting from increased hydrostatic pressure in pulmonary capillaries, or non-cardiogenic (also called low pressure oedema) caused by increased capillary permeability or a relative increase in capillary pressure.

## Causes

### Cardiogenic pulmonary oedema (see p. 88)
- Cardiac disease
  - Acute myocardial ischaemia or infarction
  - Acute decompensation of longstanding cardiac failure
  - Arrhythmia or tachycardia
  - Valvular heart disease
  - Cardiac tamponade
  - Myocarditis
  - Pulmonary embolism
- Fluid balance
  - Volume overload (sometimes iatrogenic)
  - Renal disease
  - Renal artery stenosis
- Systemic disease causing high output cardiac failure
  - Hyperthyroidism
  - Severe anaemia

### Non-cardiogenic (see p. 90)
- ARDS
- Altitude sickness
- Negative pressure pulmonary oedema
  - Laryngospasm (see p. 19)
  - Acute decompression of pneumothorax
- Neurogenic pulmonary oedema

Pulmonary oedema can be caused by many factors at the same time, e.g. infection may lead to ARDS and also provoke cardiac failure

# ☠ Cardiogenic pulmonary oedema

## Presentation and assessment

- Anxiety and sweating
- Patient often prefers sitting, standing, or leaning forward (orthopnoea)
- Increasing respiratory distress
  - Tachypnoea, dyspnoea
  - Hypoxaemia, cyanosis: often refractory to oxygen therapy
- Cough and/or frothy pink sputum
- Palpitations
- Bilateral crackles and/or wheeze
- Tachycardia
- Gallop rhythm, raised JVP
- Enlarged and tender liver, ascites, and oedema of dependent areas (e.g. legs and sacrum) may be present
- Fluid balance charts may reveal increasingly positive cumulative balance, oliguria, or volumes of fluid administered which are large in relation to patient weight or disease
- There may be evidence of decreased cardiac output
  - Tachycardia and/or hypotension
  - Oliguria
  - Delayed capillary refill
  - Decreased level of consciousness
- There may be decreased lung compliance causing increasing airway pressures in the ventilated patient[*]
- There may be a high CVP (>15 cmH$_2$O) or PCWP (>18 mmHg)

## Investigations

The range of investigations required will depend upon the underlying disease, but investigations which will help identify pulmonary oedema, differentiate between cardiogenic and non-cardiogenic causes, and serve as useful baseline measurements include

- ABGs (may show hypoxia with or without hypercapnia)
- FBC, U&Es, LFTs
- Cardiac enzymes
- ECG: tachycardia, arrhythmias, evidence of ischaemia, infarction, LV hypertrophy
- CXR: enlarged heart size, vascular redistribution, septal (Kerley B) lines, peri-hilar shadowing ("bat's wing" distribution)
- Echocardiography: LV dysfunction, valve disease, or regional wall motion abnormality may be present

## Differential diagnoses

- Non-cardiogenic pulmonary oedema
- Pneumonia
- Pulmonary embolism without cardiac failure
- Bronchospasm or anaphylaxis
- Pulmonary haemorrhage

[*] Increasing airway pressures will occur if using volume-controlled ventilation; decreasing tidal volumes will occur with pressure-controlled ventilation

**Immediate management**

- 100% $O_2$, pulse oximetry
- Rapid assessment of the likely cause is essential; the most likely cause of *de novo* pulmonary oedema is cardiac failure, cardiac arrhythmia, or acute ischaemia/infarction
- If the patient is spontaneously breathing
  - Give 100% oxygen via reservoir mask
  - Assist patient into upright sitting position
  - Consider commencing non-invasive ventilatory support: CPAP or BIPAP with a PEEP of up to 15 cmH$_2$O (see p. 50)*
  - *In extremis* consider assisting ventilation using bag and mask
  - Endotracheal intubation/mechanical ventilation may be required
  - Care with intubation: induction of anaesthesia can precipitate cardiovascular collapse
- In patients who are already intubated consider
  - Increasing FiO$_2$ to maintain adequate O$_2$ saturation
  - Adjusting position to be more upright
  - Increasing PEEP to recruit lung (PEEP may decrease cardiac output)
- Other treatments
  - Morphine 2–10 mg or diamorphine 2–5 mg IV, as a vasodilator and anxiolytic; titrated with anxiety and level of consciousness
  - Furosemide IV 20–40 mg and then double the dose if no response within 60 minutes
  - GTN IV infusion if the patient is normo- or hypertensive (1mg/ml at 0–12 ml/hour)
  - Consider dobutamine IV infusion if above measures fail or if patient is hypotensive
  - If *in extremis* consider venesecting 200–400 ml of blood whilst preparing other treatments (this can removed into a blood trans-fusion donor bag so that it can be transfused back to the patient later if required)
- If the patient is hypotensive (systolic <85 mmHg) or has evidence of low cardiac output consider
  - Dobutamine or low-dose adrenaline, IV infusion
  - Intra-aortic balloon pump insertion
- Consider initiating treatment for the following causes simultaneously
  - Arrhythmias (see pp. 136 and 140): anti-arrhythmics or cardiover-sion (because of a positive inotropic effect, digoxin may be beneficial in pulmonary oedema complicated by fast AF)
  - Acute ischaemia (see p. 128): aspirin 300 mg PO; anti-anginal measures (including analgesia and nitrates as above); consider heparinization/anti-coagulation
  - Acute MI (see p. 132): aspirin 300 mg PO, thrombolysis, or emergency angioplasty
  - Fluid overload: consider dialysis or haemofiltration to remove excess fluid

* Current evidence suggests that CPAP *may* be preferable to BIPAP

**Further management**
- Even if acute pulmonary oedema resolves rapidly consider transfer to critical care environment (HDU, CCU) for close observation
- Further investigation or history-taking may reveal acute trigger factors such as a change in medication or acute infection
- Consider withholding treatments likely to be contributing to cardiac failure including NSAIDs and β-blockers
- Consider monitoring fluid balance and inserting a urinary catheter
- Indications for considering ventilation include persistent hypoxia, persistent arrhythmias, and failure of above measures
- Further preventative treatment may be considered including regular diuretics, ACE inhibitors, digoxin, or anti-arrhythmics
- Obtain a cardiology opinion

**Pitfalls/difficult situations**
- Radiological features of cardiogenic pulmonary oedema overlap with ARDS
- Early institution of CPAP/non-invasive ventilation may help prevent tracheal intubation and ventilation
- Weaning from ventilator may be complicated by recurrence of pulmonary oedema

**Further reading**

Agarwal R, Aggarwal AN, Gupta D, Jindal SK (2005). Non-invasive ventilation in acute cardiogenic pulmonary oedema. *Postgrad Med J* **81**, 637–43.

Peter JV, Moran JL, Phillips-Hughes J, Graham P, Bersten AD (2006). Effect of non-invasive ventilation (NIPPV) on mortality in patients with acute cardiogenic pulmonary oedema: a meta-analysis. *Lancet* **367**, 1155–63.

OHEA p. 54.

# ⚠ **ARDS**

Acute respiratory distress syndrome (ARDS) can be triggered by direct insults to the lung, or can represent the pulmonary component of a system-wide insult causing multiple-organ failure (MOF). ARDS is a subset of acute lung injury (ALI) requiring higher levels of oxygen support. It is caused by increased capillary permeability and fibrosis.

---

**Definition of ARDS**

- High oxygen requirement: $PaO_2/FiO_2$ ≤26.7 kPa
- No evidence of left atrial hypertension
- PAOP (if measured) ≤18 mmHg
- CXR features consistent with ARDS: bilateral infiltrates

**The definition of ALI is as above but with $PaO_2/FiO_2$ ≤40 kPa**

---

Causes
- Pneumonia, or sepsis from any cause
- Aspiration, inhalational injury, or near-drowning
- Fat embolism, or amniotic fluid embolism
- Multiple trauma (or trauma causing lung contusion) or burns
- Pancreatitis
- Massive transfusion: transfusion-related acute lung injury (TRALI)
- High $FiO_2$
- Barotrauma, volutrauma, and shearing effects of mechanical ventilation

Presentation and assessment
The diagnosis is often one of exclusion: signs and symptoms may include
- Agitation, sweating, clamminess
- Increasing respiratory distress, tachypnoea, dyspnoea
- Tachycardia
- Hypoxaemia ($SpO_2$ <92% or $PaO_2$ <8 kPa), cyanosis, hypercapnia
- If already mechanically ventilated
  - Worsening oxygenation and/or increasing hypercapnia
  - Decreasing lung compliance

Investigations
- ABGs
- FBC, U&Es, LFTs, CRP
- ECG, CXR (shows bilateral infiltrates, absent Kerley's lines, air bronchogram, normal heart size, and no upper-lobe blood diversion)
- Echocardiogram (may reveal lack of evidence of LVF)
- Chest ultrasound or CT chest (to exclude pneumothoraces/effusions)
- There is no indication to insert a Swan–Ganz catheter, but if one is *in situ* PAOP should be ≤18 mmHg

Differential diagnoses
- Cardiogenic pulmonary oedema
- Intracardiac shunt
- Pneumonia

- Endobronchial intubation, equipment failure, or disconnection
- Pneumothorax or pleural effusions
- Pulmonary embolism
- Bronchospasm or breathing against ('fighting') the ventilator
- Foreign body, mucous plugs, or major collapse of the lung tissue

## Immediate management

- Titrate $O_2$ to blood gas result
- Consider respiratory support with non-invasive ventilation or endotracheal intubation and mechanical ventilation

### If oxygenation continues to worsen despite mechanical ventilation
- Consider altering ventilation parameters[*]
  - Increase inspiratory pressure, inspiratory time, or tidal volume if required, aiming to keep peak inspiratory pressure ≤35 cmH$_2$O
  - Increase PEEP to maintain lung recruitment
  - Consider decreasing I:E ratio to 1:1.5 or 1:1, or even inverting ratios
- Accept lower than normal levels of oxygenation, aiming for $PaO_2$ ≥8 kPa and $SaO_2$ ≥90% (80–85% may be considered acceptable in extreme cases)
- Consider increasing sedation or adding muscle relaxation
- Consider advanced airway manoeuvres or oxygenation techniques:
  - Alveolar recruitment measures (see p. 63)
  - Consider positioning the patient prone, or if lung pathology is worse on one side try positioning bad lung uppermost
  - Inhaled nitric oxide or nebulized prostacyclin
  - High-frequency oscillatory ventilation
  - ECMO
- Once **A**irway and **B**reathing are stabilized, continue **ABC** approach
- Cardiovascular optimization may improve oxygen delivery

[*] Follow a lung-protective strategy where possible (see p. 50)

## Further management

- Treat the underlying cause
- In some centres steroids are given, once ARDS has been established for 7 days, as a means of minimizing lung fibrosis

## Pitfalls/difficult situations

- Barotrauma is common; pneumothoraces may be occult
- Careful control of fluid balance and judicious use of diuretics may improve oxygenation
- In ARDS weaning from mechanical ventilation is often prolonged

## Further reading

Hudson L, Steinberg KP (1999). Epidemiology of acute lung injury and ARDS. *Chest* **116**(Suppl), 74S–82S.

Moran I, Zavala E, Fernandez R, Blanch L, Mancebo J (2003). Recruitment manoeuvres in acute lung injury/acute respiratory distress syndrome. *Eur Respir J Suppl* **42**, 37s–42s.

Fan E, Needham DM, Stewart TE (2005). Ventilatory management of acute lung injury and acute respiratory distress syndrome. *JAMA* **294**, 2889–96.

&#x1F4D5; OHCC p. 292.

# ☠ Pulmonary embolus

Mechanical obstruction of the pulmonary arterial system by embolus resulting in cardiovascular and/or respiratory compromise.

## Causes
- Current DVT or previous thromboembolic disease
- Major surgery, especially pelvic or lower limb
- Pregnancy/post-partum/caesarean section
- Lower limb trauma
- Malignancy or pro-thrombotic disorders
- Reduced mobility
- Major medical illness

## Presentation and assessment
- May present as PEA cardiac arrest
- Dyspnoea, tachypnoea, hypoxaemia,
- Pleural rub and/or wheeze can sometimes be heard
- Pleuritic chest pain, cough, or haemoptysis
- Syncope, hypotension, tachycardia, cardiovascular collapse
- Right ventricular gallop, accentuated second heart sound, RV heave,
- Raised JVP
- Clinical evidence of a DVT

## Investigations
- ABGs (hypoxia, acidosis, increased A–a gradient, or may be normal)
- FBC, U&Es
- D-dimer: when negative in the low-risk patient excludes PE; a negative result in the high-risk patient does not exclude PE (nearly all ICU patients are high risk)
- ECG: tachycardia, right bundle branch block, right axis deviation, T-wave inversion, prominent R in V1, ST elevation or depression, right heart strain, S1 Q3 T3 (rare)
- CXR: may show focal oligaemia, infarct/consolidation, raised hemi-diaphragm, pleural effusion, or be normal
- Echocardiogram (investigation of choice in unstable patients): high RV and PA pressures, TR, RV dilatation/dysfunction, septal shift
- CT pulmonary angiogram (investigation of choice in stable patients)
- Ventilation–perfusion (VQ) scan: good negative predictive value but hard to interpret when CXR abnormalities present (e.g. consolidation)
- Pulmonary angiogram: may identify filling defects

## Differential diagnoses
- Acute myocardial infarction
- Aortic dissection
- Anaphylaxis
- Bronchospasm
- Fat embolism
- Cardiac tamponade
- Pneumonia
- Pneumothorax

Immediate management

- Give 100% oxygen via reservoir mask if spontaneously breathing
- Secure airway if required only intubate if cardiorespiratory arrest imminent: mechanical ventilation can make hypotension worse
- Once **A**irway and **B**reathing are stabilized, continue **ABC** approach
- Support circulation with IV fluid bolus and inotropes/vasopressors
- Consider arterial line/central venous line before commencing thrombolysis or heparin
- Arrange routine and definitive investigations
- If the patient is unstable arrange for urgent echo and thrombolysis
    - Thrombolysis: recombinant tissue plasminogen activator (rtPA) 100 mg over 90 minutes IV or 50 mg rt-PA IV bolus on clinical suspicion alone if cardiorespiratory arrest is imminent followed by full heparinization (see p. 135 for contraindications to thrombolysis)
    - Alternative thrombolysis: urokinase 4400 IU/kg in 10 minutes, followed by 4400 IU/kg/hour for 12 hours
- If the patient is stable: arrange an urgent CTPA, heparinize without thrombolysis
    - LMWH (e.g. enoxaparin 1.5 mg/kg daily)
    - Heparinization with unfractionated heparin (for patients with renal failure or at high risk of bleeding): loading dose of 80 IU/kg (not required in a thrombolysed patient); commence 18 IU/kg/hour as a continuous infusion; titrate the dose against APTT: aim to maintain this at a value 1.5–2.5-fold higher than the normal range.
    - APTT should be measured 4–6 hours after starting treatment to ensure adequate anti-coagulation and exclude over anti-coagulation
    - APTT 6–10 hours after every change of dose and thereafter daily

Further management

- Morphine for chest pain
- Consider embolectomy if hypotension persists for >1 hour despite medical therapy or if there are contraindications to thrombolysis or anti-coagulation
- Consider IVC filter placement in patients with recurrence despite adequate anti-coagulation or where anti-coagulation is contraindicated
- Commence oral anti-coagulation with warfarin when PE has been reliably confirmed (target: INR 2.0–3.0); stop heparin when levels are therapeutic

Pitfalls/difficult situations

- Thrombolytic therapy is equally effective via a peripheral vein or pulmonary artery catheter
- Intubation and ventilation can worsen cardiovascular compromise
- Where diagnosis is unsure strongly consider anti-coagulation if there are no contraindications

- Where haemodynamic compromise is present failure to thrombolyse may greatly increase mortality
- Right ventricular dysfunction with normotension: opinions are divided as to whether thrombolysis is appropriate; seek expert help
- Pregnancy
  - If thrombolysis is required seek expert help
  - Unfractionated heparin can easily be reversed and is favoured in late pregnancy
  - Warfarin is contraindicated during pregnancy
- Cancer: high risk of recurrence but also high risk of bleeding

## Further reading

Wood KE (2002). Major pulmonary embolism: review of a pathophysiologic approach to the golden hour of hemodynamically significant pulmonary embolism. *Chest* **121**, 877–905.

BTS (2003). Guidelines for the management of suspected acute pulmonary embolism. *Thorax* **58**, 470–84.

BTS Standards of Care Committee (1997). Suspected acute pulmonary embolism: a practical approach. *Thorax* **52**(Suppl), S1–24.

Kearon C (2003). Diagnosis of pulmonary embolism. *Can Med Assoc J* **168**, 183–94.

&#x1F4D5; OHCC p. 308, OHEA p. 34.

# ⚙ Fat embolism

Fat embolism syndrome (FES) occurs when fat is embolized into the systemic circulation, typically following orthopaedic injury. Classical features of FES include cardiorespiratory effects as well as other multi-system complications. The diagnosis is often one of exclusion.

## Causes
- Orthopaedic trauma/surgery, especially involving pelvis or long bones
- Also reported following pancreatitis, burns, liposuction, sickle cell crisis, and parenteral lipid infusion

## Presentation and assessment
- May present as acute cardiovascular collapse
- More commonly presents 12–36 hours after injury
- Definitions vary but features may include
  - Cardiovascular compromise: tachycardia, hypotension
  - Respiratory distress: tachypnoea, dyspnoea
  - Hypoxaemia with $PaO_2$ <8 kPa, shunt, and increased A–a difference
  - Hypercapnia
  - Anaemia and coagulopathy
  - Neurological sequelae: delirium, seizures, coma
  - Dermatological changes: reddish-brown non-palpable petechiae, subconjunctival and oral haemorrhages
  - Renal dysfunction

## Investigations
None are diagnostic
- ABGs
- FBC, coagulation studies: anaemia, thrombocytopenia, low fibrinogen
- U&Es, LFTs
- CXR (or CT): shows features of ARDS and/or PE

## Differential diagnoses
- Pulmonary embolism
- Anaphylaxis
- Septic shock with DIC
- Thrombotic thrombocytopenic purpura

### Immediate management

Treatment is supportive:
- Titrate $O_2$ to blood gas result
- Consider respiratory support with non-invasive ventilation or endotracheal intubation and mechanical ventilation
- Once **A**irway and **B**reathing are stabilized, continue **ABC** approach
- Provide cardiovascular support with fluids and/or inotropes
- Support and correct any coagulopathy

**Further management**
- Early fixation of fractures
- Ensure adequate analgesia

**Pitfalls/difficult situations**
- ARDS may result from fat embolism

**Further reading**

Mellor A, Soni N (2001). Fat embolism. *Anaesthesia* **56**, 145–54.

# Circulation

# ☠ **Cardiac arrest**

*Unexpected* cardiac arrest in ICU or HDU is relatively uncommon as cardiac arrests are often preceded by prolonged attempts to resuscitate or support failing organs. When CPR is required BLS and ALS guidelines should be followed (see pp. 104 and 105).

## Causes

Although cardiac arrests are often cardiogenic in origin, hypoxia, hypoperfusion, neurological, or metabolic causes are all common in critical care settings. Potentially reversible causes, or factors which may alter the ongoing management of a cardiac arrest, include
- Hypoxia
- Hypovolaemia
- Hypo/hyperkalaemia (and other metabolic disorders)
- Hypothermia
- Hypoglycaemia
- Tension pneumothorax
- Cardiac tamponade
- Toxins
- Thrombosis (coronary or pulmonary)
- Severe acidaemia

## Presentation and assessment
- Within-hospital arrests are commonly preceded by a period of physiological deterioration. Early-warning scores may identify patients at risk (see p. 9)
- One-third of in-hospital cardiac arrests present with pulseless electrical activity (PEA), one-third with asystole, and one-third with ventricular fibrillation (VF)/pulseless ventricular tachycardia (VT)
- Any patient who has features consistent with a cardiac arrest should be assessed immediately
  - Sudden loss of consciousness
  - Impalpable pulse or loss of arterial pressure trace
  - Obvious apnoea or terminal gasping
  - ECG trace of VT, VF, asystole, profound bradycardia or tachycardia

## Investigations
Investigations which may affect an ongoing cardiac arrest include
- U&Es and blood glucose: to identify patients with hypo/hyperkalaemia, or hypoglycaemia. The fastest way of measuring this within the ICU/HDU is often via a blood gas analyser. An arterial *or* venous sample will suffice. Also look up the result of the most recent U&E sample
- ABGs: to identify profound acidosis that might benefit from a bolus of sodium bicarbonate
- Echocardiography: to diagnose cardiac tamponade

## Differential diagnoses
- Equipment failure: commonly ECG electrode failure or damped arterial pressure trace

Immediate management

- A **SAFE** approach should be adopted (**S**hout for help, **A**pproach with caution, **F**ree from danger, **E**valuate ABC)
- Manually confirm that the pulse is absent; do not rely on arterial pressure trace alone
- ALS algorithms (see p. 105) should be followed; do not delay defibrillation if appropriate
- Obtain information about the patient as soon as possible from notes, staff, or relatives. This may help to identify underlying cause and will clarify the resuscitation status of the patient. **Where doubt exists about the patient's resuscitation status CPR should be commenced**
- Within the ICU/HDU
  - Consider a precordial thump if arrest witnessed
  - Check airway, and if in doubt about ETT or tracheostomy consider re-intubating or reverting to bag and mask ventilation
  - If mechanically ventilated turn the ventilator oxygen to 100%; consider switching to a self-inflating bag
  - Do not disconnect ventilator tubing during defibrillation
  - Arterial pressure traces can be used to guide CPR; aim for diastolic pressure >40 mmHg
- Drugs
  - Whilst waiting for adrenaline bolus to be available consider increasing adrenaline/noradrenaline infusion rates
  - Central IV administration is usually the best route for drug delivery and is often available in ICU patients
  - If peripheral IV access cannot be established, consider using the endotracheal tube (if available); the adrenaline dose using the tracheal route is 3 mg diluted to at least 10 ml with sterile water
  - Amiodarone 300 mg IV is advised for VF/VT which persists despite three attempts at defibrillation
  - Consider atropine 3 mg IV for asystole or PEA with bradycardia
  - Magnesium sulphate IV 8 mmol for torsade de pointes, digoxin toxicity, refractory VF or VT with hypomagnesaemia
  - Sodium bicarbonate* 50 mmol for hyperkalaemia, tricyclic antidepressant overdose, or marked acidaemia (pH <7.1)
  - Calcium chloride* IV 10 ml 10% for PEA associated with hyperkalaemia, hypocalcaemia, or overdose of magnesium- or calcium-channel antagonists
- Other treatments
  - IV fluids: if hypovolaemia is suspected give colloid, saline or Hartmann's solution rapidly
  - Thrombolysis (see p. 92): where PE is strongly suspected consider giving a thrombolytic immediately
  - Needle thoracocentesis/pericardiocentesis: for tension pneumo-thorax or cardiac tamponade (see pp. 78 and 490, 146 and 504)
  - Open-chest cardiac compression should be considered following cardiothoracic surgery or chest trauma

* Do not give calcium solutions and sodium bicarbonate simultaneously via the same line

**Further management**

- Following the return of spontaneous circulation (ROSC) consider
  - ICU/HDU/CCU admission: it may be appropriate to admit the patient to a critical care setting for management of their underlying condition or post-arrest stabilization. Conversely, the patient's underlying condition may make any further interventions futile. Any decision not to admit the patient following ROSC should be made by senior clinicians, where possible with the involvement of the patient's relatives (and in light of the patient's views, if known). Transfer to a critical care environment is unlikely to be successful unless there is a sustained period of cardiovascular stability
  - Surgical intervention: on rare occasions it is necessary to proceed directly to surgery following ROSC (e.g. following trauma or ruptured ectopic pregnancy). Cases must be discussed with surgeons and a decision taken whether to operate within the current environment, if that is possible, or to transport to theatre
  - Continued mechanical ventilation: where this is considered appropriate aim for a $PaO_2$ >10 kPa and a $PaCO_2$ of 4–5 kPa
  - Sedation: if required consider short-acting drugs such as propofol so that neurological status can be assessed shortly after discontinuing sedation
  - Continued circulatory support: inotropic support or fluid therapy may be required. If LVF is present consider specific treatment (see p. 124)
  - Continued neurological support: employ measures to combat raised ICP including sedation, seizure control, $PaCO_2$ control, glycaemic control, avoidance of hypoxia and hypotension, and raising the bed head to improve venous drainage
  - Therapeutic hypothermia: cooling unconscious adult patients to 32–34°C for 12–24 hours following return of spontaneous circulation from out-of-hospital VF cardiac arrest is advised. It may also be beneficial following out-of-hospital cardiac arrests due to non-shockable rhythm, or after cardiac arrest in hospital
  - Treatment of hyperthermia: treat with antipyretics
  - Glycaemic control: avoid hypo- and hyperglycaemia; aim for blood sugars between 4.4 and 6.1 mmol/L
  - Electrolytes: correct any hypomagnesaemia and maintain potassium at 4-4.5 mmol/L
  - Thrombolysis: consider if there is evidence of PE or coronary occlusion (consider also angioplasty)
- Post cardiac arrest investigations
  - ABGs
  - FBC
  - U&Es, LFTs
  - Blood glucose
  - Cardiac enzymes
  - ECG
  - CXR
  - Later investigations may also include echocardiography to assess cardiac damage and CT head to assess neurological damage

**Pitfalls/difficult situations**

- ALS is unlikely to be successful in cases where maximal supportive therapy is already being provided
- In patients who are hypothermic, or undergoing general anaesthesia, prolonged CPR may still be successful
- After CVC insertion, chest trauma, or chest surgery do not forget to exclude tension pneumothorax or tamponade
- Hypo/hyperkalaemia and hypo/hypermagnesaemia are relatively common in critical care environments
- Pregnancy (see p. 414): use a wedge or tilt to decrease aortocaval compression where possible; urgently arrange for obstetric help (caesarian section may facilitate resuscitation and save the fetus)
- Hypothermia (see p. 260): if first attempt at defibrillation is ineffective withhold further attempts until temperature is >30°C. Actively rewarm using techniques listed on p. 262. Prolonged resuscitation may be effective.
- Drowning (see p. 410): consider the possibility of cervical spine trauma, and drug or alcohol intoxication

**Further reading**

Nadkarni VM, Larkin GL, Peberdy MA, et al. (2006). First documented rhythm and clinical outcome from in-hospital cardiac arrest among children and adults. *JAMA* **295**, 50–7.

Morris S, Stacey M (2003). Resuscitation in pregnancy. *BMJ* **327**, 1277–9.

📖 OHCC p. 272, OHEA pp. 2–6, OHEC p. 4.

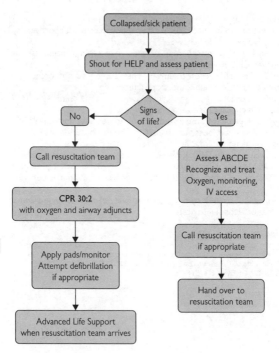

**Fig. 4.1** In-hospital resuscitation. UK Resuscitation Council guidelines 2005 (Reproduced with kind permission of the RCUK.)

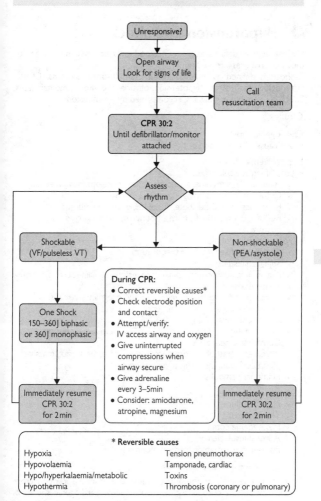

**Fig. 4.2** Adult Advanced Life Support algorithm. UK Resuscitation Council guidelines 2005. (Reproduced with kind permission of the RCUK.)

## ☼ Hypotension and shock

Hypotension is defined as systolic blood pressure <90 mmHg and/or mean arterial pressure <60 mmHg.

Shock is defined as underperfusion of multi-organ systems. Clinical signs include tachycardia, hypotension, oliguria, and altered mental status. Shock is often, but not always, accompanied by hypotension.

### Causes

#### Cardiogenic shock
- See causes listed on see p. 124

#### Hypovolaemic shock
- Loss of intravascular volume
  - Haemorrhage: trauma, aortic dissection, post-operative bleeding
  - GI loss of fluids: vomiting, diarrhoea, stomas
  - Renal loss of fluids: diabetes insipidus, excessive diuretics
  - Redistribution of fluids: burns, trauma, major surgery, sepsis, posture
- Venous pooling of blood
  - Overdose of sedatives or vasodilators
  - Spinal anaesthetic
  - Autonomic neuropathy: spinal cord lesion, Guillain–Barré syndrome
  - Anaphylaxis
  - Compression over major veins: tumour, pregnancy, ascites, extensive intra-abdominal surgery
- Impaired ventricular filling
  - Cardiac tamponade: pericardial bleeding, pericardial effusion
  - Constrictive pericarditis
  - Increased intrathoracic pressure: tension pneumothorax, massive pleural effusion, mechanical ventilation
  - Pulmonary embolism

#### Miscellaneous causes
  - Hepatic failure
  - Thyrotoxicosis
  - Myxoedema coma
  - Adrenal insufficiency
  - Poisoning, e.g. cyanide, carbon monoxide

### Presentation and assessment

Presentation depends on the primary cause and other associated factors. Shock may be low output (e.g. hypovolaemic or cardiogenic shock) or high output (e.g. sepsis or hepatic failure).
- General findings may include:
  - Anxiety and sweating
  - Tachypnoea, dyspnoea, Kussmaul breathing: significant hypotension leads to reduced tissue perfusion and a metabolic (lactic) acidosis with respiratory compensation
  - Hypoxaemia, cyanosis

- Cardiovascular findings may include:
  - Hypotension (systolic blood pressure <90 mmHg, or >30 mmHg below normal resting pressure, or MAP <60 mmHg)
  - Tachycardia, although bradycardia may be a pre-terminal sign
  - Arrhythmias, particularly AF, atrial flutter, or VT
- Organ perfusion may be impaired:
  - Cardiac: angina or ischaemia on ECG
  - Renal: oliguria, raised urea and creatinine
  - Neurological: syncope, decreased consciousness or confusion
- In low-output shock expect
  - Cold peripheries, poor peripheral perfusion and delayed capillary refill
  - Thready pulse with reduced pulse pressure
  - Decreased cardiac output
  - Increased systemic vascular resistance
  - In hypovolaemic shock JVP/CVP is decreased; there may be evidence of fluid or blood loss, or venous pooling; lungs and heart are otherwise normal; CXR and ECG are usually normal
  - In cardiogenic shock JVP/CVP may be increased; S3 may be present; examination of the lungs may show evidence of pulmonary oedema; CXR and ECG are often abnormal with evidence of pulmonary oedema, enlarged heart, and/or arrhythmia
- In high-output shock expect
  - Warm peripheries and brisk capillary refill
  - Bounding pulse with wide pulse pressure
  - Strong apical cardiac impulse
  - Normal or increased cardiac output
  - Decreased systemic vascular resistance
  - Pyrexia and raised white cell count where there is associated sepsis

If the primary survey presents a conflicting picture and the presentation does not fit a pattern, mixed shock should be considered (e.g. sepsis with myocardial dysfunction).

**Investigations**
- ABGs
- FBC, coagulation screen
- U&Es, LFTs
- Cardiac enzymes
- 12-lead ECG
- CXR
- CVP measurement
- More information from echocardiography and/or pulmonary artery catheterization (or TOD or pulse contour analysis) will be required for accurate diagnosis

**Differential diagnoses**
- Equipment malfunction: damped arterial pressure traces or poorly fitting blood pressure cuffs can give spurious readings; if in doubt re-check manually
- Mild hypotension may be a normal finding in fit healthy individuals

Immediate management

- Give 100% oxygen
- Airway may be compromised secondary to severe hypotension leading to impaired conscious level: place patient in recovery position or intubate trachea as appropriate
- Ensure breathing/ventilation is adequate
  - Fatigue may lead to respiratory failure requiring ventilatory support; in alert patients with respiratory distress, CPAP and/or non-invasive BiPAP may be indicated
  - In severe shock ventilatory support may be needed to optimize oxygenation
  - If acute pulmonary oedema is present treat with appropriate therapies (see p. 86)
- Assess hypotension: questions which need to be answered include:
  - Is this blood pressure low for this patient? (What is their normal blood pressure?)
  - Does this degree of hypotension, in this patient, have the potential to lead to morbidity?
  - Is there evidence of, or potential for, impaired cerebral perfusion, cardiac ischaemia, oliguria?
- Primary survey aims to determine the cause and the severity of presenting problem. Treat any identifiable underlying cause requiring immediate attention
  - Rule out tension pneumothorax (see p. 78) or arrhythmias (see pp. 136 and 140) as the cause for shock; treat as appropriate
  - Consider anaphylaxis, tamponade, haemorrhage
- Take a focused clinical history, carefully examine the patient, and review notes/charts where possible. Identify the likely cause of the low blood pressure: hypovolaemia, vasodilatation, or pump failure?
- Commence circulatory support
  - Ensure IV access (typically two large-bore cannulae)
  - Initial resuscitation is usually in the form of crystalloids/colloids (or warmed blood in the case of haemorrhage (see p. 114)) given rapidly until signs of adequate filling are obvious (adequate JVP/CVP). The exception to aggressive fluid therapy is cardiogenic shock, although up to 500 ml can be given initially
- **Hypovolaemia or haemorrhage** (see p. 114): treat underlying cause and fluid resuscitate; surgical intervention may be required
- **Vasodilatation** (see p. 118): treat underlying cause and commence fluid resuscitation with/without vasopressor therapy
- **Pump failure** (see p. 124): record 12-lead ECG and compare with previous ECGs; where there is evidence of myocardial infarction/ischaemia follow the appropriate treatment protocols (see pp. 128 and 132), treat cause, and commence inotropic support
- **Intropes/vasoactive agents**: noradrenaline is indicated in septic shock and dobutamine in cardiogenic shock. In the case of mixed picture adrenaline or dopamine may be started until a clearer diagnosis is possible

**Further management**

- Admit the patient into a suitable critical care facility
- Continue respiratory support until cardiovascular stability is achieved
- Perform arterial and/or central venous cannulation
- Monitor to obtain information about
  - Ventricular filling: CVP, echocardiography
  - Cardiac output and systemic vascular resistance: echocardiography, Doppler flowmetry, LidCO, pulmonary artery catheterization
- Optimize preload using colloids or blood. Keep CVP >5mmHg, haematocrit >35%
- Optimize cardiac contractility using inotropes (adrenaline, dobutamine)
- Optimize SVR using vasoconstrictors (noradrenaline) or vasodilators (glyceryl trinitrate)
- Correct any metabolic acidosis and use haemofiltration if necessary
- Correct electrolyte imbalance
- Treat pyrexia by using antipyretics and/or peripheral cooling
- If there is no response to volume replacement consider the possibility of spinal shock (see p. 401) or adrenal insufficiency (see p. 244)

---

**Interpretation of CVC variables**

**Central venous pressure (CVP)**

- There is no normal or average CVP number; the measurement is determined by venous return and right ventricular compliance. CVP should be regarded as a trend
- It is conventional to volume load an under-resuscitated patient to a target CVP of
  - ~8–10 mmHg in non-ventilated patients
  - ~12–16 mmHg in ventilated patients
- CVP monitoring should be dynamic, i.e. the patient should be volume loaded until the raise to the target CVP is sustained
  - Repeated fluid challenges are likely to be required in shocked patients with low intravascular volume with compensatory vasoconstriction; any initial rise in CVP is likely to be transient
  - Vasodilatory challenges (e.g. general anesthesia) will cause the CVP to fall
- Complete heart block, AF, tricuspid stenosis, and tricuspid regurgitation will lead to difficulty in interpreting CVP readings

**Central venous O$_2$ saturations (ScvO$_2$)**

- ScvO$_2$ may be measured on blood drawn from a CVC (mixed venous blood, S$\bar{v}$O$_2$) must be drawn from a PAFC)
- Low values (<65%) are associated with a worse outcome in trauma, severe sepsis, myocardial infarction, and cardiac failure
- ScvO$_2$ is affected by O$_2$ content, O$_2$ consumption, and cardiac output
- ScvO$_2$ may be 'artificially' high in the presence of a significant shunt
- It is conventional to resuscitated patients to a target ScvO$_2$ of >70%
- Monitoring should be dynamic to ensure that any rise is sustained

### Causes of increased/decreased systemic vascular resistance

Increased systemic vascular resistance
- Hypothermia
- Vasoconstriction
- Sympathetic stimulation
- Vasoconstrictive drugs: noradrenaline

Decreased systemic vascular resistance
- Sepsis
- Hyperthermia
- Hyperthyroidism
- A–V shunts
- Liver failure
- Vasodilators
- Spinal/epidural block

### Flow rates of different gauge cannulae[*]

- 14G (orange)          250–360 ml/min
- 16G (grey)            130–220 ml/min
- 18G (green)           75–120 ml/min
- 20G (pink)            40–80 ml/min
- 22G (blue)

* At 10 kPa via 110 cm tubing (internal diameter 4 mm) (Yentis S, Hirsch N, Smith G. *A to Z of Anaesthesia and Intensive Care* (2nd edn), Butterworth-Heinemann, Oxford, 2000.)

### Pitfalls/difficult situations

- A MAP of 65 mmHg in a young fit patient (e.g. due to a functioning epidural) may cause no tissue hypoperfusion, whereas in an elderly patient with background vascular disease it may lead to myocardial ischaemia (coronary blood occurs mainly in diastole), cerebral ischaemia, or acute pre-renal failure
- Overlapping aetiologies and mixed picture occur (e.g. sepsis with myocardial failure)
- Shock due to overwhelming sepsis can be resistant to resuscitation
- Increased CVP and lack of reponse to inotropes in suspected cardiogenic shock could be due to cardiac temponade, pulmonary hypertension/embolism, or right ventricular infarction; use of echocardiography or right heart catheter (or radiological examination for pulmonary embolism) may be required for correct diagnosis

### Further reading

Edwards JD (2000). Some aspects of circulatory failure and shock. Part1. *Int J Intensive Care* **7**, 68–72.

Rady MY (2005) Bench-to-bedside review: Resuscitation in the emergency department. *Crit Care*; **9**,170–6.

📖 OHCC p. 312, OHEA p. 24, 302, OHEC p. 4–13.

**Table 4.1** Drugs used to treat hypotension

| Drug | Dose | Comments |
| --- | --- | --- |
| Adrenaline | 0.5–1 mg IM in anaphylaxis<br>0.5–1 mg IV/ET in cardiac arrest<br>0.05–3 μg/kg/min IV infusion | β- and α-agonist: increases myocardial contractility, heart rate, and SVR<br>Agent of choice in anaphylaxis, cardiac arrest, and severe hypotension of undiagnosed cause |
| Noradrenaline | 0.05–3 μg/kg/min IV infusion | Predominantly α-agonist (increases SVR); agent of choice in high-output and/or septic shock<br>Should be avoided in hypovolaemic shock and cardiogenic shock |
| Dopamine | 0.5–10 μg/kg/min IV infusion | <5 μg/kg/min: predominantly dopaminergic effects, increases renal/splanchnic perfusion<br>5–10 μg/kg/min: mainly β and some α-agonism, increases heart rate, contractility and SVR<br>Often used as first line agent for moderate hypotension until the cause is established |
| Dobutamine | 0.5–10 μg/kg/min IV infusion | Predominantly β-agonistic: increases heart rate and myocardial contractility, and reduces systemic vascular resistance by dilating vascular supply to the muscles<br>Drug of choice in treating pump failure in cardiogenic shock<br>Can worsen hypotension if given in hypovolaemia |
| Metaraminol | Bolus 0.5 mg over 2–3 min | Used to increase systemic vascular resistance in high-output failure; boluses can be repeated until IV infusion of nor-adrenaline is established |
| Phenylephrine | Bolus 0.1 mg–0.5 mg over 2–3 min | Same as metaraminol |
| Vasopressin | 0.01–0.04 units/min IV infusion | Used to increase SVR in severe refractory septic shock |
| Terlipressin | 1 mg IV 8-hourly | Same as vasopressin |

# ☠ Anaphylaxis

Anaphylaxis is an exaggerated response to a substance to which an individual has become sensitized. Basophils and mast cells release histamine, serotonin, and other vasoactive substances in an IgE-mediated reaction.

## Causes

- Insect bites (particularly wasp and bee stings)
- Foods and food additives (particularly peanuts, fish, eggs)
- Drugs and IV infusions (blood products, vaccines, antibiotics, aspirin, contrast media, Pabrinex®, parenteral vitamin K)
- Anaesthetic drugs, particularly muscle relaxants, are common causes of anaphylaxis occurring in hospitals

## Presentation and assessment

*Any* combination of:
- Cardiovascular collapse (88% of cases): cardiac arrest or tachycardia, hypotension, and other signs of shock (see p. 106)
- Bronchospasm (40%): wheeze, cough, and/or accompanying desaturation, tachypnoea and dyspnoea
- Angio-oedema (24%): leading to laryngeal oedema and/or airway obstruction/stridor
- Erythema (48%), cutaneous rash (13%), urticaria (8%)

## Investigations

- Take 3× 5–10 ml blood samples for mast cell tryptase level
  - Immediately after treatment of initial reaction
  - 1 hour after the reaction
  - 6–24 hours after the reaction
- ABGs
- FBC, clotting studies, fibrinogen
- U&Es, LFTs, magnesium
- CXR

Tryptase samples should be stored at −20°C until they can be analysed. Concentrations peak 1 hour after the reaction and concentrations of >20 ng/ml can be seen. A negative test does not entirely exclude anaphylaxis. Urinary methylhistamine can also be measured although its usefulness remains controversial.

## Differential diagnoses

- Airway or ETT obstruction, or endobronchial intubation
- Tension pneumothorax
- Air embolus/amniotic fluid embolus/fat embolus
- Severe bronchospasm/asthma
- Type IV allergy: T-cell mediated, not life threatening, and causes localized cutaneous reactions 6–48 hours after allergen exposure
- Thyroid crisis
- Septic shock
- Hereditary angioneurotic oedema
- Carcinoid syndrome

## Immediate management

- Stop trigger agents and call for help
- Give 100% oxygen
- Secure the airway and ensure breathing/ventilation is adequate; endotracheal intubation may be required
- If intubated exclude airway/breathing system obstruction
- Lie patient flat with legs elevated
- Give adrenaline: either IM or IV
  - IM dose 0.5–1 mg (0.5–1 ml of 1:1000) up to every 10 min
  - IV dose 50–100 µg (0.5–1 ml of 1:10 000) over 1 min, and repeat as necessary
  - Continuous ECG monitoring is advisable whilst giving adrenaline
- Ensure IV access and commence rapid infusion of crystalloid/colloid (may need up to 4 L)

## Further management

- Give $H_1$ and $H_2$ antagonists (chlorphenamine 10–20 mg IV slowly and ranitidine 50 mg IV)
- Give corticosteroids (hydrocortisone 200 mg IV 6-hourly)
- If bronchospasm persists consider salbutamol 250 µg IV or 2.5–5 mg via nebulizer and/or aminophylline 250 mg IV slowly (up to 5 mg/kg) if not already on theophylline
- If hypotension persists or relapses (5%) consider inotrope infusions
- Let the endotracheal tube cuff down prior to extubation in order to ascertain a leak (to gauge the degree of airway oedema)
- Refer the patient to an allergist when convenient; include copies of the notes, drug chart, and a full description of the reaction chronology
- Skin-prick tests will be performed to any suspected drugs
- Report anaphylactic reactions on a CSM 'yellow card'
- If this was a 'wrong blood' reaction, send all products back to the laboratory and involve a haematologist

## Difficult situations

- Watch for the development of ARDS; this can manifest hours later
- Myocardial infarction and dysrhythmias can occur, especially if there is pre-existing ischaemic heart disease, or if hypoxia/acidosis is present
- Latex anaphylaxis: may present up to 30–60 minutes after contact because of delayed airborne exposure or mucous membrane contact. If latex allergic, use non-latex gloves, avoid drugs from vials with latex bungs (or uncap vials prior to drawing up), and use breathing circuit filters
- Stridor may be mistaken for bronchospasm, and vice versa
- Do not forget that latex and colloids can cause anaphylaxis

## Further reading

AAGBI and British Society for Allergy and Clinical Immunology (2003). Suspected anaphylactic reactions associated with anaesthesia. Available online at: www.aagbi.org

UK Resuscitation Guidelines. Available online at: www.resus.org.uk/pages/reaction

Gruchalla RS, Pirmohamed M (2006). Antibiotic allergy *N Engl J Med* **354**, 601–9.

📖 OHCC p. 496, OHEA pp. 126, 242.

# :⚙: Haemorrhagic shock

Hypotension and underperfusion of organs can occur secondary to intra-vascular loss of blood. Initially the body responds to hypovolaemia by peripheral vasoconstriction and tachycardia. Oliguria (urine <0.5 ml/kg/hour), thirst, and signs of organ failure (e.g. dyspnoea, myocardial failure, drowsiness) appear later.

## Causes

- Trauma
- Gastro-intestinal bleeding
- Post-operative (or post-procedure) bleeding
- Bleeding in response to trivial trauma can occur in association with
  - Coagulation factor abnormality – e.g. haemophilia
  - Thrombocytopenia
  - Splenomegaly
- Other occult bleeding:
  - Thoracic, intra-abdominal or retroperitoneal, e.g. ruptured abdominal aortic aneurysm or ruptured ectopic pregnancy

## Presentation and assessment

- There may be overt evidence of bleeding from a bleeding site or from post-operative drains
- Certain mechanisms of trauma predispose to occult bleeding (see p. 398)
- Certain patients are more likely to have a coagulopathy (see p. 306):
  - Patients with a history of congenital disease (may carry a card)
  - Patients being treated for haematological malignancy

In a healthy individual the physiological response to haemorrhage varies according to the volume of blood lost.

- ≤15% (0.75L*)of total blood volume (TBV) results in
  - Slight tachycardia
  - Mild peripheral vasoconstriction with thirst as accompanying symptom
- 15–30% (0.75–1.5 L) TBV
  - Pulse rate increases to 100–120 beats/minute (see Pitfalls/difficult situations)
  - Capillary refill is sluggish (>2 seconds)
  - Oliguria develops
  - Patient may be anxious
- 30–40% (1.5–2 L) TBV:
  - Hypotension develops
  - Pulse becomes thready
  - Dyspnoea develops
- >40% TBV (≥ 2 L*):
  - Severe hypotension
  - Thready pulse
  - Anuria
  - Ashen complexion
  - Drowsiness or unconsciousness

* Assuming a total blood volume of about 5 L (70–80 ml/kg)

## Investigations

Investigations can be divided into those which are diagnostic (mainly for identifying the source of suspected concealed bleeding), and those which monitor the degree of bleeding and the development of associated complications.

*Diagnostic*
- Plain radiographs, especially of pelvis and chest
- Abdominal ultrasound may identify free blood, ruptured ectopic pregnancy, or aortic aneurysm
- CT scan of pelvis, abdomen, or chest according to clinical indication
- Peritoneal lavage
- GI endoscopy
- Angiography
- Radio-labelled bleeding scan
- β-HCG (urine or blood) may aid in the diagnosis of ectopic pregnancy

*To monitor progress:*
- ABGs
- FBC, including haematocrit (bedside testing of Hb may also be useful, e.g. Haemacue)
- Coagulation studies, including fibrinogen (DIC screen)
- U&Es, LFTs
- ECG

Blood samples for cross-matching or blood typing should also be taken (see Immediate management)

## Differential diagnoses

Any cause of shock must be considered, particularly
- Other causes of shock associated with trauma
  - Tension pneumothorax
  - Cardiac tamponade
  - Cardiac contusion
  - Spinal cord lesion
- Sepsis
- Anaphylaxis
- Cardiogenic shock

## Immediate management

- Give 100% oxygen
- In cases of trauma ensure cervical spine protection
- Secure the airway and ensure breathing/ventilation is adequate; endotracheal intubation may be required
- Assess the degree of blood loss
- Control haemorrhage if possible
  - Establish the cause of bleeding without interrupting ongoing fluid resuscitation
  - Consider compression/elevation of external bleeding sites
  - Consider if patient requires life-saving surgery (e.g. ectopic pregnancy, ruptured spleen)
- Commence circulatory support
  - Consider head-down tilt (Trendelenburg)
  - Two large-bore intravenous cannulae (14 G) inserted in antecubital fossa; in case of difficulty use femoral veins, external jugular veins, or cutdown at ankle or antecubital fossa.
  - Take sample for blood cross-matching when inserting cannulae
  - Start restoring intravascular volume (see table on p. 117)
  - Blood transfusion* alongside crystalloids/colloids as soon as possible if bleeding is >30% TBV, >1.5 L (or Hb <8 g/dl); use O-negative or type-specific blood in these circumstances while waiting for cross-matched blood
- Serial physical examinations may be require to assess progress

* Adhere strictly to the cross-checking procedures for blood replacement to prevent inadvertent mismatched transfusion.

## Further management

- Continue with respiratory support until cardiovascular stability is established
- Where there is massive blood loss (≥6 units of blood or ≥30% TBV lost) involve haematologists for guidance on appropriate blood and component therapy. Common protocols include the following
  - FFP (12 ml/kg) if PT or APTT >1.5 times normal, or if more than 4–6 units of stored blood is transfused
  - Platelet concentrates (one pack/10 kg body weight) if the count is <50 × 10$^9$/L
  - Cryoprecipitate (one pack/10 kg body weight) if fibrinogen <0.8 g/L
- Look for and treat complications of massive blood transfusion: hypothermia, hypocalcaemia, hyperkalaemia, coagulation factor depletion, thrombocytopenia, metabolic acidosis
- Consider the following monitoring
  - CVP line to assess intravascular fluid status
  - Urinary catheterization to allow urine output measurements
  - Arterial line insertion/invasive blood pressure measurements
  - CO monitoring to assess cardiac contractility
- Inotropic support may be required initially. Adrenaline, noradrenaline, or dopamine are the agents of choice; these should be discontinued as soon as volume replacement and the control of bleeding allows

**Pitfalls/difficult situations**

- Lack of clinical improvement despite adequate resuscitation may indicate ongoing bleeding
- Elevated CVP may indicate pneumothorax, cardiac tamponade, or cardiac contusion; these can also occur alongside major haemorrhage
- Where concealed bleeding is suspected, get early help from surgeons, radiologists, or GI endoscopists; endoscopic cautery, sclerotherapy, or open surgery may be required to stop bleeding
- Long-bone fractures can be a source of occult blood loss
- The use of inotropes may mask the extent of hypovolaemia
- Wound drains can become blocked or displaced, leading to underestimation of blood loss
- Tachycardia does not always develop: up to 10% of patients with intra-abdominal bleeding respond with bradycardia; elderly patients and those on β-blockers do not develop tachycardia and may develop hypotension at relatively lesser blood loss
- Patients with cardiac illness or severe coexisting morbidity do not compensate well for hypovolaemia.

---

**Fluids suitable for use in haemorrhage**

- Crystalloids: normal saline*, Hartman's solution[†]
  - Often used as first-line fluid until diagnosis becomes clear
  - Only one-third of the volume remains intravascular; 3 L of crystalloid are needed to replace every litre of blood lost
  - Consider colloids/blood if the requirement is >2 L
- Colloids: Haemaccel, Gelofusine, starch[‡], human albumin solution (HAS)
  - Most remains intravascular for 4–6 hours; therefore blood volume can be replaced on one-for-one basis
  - Can cause coagulopathies if >1.5 L is given
- Blood[§]
  - Consider if blood loss is >30% TBV, >1.5 L, or Hb <8 g/dl
  - If a massive blood transfusion is required (≥6 units of blood), look for and prevent coagulopathies and problems related to massive blood transfusion

* Also known as saline 0.9%
[†] Also known as compound sodium lactate (CSL); Ringer's lactate is equivalent
[‡] There are many starch-containing colloids; the most common are hetastarch, pentastarch, and Voluven
[§] Blood available for transfusion is likely to be packed red cells (PRC), rather than whole blood

---

**Further reading**
📖 OHEA p. 326.

## :⚙: Septic shock

Septic shock occurs when severe infection leads to profound vasodilatation with or without myocardial depression. The resulting hypoperfusion results in organ damage.

---

**Definitions relating to septic shock**

- **Systemic inflammatory response syndrome** (SIRS): response to a variety of clinical insults manifested by two or more of the following
  - Temperature >38°C or <36°C
  - Heart rate >90 beats/min
  - Respiratory rate >20 breaths/min or $PaCO_2$ <4.3 kPa
  - White cell count >12000 cells/mm$^3$, <4000 cells/mm$^3$, or >10% immature (band) forms
- **Sepsis**: SIRS criteria in presence of infection
- **Severe sepsis**: Sepsis associated with organ dysfunction, hypoperfusion abnormalities, or hypotension (hypoperfusion abnormalities include, but are not limited to, lactic acidosis, oliguria, or an acute alteration in mental status)
- **Septic shock**: Sepsis-induced hypotension despite fluid resuscitation, with perfusion abnormalities

---

### Causes

Most infections have the potential to cause septic shock, and variations will occur according to the case mix of individual hospitals

- Site of infection
  - Respiratory (~38%)
  - Primary bacteraemia (~15%)
  - Device related (~5%)
  - Wound/soft tissue (~9%)
  - Genitourinary (~9%)
  - Abdominal (~9%)
  - Endocarditis (~1.5%)
  - CNS (~1.5%)
  - Other/unidentified (~12%)
- Type of organism
  - Bacterial (Gram positive more common than Gram negative)
  - Fungal (may account for up to 5–10%)
  - Viral
- Predisposing factors
  - Extremes of age
  - Major surgery
  - Loss of tissue coverage (e.g. burns or trauma)
  - Chronic disease: heart failure, COPD, diabetes, chronic renal failure
  - Immunocompromise: HIV, chemotherapy, haematological malignancy, neutropenia, malnutrition, alcoholism, and/or hepatic failure

**Presentation and assessment**
- Anxiety and sweating
- Tachypnoea, dyspnoea
- Hypoxaemia, cyanosis
- Cardiovascular findings may include
  - Hypotension (systolic blood pressure <90 mmHg, or >30 mmHg below normal resting pressure, or MAP <60 mmHg)
  - Tachycardia, although bradycardia may be a pre-terminal sign
  - Arrhythmias, particularly AF, atrial flutter, or VT
  - Decreased JVP or CVP
- Swan–Ganz catheterization or cardiac output monitoring may reveal
  - Increased cardiac output, although it may decreased in severe sepsis
  - Decreased PAOP and decreased systemic vascular resistance
- Organ perfusion:
  - Skin: peripheries may initially be warm and well perfused, even flushed. Later poor peripheral perfusion may occur
  - Cardiac: angina or ischaemia
  - Renal: oliguria, raised urea and creatinine
  - Neurological: syncope, decreased consciousness or confusion
- There may be evidence of infection
  - Pyrexia (or relative hypothermia) or rigors
  - High or low WCC, or raised CRP
  - Obvious abscesses, frank pus in wounds, wound drains, or urine
  - Symptoms vary according to the system(s) affected: respiratory (see p. 332), abdominal (see p. 346), wound/soft tissue (see p. 348), genitourinary (see p. 344), endocarditis (see p. 336), CNS (see p. 340)
  - Examination of devices and lines which have been inserted (e.g. new prosthesis, central venous catheters, epidural catheters) may reveal evidence of inflammation around entry site

**Investigations**
- ABGs and lactate (arterial or venous)
- FBC, clotting screen, fibrinogen
- U&Es, LFTs, blood glucose, magnesium, calcium, and phosphate
- Full septic screen: 2 × blood cultures, urine and sputum culture
- CRP and/or ESR (procalcitonin may be available in some centres)
- ECG
- CXR
- Echocardiography (TTE or TOE) if endocarditis suspected or to assess any LV dysfunction
- Other investigations for locating septic focus may include
  - CT abdomen, pelvis, chest, or head
  - Lumbar puncture
  - Wound swabs, throat swabs, or speculum examination and vaginal swabs
  - Broncho-alveolar lavage
  - Stool culture

**Differential diagnoses**
- Any cause of shock, especially cardiogenic shock

Immediate management

- Give 100% oxygen
- Secure the airway; endotracheal intubation may be required
- Ensure breathing/ventilation is adequate
  - Fatigue may lead to respiratory failure; CPAP and/or non-invasive BiPAP may be indicated
  - In severe shock, full ventilatory support may be needed to optimize oxygenation
- Ensure IV access (typically two large-bore cannulae)
- Commence circulatory support in patients with hypotension or elevated serum lactate
- Arterial and/or central venous cannulation
- Resuscitate with crystalloids/colloids, aiming for
  - CVP 8–12 mmHg
  - MAP ≥65 mmHg
  - Urine output ≥0.5 ml/kg/hour
  - Central venous or mixed venous oxygen saturations ≥70%
- Consider transfusing packed red blood cells to achieve a haematocrit of ≥30% if venous oxygen saturation <70% despite a CVP of 8–12 mmHg
- Consider dobutamine up to 20 µg/kg/min if venous oxygen saturation <70%, or if cardiac output is low despite fluid resuscitation
- Vasopressor therapy with noradrenaline 0.05–3 µg/kg/min or dopamine 0.5–10 µg/kg/min (via a central catheter) is indicated when fluid challenge fails to restore adequate blood pressure and organ perfusion or until fluid resuscitation restores adequate perfusion
- Treat any identifiable underlying cause, make a full survey for likely sources of infection, take a focused clinical history, and review notes and charts where possible
- Take all appropriate cultures; ensure one or two percutaneous blood culture samples; also sample blood from each intravascular catheter
- Commence appropriate antibiotics ideally within first hour of treatment: respiratory (see p. 332), abdominal (see p. 346), wound/soft tissue (see p. 348), genitourinary (see p. 344), endocarditis (see p. 336), CNS (see p. 340)
- Remove intravascular access devices that are a potential infection source after establishing other vascular access
- Arrange surgery, if required, to remove focus of infection

Further management

- Admit the patient to a suitable critical care facility
- Consider instituting monitoring to obtain information about
  - Ventricular filling: CVP insertion, echocardiography
  - Cardiac output and systemic vascular resistance: echocardiography, Doppler flowmetry, LidCO, pulmonary artery catheter
- Correct electrolyte imbalance
- Consider treating pyrexia: use antipyretics and/or peripheral cooling

- Consider vasopressin 0.01–0.04 units/minute in patients with refractory shock
- Consider steroids: hydrocortisone 50–75 mg IV 6-hourly for 7 days (with or without fludrocortisone 50 µg PO OD)
- Consider performing a short synacthen test (250 µg ACTH) stimulation test); discontinue steroids in patients where cortisol increase is >9 µg/dl
- Consider activated protein C (see pp. 122 and 123 for dose and indications/contraindications); may not be appropriate in patients with severe comorbidities, or where treatment is likely to be futile
- Reassess antimicrobial regimen within 72 hours and adjust according to culture results
- Consider combination therapy for neutropenic patients and those with *Pseudomonas* infections

*Treat or prevent complications*
- Respiratory
  - ARDS: use a lung-protective ventilation strategy (see p. 50)
  - Ventilator associated pneumonia: raise the bed head 45° unless contraindicated
  - Use a weaning protocol
- Renal
  - Do not use 'renal dose' dopamine
  - Correct any metabolic acidosis; use continuous veno-venous haemofiltration (CVVH) or intermittent haemodialysis if necessary
  - Avoid bicarbonate therapy for lactic acidaemia if pH ≥7.15
- Haematology
  - Do not use erythropoietin to treat sepsis-related anaemia
  - Do not use fresh frozen plasma to correct laboratory clotting abnormalities unless there is bleeding or invasive procedures are planned
  - DIC: correct fibrinogen if bleeding or risk of bleeding
  - ARDS: minimize the use of blood products by following a restrictive transfusion policy for blood (see p. 310) (aim for ≥7.0 g/dl where there is no bleeding or coronary artery disease) and for platelets (transfuse if <5 × $10^9$/L, OR if 5–30 × $10^9$/L and there is a bleeding risk, OR if <50 × $10^9$/L and surgery or invasive procedures are planned)
  - Do not use antithrombin therapy
- Other measures:
  - Provide stress ulcer prophylaxis (e.g. ranitidine 50 mg IV 8-hourly).
  - Sedation: use a protocol and sedation score and avoid neuro-muscular blockers if possible
  - Consider DVT prophylaxis with low-dose unfractionated heparin or low-molecular-weight heparin; compression stockings or an intermittent compression device, where heparin is contraindicated
  - Maintain strict glycaemic control where possible
  - Initiate enteral feeding where possible as soon as practicable

**Pitfalls/difficult situations**
- Mixed pictures of shock often occur with sepsis coexisiting with other causes such as cardiac failure
- New infections are common in patients already admitted to critical care and are often picked up via routine blood sampling (e.g. raised white cell count on FBC) or on X-rays performed for other reasons (e.g. CXR to check CVC position). Have a low threshold for suspecting vascular access catheters as a source for bacteraemia
- Organsims are often not found in culture (in up to 40% of cases)

---

**Indications for activated protein C infusions**

**Dose: 24 µg/kg/hour IV for 96 hours**
- Evidence of SIRS (≥three criteria)
  - Temperature >38°C or <36°C
  - Heart rate >90 beats/min
  - Respiratory rate >20 breaths/min or $PaCO2$ <4.3 kPa
  - White cell count >12 000 cells/mm$^3$, <4000 cells/mm$^3$, or >10% immature (band) forms
- Proven or suspected infection, e.g. positive cultures, perforated viscus, CXR, or clinical evidence of pneumonia
- Evidence of sepsis-induced multiple-organ failure within past 72 hours
  - Cardiovascular: sustained (>1 hour) systolic blood pressure ≤90 mmHg or MAP ≤70 mmHg despite adequate fluid resuscitation; OR vasopressors required to maintain systolic blood pressure ≤90 mmHg or MAP ≤70 mmHg
  - Renal: urine output <0.5 ml/kg/hour for >1 hour despite adequate fluid resuscitation
  - Respiratory: $PaO_2/FiO_2$ ≤30 kPa
  - Haematology: platelet count <80 × 10$^9$/L (or 50% decrease from peak level in past 72 hours)
  - Metabolic: pH ≤7.3 or base excess more negative than −5mmol/L with plasma lactate >2.5 mmol/L

---

**Further reading**

Angus DC, Linde-Zwirble WT, Lidicker J, et al. (2001). Epidemiology of severe sepsis in the United States: Analysis of incidence, outcome, and associated costs of care. *Crit Care Med* **29**, 1303–10.

Dellinger RP, Carlet JM, Masur H, et al. (2004) Surviving Sepsis Campaign: guidelines for management of severe sepsis and septic shock. *Intensive Care Med* **30**, 536–55.

Rivers E (2006). The outcome of patients presenting to the emergency department with severe sepsis or septic shock. *Crit Care* **10**, 154.

Rivers E, Nguyen B, Havstad S, et al. (2001). Early goal-directed therapy in the treatment of severe sepsis and septic shock. *N Engl J Med* **345**, 1368–77.

www.survivingsepsis.org

📖 OHCC p. 486.

**Contraindications to activated protein C infusions**

**Absolute contraindications**
- Active internal bleeding
- Recent trauma likely to increase risk of major bleeding
- Recent (<3 months) severe head trauma, intracranial/intraspinal surgery, haemorrhagic stroke
- Intracranial neoplasm, CNS mass lesion, or cerebral herniation
- Intracerebral AVM or cerebral aneurysm present
- Known bleeding diathesis
- Epidural catheter *in situ*
- Major GI bleed within last 6 weeks, unless definitive surgery performed
- Chronic severe hepatic disease
- Known hypersensitivity to activated protein C
- Surgery requiring general/spinal surgery within preceding 12 hours
- Active post-operative bleeding
- Platelets <30 × $10^9$/L (if platelet transfusion given and levels rise to >30 × $10^9$/L within 6 hours, treat as *relative* contraindication)
- Concurrent treatment dose of LMWH or IV heparin

**Relative contraindications**
- Recent ( <7days) administration of aspirin, clopidogrel, dipyridamole, glycoprotein 2b3a inhibitors, or warfarin
- Raised INR
- Recent (<3 months) ischaemic stroke
- Recent (<3 days) administration of thrombolysis
- Pregnant or breastfeeding patients
- Recent (<3 months) DVT or PE: confirmed or strongly suspected
- Hypercoagulable condition (e.g. hereditary protein C/S deficiency)
- Acute pancreatitis with no infective source
- Anticipated (within 2–4 days) surgery requiring general/spinal anaesthesia
- HIV with a CD4 count <50
- History of bone marrow or solid organ transplantation
- CRF requiring haemodiaysis or peritoneal dialysis

Modified from Mid-Trent Critical Care Network drotrecogin alfa (activated) prescription (adult patients) protocol.

# ✪ Cardiogenic shock/ventricular failure

Cardiogenic shock occurs when cardiac output fails to provide adequate organ perfusion. The most commont causes are chronic heart failure and myocardial stunning associated with myocardial infarction or ischaemia.

## Causes
### Left ventricular failure
- Pump failure
  - Myocardial ischaemia/infarction
  - Cardiomyopathies: hypertrophic, dilatory, restrictive
  - Myocardial injury or infection
- Outflow obstruction
  - Aortic stenosis or coarctation of aorta
  - Malignant hypertension
  - Hypertrophic cardiomyopathy
- Valve abnormalities

### Right ventricular failure
- Pump failure
  - Ischaemia, infarction
- Outflow obstruction
  - Pulmonary embolism or pulmonary hypertension (caused by chronic lung disease, hypoxia, ARDS, or vasculitis)
- Valve abnormalities

## Global myocardial depressant factors
- Metabolic: hypoxia, acidosis, hypocalcaemia, hypophosphatemia, thyroid disease
- Drugs: β-blockers, calcium-channel blockers, alcohol
- Sepsis

## Arrhythmias
- Severe bradycardia or tachycardia
- Loss of atrial contribution to ventricular filling in acute atrial fibrillation may provoke cardiogenic failure if there is underlying cardiac disease

## High-output states
- Hyperthyroidism
- Heart disease with anaemia or pregnancy
- Arterio-venous shunts
- Paget's disease
- Beri-beri

## Presentation and assessment
Acute cardiogenic shock is often associated with pulmonary oedema (see p. 86). In situations where it is not, or where pulmonary oedema has been successfully treated, the predominant symptoms are of cardiac stress, hypo-perfusion, or fluid accumulation (which may not have had time to develop).

Signs and symptoms may include:
- Anxiety and sweating
- Chest pain (not always present)
- Tachypnoea, dyspnoea, hypoxaemia, cyanosis
- If pulmonary oedema is present
  - Patient may prefer sitting, standing, or leaning forward (orthopnoea)
  - Cough and/or frothy pink sputum
  - Bilateral crackles and/or wheeze
  - May resulting in difficulty ventilating patients on IPPV
- Poor perfusion may result in
  - Cold peripheries and poor peripheral perfusion
  - Delayed capillary refill (>2 seconds)
  - Dizziness, syncope, decreased consciousness
  - Oliguria
- Cardiovascular findings may include
  - Hypotension (systolic blood pressure <90 mmHg, or >30 mHg below normal resting pressure, or MAP <60 mmHg)
  - Tachycardia, although bradycardia may precipitate cardiogenic shock, or be a pre-terminal sign associated with it
  - Raised JVP (>4 cm from sternal angle) or CVP (>15 cmH$_2$O)
  - Gallop rhythm; S3 may be present
  - Enlarged and tender liver; ascites and oedema of dependent areas (e.g. legs or sacrum) may be present
- PAFC catheterization or cardiac output monitoring may reveal
  - Decreased cardiac output (cardiac index < 2 L/min/m$^2$)
  - PAOP may be increased (>18 mmHg)
  - Increased systemic vascular resistance

Investigations
- ABGs (hypoxia and acidosis are common)
- FBC
- U&Es, LFTs, blood glucose
- Serum magnesium, calcium, and phosphate
- Cardiac enzymes
- TFTs
- ECG (tachycardia, arrhythmias, evidence of ischaemia, infarction, LV hypertrophy)
- CXR (enlarged heart size, evidence of pulmonary oedema)
- Echocardiography (LV dysfunction, valve disease)

Differential diagnoses
- Any cause of hypotension and shock, but especially:
  - Tension pneumothorax
  - Cardiac tamponade or aortic dissection
  - Sepsis
  - Hypovolaemic shock or haemorrhage
  - Anaphylaxis
- Pulmonary oedema not associated with cardiac disease
  - Neurogenic pulmonary oedema
  - Fluid overload

## Immediate management

- Give 100% oxygen
- Secure the airway and ensure breathing/ventilation is adequate; endotracheal intubation may be required
- Ensure IV access
- Treat any identifiable underlying cause
- In cardiogenic shock following cardiac surgery always consider the possibility of bleeding or cardiac tamponade
- Treat acute pulmonary oedema with appropriate therapy (see p. 86)
  - Non-invasive ventilation with PEEP of up to 15 cmH$_2$O is likely to improve oxygenation
  - Use diuretics and therapies which may worsen hypotension with extreme caution
- Record 12-lead ECG and compare with previous ECGs
  - Treat any arrhythmias (see pp. 136 and 140)
  - Where there is evidence of myocardial ischaemia follow the appropriate treatment protocol (see p. 128), avoiding any measures which will worsen hypotension (e.g. vasodilators, β-blockade, aggressive sedation)
  - Where there is evidence of myocardial infarction follow appropriate reperfusion strategies (see p. 132)
- If possible obtain an echocardiogram to aid in diagnosis
- Where angioplasty, revascularization surgery, or valvular dysfunction are involved discuss with a cardiologist
- Correct any electrolyte imbalance
- Arterial and/or central venous cannulation should be considered, and if thrombolysis or anti-coagulation are likely then they should be performed early by an experienced operator, avoiding the subclavian route
- In some situations it may be of benefit to attempt to optimize filling pressures
  - Volume loading as above may be required where there is evidence of coexisting hypovolaemia or evidence of a right ventricular/inferior MI
  - If CVP is low (<5 cmH$_2$O)or PAOP is low (<15 mmHg) small fluid boluses (100–200 ml) may be given according to response; aim for a PAOP of 15-20 mmHg
- Consider inotropic support if hypotension persists despite the above measures
  - When using inotropes titrate according to organ response/ perfusion, or aim for a systolic blood pressure of 90–100 mmHg, or MAP ≥60 mmHg
  - Dobutamine 0.5–10 µg/kg/min IV infusion is the first-line inotrope in treating pump failure in cardiogenic shock;[*] can be given via peripheral or central IV access. Occasionally dobutamine worsens hypotension, especially if hypovolaemia present

- Adrenaline 0.05–3 µg/kg/min IV infusion may improve organ (including cardiac) perfusion, but may also increase heart rate, peripheral vascular resistance, and myocardial oxygen demand
- Dopamine 0.5–10 µg/kg/min as IV infusion may have the same effects as adrenaline, particularly at higher doses
- Milrinone or enoximone may be considered in refractory cardiogenic shock
- Intra-aortic balloon pump (IABP) counter-pulsation should be considered for patients with refractory cardiogenic shock, especially where it can be used as a bridge to further treatment

\* When using inotropes in patients with cardiogenic shock following cardiac surgery follow the advice of cardiac surgeons or cardiac anaesthetists.

## Further management

- In certain circumstances (e.g. cardiac failure secondary to viral myocarditis) cardiac surgeons may be able to offer insertion of a left ventricular assist device (LVAD) as a bridge to recovery or cardiac transplantation
- Perform serial ECGs and monitor cardiac enzymes for evidence of an evolving infarct
- Once stable, consider starting long-term therapies for heart failure
  - Diuretics
  - ACE inhibitors
  - β-Blockers
  - Digoxin (commonly used if there is coexisting atrial fibrillation, but may be used in the absence of AF)
- Monitor and treat any of the complications associated with hypotension, e.g. renal failure

## Pitfalls/difficult situations

- Cardiogenic shock often occurs in combination with other diseases such a sepsis, providing a mixed diagnostic picture
- Early revascularization is particularly important in patients with myocardial infarction complicated by cardiogenic shock

## Further reading

Young R, Worthley LIG (2004). Current concepts in the management of heart failure *Crit Care Resusc* **6**, 31–53.
📖 OHCC p. 324, OHEC pp. 67–82.

# :⚙: **Myocardial ischaemia**

Myocardial ischaemia occurs when myocardial oxygen supply cannot meet the oxygen demands of its work.

## Causes

- Decreased supply
  - Severe pre-existing coronary artery disease (coronary atheroma)
  - Prinzmetal angina or drug-induced coronary vasoconstriction
  - Decreased arterial oxygen content (e.g. hypoxia or anaemia)
  - Decreased coronary perfusion pressure (CPP = DAP – LVEDP) caused by hypotension or raised LV wall tension (hypertrophy, dilatation)
  - Vasodilator drugs causing coronary steal
  - Heart valve disease (particularly aortic stenosis)
- Increased demand
  - Sustained tachycardia, arrhythmias (also decreases diastolic time)
  - Hypertension
  - Sympathetic stimulation (e.g. pain, agitation, or inadequate sedation)
  - Hyperdynamic states (pregnancy, hyperthyroidism, sepsis, or inotropes including β-agonists, calcium, phosphodiesterase inhibitors)
  - Ventricular hypertrophy

## Presentation and assessment

- Agitation/feeling of impending doom
- Vomiting, pallor, and diaphoresis
- Central crushing chest pain often radiating to the left arm or jaw
- Hypertension or hypotension
- Tachycardia, bradycardia, palpitations, ventricular arrhythmias
- Pulmonary oedema (resulting in difficulty ventilating patients on IPPV)
- ECG shows ST segment depression/elevation or T-wave inversion[*]

## Investigations

- ABGs
- FBC, clotting screen, and D-dimer (to rule out PE)
- 12-lead ECG
- CXR
- U&Es, LFTs magnesium, calcium, and phosphate, TFTs, blood glucose
- Cardiac enzymes (serial), particularly CK and troponin I/T (12 hours post onset of chest pain)
- Consider ECHO (ischaemic section of myocardium may be dyskinetic)

## Differential diagnoses

- Pericarditis
- Dissecting aortic aneurysm
- Pulmonary embolism
- GI tract disease: oesophageal reflux, spasm, or rupture; biliary tract disease; perforated peptic ulcer; pancreatitis
- Bundle branch block may be confused with ST segment changes that accompany ischaemia

[*] True analysis should be done using a 12-lead ECG as single-lead analysis may be misleading

## Immediate management

- Give 100% oxygen
- Secure the airway and ensure breathing/ventilation is adequate; endotracheal intubation may be required
- Ensure IV access
- Record 12-lead ECG
- Restore oxygen supply to myocardium
  - Give aspirin 300 mg to chew, or via NGT
  - If hypovolaemic, administer fluid cautiously; minimum volume aiming for maximum intravascular volume expansion
  - If severe anaemia is present give blood (with diuretic cover if required); aim for Hb concentration of around 7–9 g/dl
  - If hypotensive with persistent ischaemia consider vasopressor
  - If blood pressure restored but cardiac output poor consider inodilator (dobutamine)
  - Stop any vasopressor drugs if suspected as the precipitant
- Reduce oxygen demand by myocardium
  - Treat any tachyarrhythmias (p. 140); if still tachycardic, reduce heart rate using β-blocker (metoprolol 1–2 mg at a time, or esmolol 0.5 mg/kg loading dose then 50–200 µg/kg/min)
  - If pain is the cause, administer cardiostable analgesia (diamorphine, fentanyl, morphine)
  - If inadequate sedation is a suspected precipitant, consider careful titration of sedation
  - If hypertensive, treat any causes and consider GTN infusion to reduce afterload (50 mg/50 ml IV starting at 3 ml/hour, titrating to effect): GTN may be delivered sublingually to 'buy time'

## Further management

- Once stabilized on other therapy wean off GTN
- High-dose statins may reduce long- and short-term mortality
- Consider adding calcium-channel antagonist for continuing angina
- Start a low molecular weight heparin or clopidogrel (75 mg PO) unless contraindicated. Stop when stabilized or pain free for 24 hours
- Consider unfractionated heparin instead, and/or early angiography if the patient has recently undergone surgery
- Check serial ECGs and cardiac enzymes for 3 days
- Consider administering GP2b3a inhibitor (tirofiban or eptifibatide)
- Consider inserting an arterial line, CV catheter, and/or PAFC/TOD in order to measure cardiac output
- Consider BiPAP/CPAP if ventilation is inadequate

## Pitfalls/difficult situations

- Sedated patients will not manifest the classic symptoms of ischaemia; have a high index of suspicion, guided by other tests/ECG analysis
- If β-blockade is contraindicated (asthma, LVF, bradycardia), consider a rate-limiting calcium-channel blocker (verapamil, diltiazem)
- The risk of fatal haemorrhage is high if surgery is required for an ICU patient who has received GP2b3a inhibitors or clopidogrel

- Nitrate therapy tolerance: a nitrate-free period is needed if the patient is on continuous therapy. Alternatively, switch to slower-release preparations once stabilized
- Where possible invasive lines should not be performed until 7 days after clopidogrel or 48 hours after GP2b3a inhibitors; however, in patients with ongoing ischaemia/recent coronary stents these drugs should not be stopped

## Further reading

Yeghiazarians Y, Braunstein JB, Askari A, Stone PH (2000). Medical progress: unstable angina pectoris. *N Engl J Med* **342**, 101–14.

Thadani U, Davidson C, Singleton W, Taylor SH (1979). Comparison of the immediate effects of five beta-adrenoreceptor-blocking drugs with different ancillary properties in angina pectoris. *N Engl J Med* **300**, 750–5.

OHCC p. 320, OHEA pp. 30, 294, OHEC pp. 46–65.

# ☼ Myocardial infarction

Myocardial infarction (MI) occurs when acute ischaemic injury results in irreversible damage to the myocardium.

## Causes
- Coronary artery thrombosis
- Atherosclerotic plaque rupture and thrombus formation
- Severe stress-induced coronary artery spasm

## Presentation and assessment
Acute MI is diagnosed by history, ECG changes, and elevated cardiac enzymes. Presentation is as with myocardial ischaemia (see p. 128), but also includes
- STEMI: ECG shows hyper-acute T waves, ST elevation, or new LBBB
- NSTEMI: ECG shows ST depression, T-wave inversion, or normal
- Silent (diabetic patients, elderly, epidural *in situ*, patients on NSAIDs)
- Acute pulmonary oedema
- Syncope or acute confusional state
- Epigastric pain and vomiting
- DKA
- Stroke
- Oliguria
- Cardiogenic shock

## Investigations
- ABGs
- Serial 12-lead ECGs
- FBC, clotting screen, and D-dimer (to rule out PE)
- U&Es, LFTs, magnesium, calcium, phosphate, TFTs, blood glucose
- Random lipids
- Cardiac enzymes (serial), particularly CK and troponin I/T (12 hours post onset of chest pain)
- CXR

## Differential diagnoses
- Old LBBB
- Old LV aneurysm (may result in persistent ST elevation)
- Pericarditis (saddle-shaped ST segments)
- Prinzmetal angina
- Normal high take-off or single rhythm strip ST elevation which is NOT indicative of MI in isolation
- Pulmonary embolism
- Brugada syndrome (inherited condition with ST elevation in leads V1–V3 and RBBB)

Immediate management

- Give 100% oxygen
- Secure the airway and ensure breathing/ventilation is adequate; endotracheal intubation may be required
- Record 12-lead ECG and compare with previous ECGs
- Ensure IV access
- Give aspirin 300 mg to chew, or via NGT
- Diamorphine 2.5–5 mg IV (consider also giving an anti-emetic)
- GTN two puffs sublingually
- Give β-blocker (metoprolol IV 1–2 mg at a time, or esmolol 0.5 mg/kg IV loading dose then 50–200 µg/kg/min)
- Thrombolysis
  - 'Time is muscle': assess suitability for thrombolysis urgently; thrombolysis should be administered to eligible patients within 20 min
  - Streptokinase (1.5 million units in 500 ml normal saline over 1 hour) is the usual thrombolytic agent; not to be repeated unless within 4 days since first dose
  - Rt-PA is indicated if SK already received (15 mg IV bolus, then 50 mg over 30 min, then 35 mg over 60 min); benefit within 6 hours, especially in young patients with anterior MI. Follow this with heparin infusion. This regime is preferred if invasive procedures and/or surgery are needed.
  - Arterial or central venous cannulation should not be delayed if clinically indicated and should be performed by an experienced operator to minimize bleeding risk; avoid the subclavian route
- Inform cardiologist early with a view to early angioplasty or revascularization surgery, particularly if the patient has cardiac failure, continuing pain, or valvular dysfunction

Further management

- Coronary angiography with angioplasty and/or stenting is preferable to thrombolysis in the post-operative setting, and also in pregnant patients
- Where thrombolysis has been performed repeat the 12-lead ECG after thrombolysis to ensure >50% resolution of ST changes; if it does not rescue angioplasty should be considered
- Be vigilant to the further complications of bradycardia and heart block, tachyarrhythmias, LVF, pericarditis, DVT and PE, cardiac tamponade, MR, VSD, Dressler's syndrome, and LV aneurysm
- Repeat 12-lead ECGs for new ST-segment and T-wave changes (normal ECG does not exclude MI in 10–20% of cases) or left bundle branch block
- Observe for the formation of pathological Q waves (hours to days)
- Cardiogenic shock may be managed by commencing dobutamine
- Continuing chest pain may occur: may be ischaemic or pericarditic in origin (consider urgent angiography with/without angioplasty or stenting)

- Mitral valve dysfunction may be secondary to papillary muscle rupture
- DC cardioversion must be considered to treat tachyarrhythmias complicated by hypotension
- Temporary pacing may be needed for bradyarrhythmias complicated by hypotension
- Arrange for TTE/TOE post infarction to assess LV function and valve status

## Pitfalls/difficult situations

- Cardiopulmonary arrest: intrathoracic haemorrhage can occur with vigorous chest compressions in the thrombolysed patient
- Cardiac failure is common and cardiogenic shock can be difficult to recognize in the patient with pre-existing septic shock
- Hypotension is not always cardiogenic shock; consider reaction to thrombolysis or hypovolaemia
- Pericardial tamponade can be fatal in the thrombolysed patient
- NSAIDs are very effective for pericarditic pain; however, care with gastric erosion potential in the thrombolysed patient
- Thrombolysis is usually contraindicated following surgery and is contraindicated if the patient is on activated protein C
- If invasive cardiac monitoring is contraindicated consider non-invasive alternatives

## Further reading

Zimetbaum PJ, Josephson ME (2003). Current concepts: use of the electrocardiogram in acute myocardial infarction. *N Engl J Med* **348**, 933–40.

Anderson HV, Willerson JT (1993). Current concepts: thrombolysis in acute myocardial infarction. *N Engl J Med* **329**, 703–9.

Keeley EC, Grines CL (2004). Primary coronary intervention for acute myocardial infarction. *JAMA* **291**, 736–9.

**Thrombolysis criteria in myocardial infarction:**

- History of cardiac sounding pain or dyspnoea lasting more than 20 min in the past 12 hours
- Presentation within 12 hours of onset of pain
- ECG supports clinical diagnosis:
  - >1 mm ST elevation in two consecutive limb leads
  - >2 mm ST elevation in two consecutive chest leads
  - ST depression in septal leads V2–V4 with ST elevation >1 mm in posterior leads V7–V8
  - LBBB
- No contraindications to thrombolysis

**Consider emergency coronary angiography and primary angioplasty where there is an absolute contra-indication to thrombolysis**

**Thrombolysis <u>relative</u> contraindications**

- CPR for more than 10 min
- Pancreatitis
- Pregnancy
- Severe hypertension (>180/110 mmHg)
  If hypertensive consider
  - Treating pain with IV diamorphine
  - Commencing IV Isoket
  - Giving atenolol 5 mg IV

**Thrombolysis <u>absolute</u> contraindications**

- Aortic dissection suspected
- Active GI bleeding within the past 2 weeks
- Major surgery or trauma in previous 6 weeks
- Puncture of a non-compressible vessel or organ biopsy within last 2 weeks
- Haemorrhagic stroke in previous 3 months
- History of intracranial lesion
- Anti-coagulation with INR >2
- Known bleeding disorder
- Recent central neuraxial blockade

# ⚙ Bradyarrhythmias

Bradycardia is defined as a heart rate <60 beats/minute. *Excessive* bradycardia (i.e. heart rate <40 beats/minute) is more likely to be pathological, and patients are more likely to be cardiovascularly compromised.

Bradycardia may also be relative
- Heart rate should be appropriate to circumstances, e.g. sepsis and haemorrhage would normally be expected to cause tachycardia
- In patients with poor physiological reserve even moderate bradyarrhythmias may cause symptoms

## Causes
- Sinus bradycardia
  - May be normal, especially in healthy young adults, athletes, and heavily sedated patients
  - Vagal stimulation (e.g. lung recruitment manoeuvres, ocular pressure, peritoneal stretching, vagino-cervical stimulation) may cause profound bradycardia in sedated patients
  - Hypothermia
  - Head injury, raised ICP
  - Pre-terminal sign associated with hypoxia and shock, cardiac injury
  - Drugs: β-blockers, calcium-channel agonists
  - Hypothyroidism
  - Myocardial ischaemia or infarction
  - Bradycardia/tachycardia syndrome
- Heart block
  - Myocardial ischaemia or infarction, particularly inferior infarcts
  - Following cardiac surgery
  - Electrolyte abnormalities, especially hyperkalaemia
  - Drugs, e.g. β-blockers, calcium-channel inhibitors, digoxin
  - Cardiac contusion
  - Myocarditis/infection, e.g. Lyme disease
  - Amyloid or sarcoid infiltratrion
  - Idiopathic or congenital (with or without structural abnormality)

---

**Types of heart block**

- First degree: PR interval >0.2 seconds (does not require treatment)
- Second degree
  - Mobitz type I (Wenkebach): PR interval gradually lengthens with each beat until there is an absent QRS following a P wave. The cycle then repeats
  - Mobitz type II: PR interval remains the same; intermittently there is failure of AV conduction and no QRS follows a P wave
- Complete heart block: there is complete dissociation between P waves and QRS complexes. Where the ventricle establishes its own 'escape' rhythm the QRS complexes are wide (>0.12 seconds) and the heart rate is typically 20–40 beats/min. Occasionally a nodal escape rhythm is established and QRS complexes may be narrow

---

**Presentation and assessment**

Asymptomatic
- Physiological bradycardia may be asymptomatic
- Occasionally second-degree heart block, or complete heart block, is an incidental finding
- In anaesthetized or sedated patients evidence of symptoms such as angina or myocardial ischaemia may be hard to identify

Symptomatic
- Anxiety and sweating
- The patient may have chest pain
- Tachypnoea, dyspnoea
- Hypoxaemia, cyanosis
- Angina or ischaemia on ECG
- Hypotension (systolic blood pressure <90 mmHg)
- Poor perfusion may result in
  - Cold peripheries and poor peripheral perfusion
  - Delayed capillary refill (>2 seconds)
  - Dizziness, syncope, decreased consciousness
  - Oliguria
- If heart failure is present
  - Raised JVP (>4 cm from sternal angle) or CVP (>15 cmH$_2$O)
  - Cannon A waves may be seen in ventricular tachycardia (these are a sign of AV dissociation and are also seen in asymptomatic individuals in the absence of heart failure)
  - Gallop rhythm; S3 may be present
  - Enlarged and tender liver; ascites and oedema of dependent areas (e.g. legs or sacrum) may be present
- Haemodynamic measurements may reveal decreased cardiac output and increased systemic vascular resistance
- If pulmonary oedema is present
  - Patient may prefer sitting, standing, or leaning forward (orthopnoea)
  - Cough and/or frothy pink sputum
  - Bilateral crackles and/or wheeze
  - May result in difficulty ventilating patients on IPPV

**Investigations**

In symptomatic individuals, or if heart block is second degree or worse
- 12-lead ECG with rhythm strip
- ABGs
- FBC
- U&Es, LFTs, TFTs, magnesium, calcium
- Cardiac enzymes
- CXR
- Consider echocardiography once stable

**Differential diagnoses**
- Equipment failure
- Any cause of shock, heart failure, or a terminal bradycardia, e.g. bronchospasm, head injury, tension pneumothorax

## Immediate management

- Give 100% oxygen; secure the airway and ensure breathing/ventilation is adequate; endotracheal intubation may be required
- Record 12-lead ECG
- Ensure IV access
- Correct any electrolyte abnormalities
- Temporary pacing wires are often left *in situ* following cardiac surgery; pacing via these is first-line therapy

### Asymptomatic or mild symptoms

- If the risk of asystole is low (see Fig. 4.3), investigate and treat underlying cause
- Atropine 300–600 µg IV may be useful for minor symptoms, or if bradycardia is likely to worsen; rebound tachycardia may occur
- Glycopyrronium bromide 200–600 µg IV may be considered as an alternative to atropine and is less likely to cause tachycardia

### High risk of asystole (see Fig. 4.3)

- Assess the symptoms; consider using drugs to increase heart rate
- Ensure transcutaneous pacing facility immediately available
- Arrange for cardiology assessment for transvenous pacing

### Adverse signs or severe symptoms (see Fig. 4.3)

- Atropine 500 µg IV; repeat as necessary to a maximum of 3 mg
- Consider an adrenaline infusion 2–10 µg/min IV, titrate to response
- Percussion pacing (repeated precordial thumps) may 'buy time'
- Transcutaneous pacing
  - Use a defibrillator with transcutaneous pacing function
  - Ensure pads are attached to clean dry skin if possible (sternum and apex, or anterior and posterior)
  - Choose *fixed* mode (consider *demand*, if available, once stable)
  - Increase the *output* (in mA) until *capture* occurs; pacing spikes are seen and QRS complexes are triggered by them
  - Set the rate for 50–70 beats/min and ensure there is a pulse present with QRS complexes; otherwise treat for PEA
  - Muscle twitching is normal; sedation or analgesia may be required if there is associated pain.
- Glucagon 1–5 mg IV (slow), or 1–7.5 mg/hour, may be useful if bradyarrhythmia is caused by β-blockers or calcium-channel blockers
- Dopamine dose 5–20 µg/kg/min IV is an alternative to adrenaline
- Aminophylline 0.5 mg/kg/hour IV is an alternative to adrenaline
- Isoprenaline 1–10 µg/min IV is an alternative to adrenaline
- Arrange for transvenous pacing

## Further management

- Look for any other coexisting conditions, especially if signs and symptoms fail to respond to correction of heart rate
- Monitor for an evolving infarct with cardiac enzymes and serial ECGs

### Pitfalls/difficult situations

- Complete heart block only rarely responds to drug therapy
- In arrest situations bradyarrhythmia with a rhythm normally compatible with supporting circulation should be treated as PEA (see p. 105); pacing should be considered if complete heart block is present. There is no benefit to be derived from pacing asystole

### Further reading

Durham D, Worthley LIG (2002). Cardiac arrhythmias: diagnosis and management. The bradycardias. *Crit Care Resusc* **4**, 54–60.

OHCC p. 318, OHEA p. 8, OHEC pp. 126–34

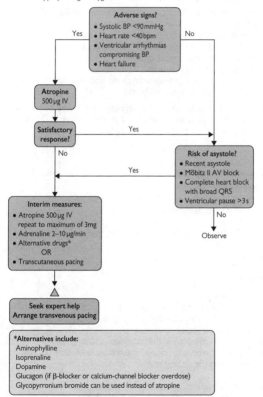

If appropriate, give oxygen, cannulate a vein, and record a 12-lead ECG

**Adverse signs?**
- Systolic BP <90mmHg
- Heart rate <40bpm
- Ventricular arrhythmias compromising BP
- Heart failure

Yes → **Atropine** 500µg IV

**Satisfactory response?** — Yes →

No →

**Risk of asystole?**
- Recent asystole
- Möbitz II AV block
- Complete heart block with broad QRS
- Ventricular pause >3s

Yes →

No → Observe

**Interim measures:**
- Atropine 500µg IV repeat to maximum of 3mg
- Adrenaline 2–10µg/min
- Alternative drugs*
  OR
- Transcutaneous pacing

**Seek expert help Arrange transvenous pacing**

**\*Alternatives include:**
Aminophylline
Isoprenaline
Dopamine
Glucagon (if β-blocker or calcium-channel blocker overdose)
Glycopyrronium bromide can be used instead of atropine

**Fig. 4.3** Bradycardia algorithm (includes rates inappropriately slow for haemodynamic state). UK Resuscitation Council guidelines 2005. (Reproduced with kind permission of the RCUK.)

# ☺ **Tachyarrhythmias**

Tachycardia is defined as a heart rate >100 beats/minute. Tachycardia is more likely to be pathological, and patients are more likely to be cardiovascularly compromised, at rates >150 beats/minute. Tachyarrhythmias can be either broad complex or narrow complex.

---

**Types of tachyarrhythmia**

- Narrow complex tachyarrhythmia (QRS <0.12 seconds)
  - Sinus tachycardia
  - Ectopic atrial tachycardia
  - Atrial fibrillation with fast ventricular response rate (fast AF)
  - Atrial flutter
  - Re-entrant tachycardias
- Broad complex tachyarrhythmia (QRS >0.12 seconds)
  - Ventricular tachycardia (monomorphic)
  - Torsade de pointes (polymorphic VT)
  - Any cause of narrow complex tachycardia with aberrant conduction (e.g. bundle branch block)

Supraventricular tachycardia (SVT) can represent any cause of narrow complex tachycardia, although in practice it most commonly refers to re-entrant tachycardia and ectopic atrial tachycardia

---

## Causes

*Sinus tachycardia*
- Physiological response to
  - Pain
  - Anxiety or inadequate sedation
  - Hypovolaemia
  - Sepsis and systemic inflammatory response, pyrexia
  - Hypoxaemia and hypercarbia
  - Anaemia
- Inotropes
- Thyrotoxicosis

*Other types of tachycardia*
- Primary cardiac disease: ischaemic heart disease, cardiomyopathy, valve disease, abnormal conduction (long QT syndrome: torsade de pointes)
- Hypoxaemia, hypercarbia, or acidaemia
- Electrolyte abnormalities, especially potassium and magnesium
- Pharmacological: inotropes (tricyclics, macrolide antibiotics, antifungals, antipsychotics—torsade de pointes)
- Hyperthyroidism
- Extremes of temperature
- Pulmonary artery catheterization/CVC line placement
- Following cardiac surgery
- Cardiac hypoperfusion, often associated with shock or sepsis

**Presentation and assessment**
Patients may be asymptomatic, present in cardiac arrest, or may show evidence of
- Anxiety and sweating
- Palpitations
- Chest pain
- Tachypnoea, dyspnoea
- Hypoxaemia, cyanosis
- Angina or ischaemia on ECG
- Hypotension (systolic blood pressure <90 mmHg) *or* hypertension
- Poor perfusion may result in
  - Cold peripheries and poor peripheral perfusion
  - Delayed capillary refill (>2 seconds)
  - Dizziness, syncope, decreased consciousness
  - Oliguria
- If heart failure is present
  - Raised JVP (>4 cm from sternal angle) or CVP (>15 cmH$_2$O)
  - Cannon a waves may be seen in ventricular tachycardia (these are a sign of AV dissociation and are also seen in asymptomatic individuals in the absence of heart failure)
  - Gallop rhythm; S3 may be present
  - Enlarged and tender liver; ascites and oedema of dependent areas (e.g. legs or sacrum) may be present
- Haemodynamic measurements may reveal decreased cardiac output and increased systemic vascular resistance
- If pulmonary oedema is present
  - Patient may prefer sitting, standing, or leaning forward (orthopnoea)
  - Cough and/or frothy pink sputum
  - Bilateral crackles and/or wheeze
  - May resulting in difficulty ventilating patients on IPPV

**Investigations**
- 12-lead ECG with rhythm strip
- ABGs
- FBC
- U&Es, LFTs, TFTs, magnesium, calcium
- Cardiac enzymes
- CXR
- Consider echocardiography once stable

**Differential diagnoses**
- Interference from equipment, e.g. haemofiltration
- Any cause of sudden hypotension, e.g. haemorrhage or anaphylaxis
- Sinus tachycardia as a response to trauma, or sepsis, is often mistaken for SVT. SVT is more likely if
  - Onset is sudden
  - Rate is very high
  - Rhythm is irregular
  - Rhythm responds to treatment

## Immediate management

- Stop any triggers (e.g. drugs or procedures)
- Give 100% oxygen; secure the airway and ensure breathing/ventilation is adequate; endotracheal intubation may be required
- Record 12-lead ECG
- Obtain IV access

If the patient has severe haemodynamic compromise
- Significant hypotension (systolic blood pressure <90 mmHg)
- Heart failure
- Chest pain or severe ischaemia on ECG
- Reduced consciousness level
- Consider precordial thump for witnessed arrhythmia
- Proceed to urgent synchronized DC cardioversion[*] with 200–360 J[†]
  - If AF or atrial flutter consider giving heparin 5000–10 000 IU IV
- Consider amiodarone as an alternative to cardioversion

If the patient is stable
- Investigate and treat underlying cause (e.g. hypoxaemia, hypotension, and sepsis) whilst instituting specific arrhythmia treatments
- Correct electrolyte and acid–base abnormalities
- Identify underlying rhythm and follow the protocol in Fig. 4.4

### If narrow complex tachycardia

- In cardiac arrest treat as PEA (see p. 105)
- Look for evidence of accessory pathway

Sinus rhythm: regular
- No specific treatment required; correct any underlying disorder

Ectopic atrial tachycardia: regular, abnormal P-wave pattern, 1:1 conduction (usually)
- Try amiodarone, esmolol, or digoxin

Re-entrant tachycardia/SVT: regular, P waves may be hidden in QRS, or conducted retrograde; a short PR interval and delta wave may be seen in ECGs with sinus rhythm prior to tachycardia
- Consider carotid sinus massage
  - Check for evidence of carotid disease: bruit, previous CVA/TIA
  - The carotid sinus lies near the upper border of the thyroid cartilage: massage first one side, then the other for up to 15 seconds
  - Stop if sinus rhythm supervenes, or if there is a prolonged ventricular pause: with compliant patients the combination of carotid sinus massage with a Valsalva manoeuvre may be effective
  - Try adenosine unless pre-excitation (i.e. Wolff–Parkinson–White syndrome) and AF/atrial flutter is suspected
  - Consider amiodarone, verapamil, esmolol, or cardioversion[*]

Atrial fibrillation: irregular, no atrial activity seen.

Atrial flutter: regular, rate often 130–150 beats/min, saw-tooth P-wave pattern (may be lost with 2:1 AV conduction, P waves may merge into QRS complexes)

- If AF <48 hours old consider cardioversion with amiodarone or synchronized DC shock* (consider heparin 5000–10 000 IU IV)
- If AF >48 hours old consider rate control with digoxin, esmolol, or verapamil, *except* where there is evidence of AF or atrial flutter *and* an accessory pathway; if there is an accessory pathway avoid adenosine, digoxin, and verapamil as these can all exacerbate the tachycardia

**Unsure of rhythm**

- Try carotid sinus massage and/or adenosine (unless AF or atrial flutter with accessory pathway suspected (see above))

**If broad complex tachycardia**

- In cardiac arrest treat as pulseless VT (see p. 105)

Ventricular tachycardia: regular broad complex AV dissociation present, fusion and capture beats, QRS concordance in precordial leads

- Treat with amiodarone or cardioversion*
- Consider lidocaine if haemodynamically stable
- Correct magnesium and potassium
- Consider overdrive pacing

Torsade de pointes: irregular rotating QRS complex

- Treat as for ventricular tachycardia, but
  - Aggressively correct magnesium and potassium
  - If QTc is prolonged when in sinus rhythm give magnesium as a bolus *and* an infusion (see below), and arrange temporary pacing

SVT with aberrant conduction (i.e. bundle branch block)

- Treat as relevant narrow complex tachycardia
- If in doubt treat as VT

* Where possible cardioversion should be performed under sedation or anaesthesia
† 200–360 J monophasic *or* 150 J biphasic

---

**Adenosine**

Dose
- 3 mg IV as rapid bolus, followed by saline flush; if no response try 6 mg then 12 mg

Side effects
- Flushing and chest tightness/bronchospasm
- Choking
- Nausea
- Bradycardia

Contraindications
- Asthma
- Sick sinus syndrome
- Second- or third-degree heart block
- AF or A flutter and pre-excitation syndromes
- In heart transplant recipients

## Other drugs

- Amiodarone: loading dose 5 mg/kg IV (~300 mg) over 15–30 min (in 100 ml 5% dextrose, via CVC if possible); maintenance dose 15 mg/kg (~900 mg) over 24 hours
- Digoxin: loading dose 0.75–1.0 mg IV over 2 hours (in 100 ml 5% dextrose); maintenance dose of 0.0625–0.25 mg/day (adjust according to age, renal function, and drug interactions)
- Esmolol loading dose 500 µg/kg IV over 1 min, then 50–200 µg/kg/min
- Lidocaine: loading dose 1 mg/kg IV over 2 min; if required repeat at 5–10 min intervals up to 200 mg
- Magnesium IV replacement infusion 20 mmol (5 g) over 1–2 hours (in 100 ml 5% dextrose) via central line; aim for a plasma concentration of 1.4–1.8 mmol/L
  - In torsade de pointes 8 mmol (2 g) in 100 ml 5% dextrose IV over 2–5 min followed by an infusion of 2–4 mmol/hour (0.5–1 g/hour)
- Potassium IV 40 mmol over 1–4 hours (in 100 ml 5% dextrose) via central line; aim for plasma concentration of 4.5–5.0 mmol/L
- Verapamil IV 2.5–5 mg over 1 min: avoid with re-entry tachycardia; may cause profound hypotension if given to misdiagnosed VT or in hypotensive patients (or patients with LV dysfunction); may cause profound bradycardia in combination with β-blockade

## Further management

- Consider referral to cardiologist for all tachyarrhythmias which are complex or do not respond to treatment
- In stable AF or atrial flutter >48 hours old where rate control has been achieved consider anti-coagulation and/or TOE to identify any atrial thrombus before proceeding to elective cardioversion
- Look for any other coexisting conditions, especially if signs and symptoms fail to respond to correction of heart rate
- Monitor for an evolving infarct with cardiac enzymes and serial ECGs
- Consider obtaining an ECHO where structural heart disease or myocardial damage is suspected

## Pitfalls/difficult situations

- Many patients in critical care settings are already sedated or anaesthetized, and proceeding directly to cardioversion may be more appropriate than drug therapy; where cardioversion has failed consider repeating after normalization of electrolytes, or after treatment with amiodarone
- CVC position is a common cause dysrhythmias; confirm the position with a CXR, aiming for above the carina
- In patients with chest disease, or after chest surgery, amiodarone may no longer be a first-line drug as it can cause lung function deterioration
- Digoxin toxicity commonly occurs in patients with renal failure
- New AF is a common post-operative occurrence and may respond to fluid loading and magnesium bolus (as for torsade de pointes but over 20–30 min); magnesium may cause flushing and hypotension
- Sodium bicarbonate (50 ml 8.4% IV) may be required for rapid correction of acidaemia, especially in tricyclic antidepressant overdose

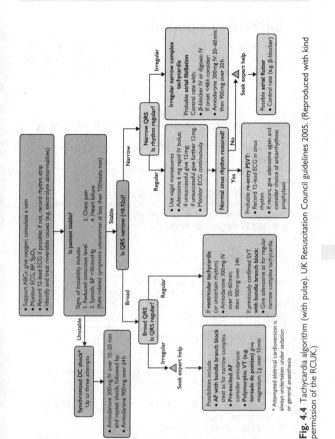

**Fig. 4.4** Tachycardia algorithm (with pulse). UK Resuscitation Council guidelines 2005. (Reproduced with kind permission of the RCUK.)

## Further reading

Durham D, Worthley LIG (2002). Cardiac arrhythmias: diagnosis and management. The bradycardias. *Crit Care Resusc* **4**, 54–60.

Reising S, Kusumoto F, Goldschlager N (2007). Life-threatening arrhythmias in the intensive care unit. *J Intensive Care Med* **22**, 3–13.

OHCC p. 316, OHEA pp. 12, 16, 20, OHEC pp. 136–66.

# :☠: Cardiac tamponade

Tamponade occurs when blood/fluid accumulates in the pericardium and impairs cardiac output; 100–200 ml accumulated rapidly may cause acute tamponade, whilst up to 1000 ml may build up in chronic tamponade.

## Causes
- Acute
  - Blunt or penetrating thoracic trauma
  - Recent cardiac surgery, cardiac catheterization, or cardiac pacing
  - Recent CVC insertion
  - Coagulopathy: thrombocytopenia/uraemia/anti-coagulation
  - Pericarditis
  - Dissecting aortic aneurysm, or cardiac rupture after acute MI
- Chronic
  - Metastatic disease or following radiotherapy
  - Pericarditis: idiopathic or secondary to uraemia, connective tissue disorders (e.g. systemic lupus erythematosus)
  - Infection: bacterial, viral, fungal, TB, HIV
  - Hypothyroidism

## Presentation and assessment
- May present as cardiac arrest
- Anxiety, restlessness, and/or palpitations
- Chest pain relieved by sitting upright and leaning forwards
- Respiratory distress: tachypnoea, dyspnoea, and cyanosis
- Cardiovascular findings include:
  - Tachycardia and hypotension
  - Dizziness, syncope, decreased consciousness
  - Oliguria
  - Poor peripheral perfusion
  - Raised JVP/CVP, especially if there is a prominent 'x' descent and loss of 'y' descent (Kussmaul's sign)
  - Peripheral oedema
  - Decreased pulse pressure, pulsus paradoxus, disappearance of radial pulse on inspiration
  - Muffled heart sounds or a pericardial rub
  - Elevated and equalized ventricular filling pressures (CVP/PCWP)

## Investigations
- ABGs
- FBC, coagulation screen
- U&Es, LFTs
- CXR: widened mediastinum or globular heart
- ECG: low voltage with electrical alternans or T-wave changes
- Echocardiography (TTE or TOE): visible pericardial fluid, small ventricles with impaired filling, diastolic collapse of right ventricle
- CT/MRI chest
- PAFC/TOD: low cardiac output, high SVR, and high PCWP
- Cytology and culture of pericardial fluid

**Differential diagnoses**
- Tension pneumothorax
- Cardiogenic shock, myocardial failure, myocardial infarction
- Pulmonary embolus
- Constrictive/restrictive pericarditis
- Volume overload
- SVC obstruction
- Anaphylaxis
- Acute severe asthma

**Immediate management**
- Give 100% oxygen
- Secure the airway and ensure breathing/ventilation is adequate; endotracheal intubation may be required
- Ensure adequate IV access
- Administer IV fluids/inotropic support
- Under no circumstances remove any penetrating foreign body
- Monitor the patient's ECG

**Imminent/actual cardiac arrest**
- Proceed to emergency sub-xiphoid aspiration/pericardiocentesis (see p. 504)

**Post cardiac surgery**
- Clear any obstruction to chest drains
- Call for surgical help, alert theatres, obtain wire cutters
- Administer anaesthesia prior to chest opening using the most cardiostable induction agents/analgesics (be prepared to open chest immediately post-induction)
- Intubate and ventilate if not already
- If it is not possible to maintain haemodynamic stability, open chest immediately
- Ensure blood and clotting factors are ready

Other situations
- Arrange urgent echocardiogram to confirm tamponade
- Proceed to immediate pericardiocentesis if
  - Echocardiogram shows >1.5 cm fluid plus diastolic collapse
- Seek cardiology advice if
  - Echocardiogram shows <1.5 cm fluid plus diastolic collapse
  - Echocardiogram shows >1.5 cm fluid but no collapse
  - Echocardiogram shows effusion with dilated LV

Perform pericardiocentesis under echocardiogram guidance where possible
- Replace blood loss and check clotting screen (replacing clotting products as required)

**Further management**
- Avoid bradycardia, maintain filling pressures and sympathetic tone
- Blood pressure may surge on relief of tamponade causing pulmonary oedema
- Correct metabolic acidosis
- IPPV may worsen hypotension and tamponade
- Antibiotic cover may be needed if the chest has been opened
- Follow up cytology and culture of pericardial fluid

**Pitfalls/difficult situations**
- Tamponade may recur; an indwelling pericardiocentesis catheter may be required
- Creation of a pericardial window or pericardiectomy may be appropriate in some patients
- Low-pressure tamponade with small amounts of fluid can occur; in these cases where JVP is not elevated, RAP is normal and the patient may respond to IV fluids
- Beware of coagulopathies, particularly in the post-MI patient who has received thrombolysis
- Ensure that wire cutters are available immediately for any post-operative cardiac surgical patients

**Further reading**

Callaham M (1984). Pericardiocentesis in traumatic and non-traumatic cardiac tamponade. *Ann Emerg Med* **13**, 924–45.
Spodick DH (2003). Acute cardiac tamponade. *N Engl J Med* **349**, 684–90.
&#x1F4D5; OHEA p. 32.

# ① **Superior vena cava obstruction**

SVC obstruction can occur because of either external compression or internal thrombus formation. It is commonly associated with lung cancer.

### Causes
- Lung cancer, especially small cell
- Mediastinal lymphoma
- Aortic aneurysm
- Mediastinal fibrosis
- TB
- Venous thrombosis secondary to Hickman, PICC, dialysis line, or other long-term CVC

### Presentation and assessment
When SVC obstruction develops slowly the collateral circulation has time to develop and signs/symptoms may be mild. Acute SVC obstruction often presents as an emergency with the following
- Tachypnoea, dyspnoea, and cough
- Headache
- Facial 'fullness' and collar tightness
- Symptoms improved by sitting upright and leaning forwards; worsened by bending over
- Upper body plethora, cyanosis, venous distension, and oedema

### Investigations
- FBC, coagulation screen
- U&Es, LFTs, $Ca^{2+}$
- CXR
- Chest CT
- Angiography
- Neck vein Doppler ultrasound

### Differential diagnoses
- Acute airway obstruction
- Cardiac tamponade
- Angio-oedema
- Thyroid goitre
- Axillary thrombosis

Immediate management

- Give 100% oxygen
- A head-up position may improve symptoms
- Secure the airway and ensure breathing/ventilation is adequate; endotracheal intubation may be required
- Ensure adequate IV access; lower limb IV access is preferable, especially when inducing anaesthesia, as severe SVC obstruction leads to a very slow arm–brain time
- IV dexamethasone (8–16 mg) may improve symptoms

*Where an oncological cause is suspected*

- Get oncology advice
- Urgent chemotherapy or radiotherapy may be advised, especially if SVC obstruction is the first presenting symptom of malignancy

*Where line thrombosis is suspected*

- Discuss with team responsible for indwelling line: line removal, anti-coagulation, or thrombolysis via CVC may be advised

Further management

- Treat the underlying cause: in most cases any mortality will be due to the malignancy responsible
- Stenting of the SVC may be considered in some cases

Pitfalls/difficult situations

- An equivalent pathology of the inferior vena cava exists although lower body swelling is often initially attributed to other causes
- Patients may be so agitated that induction of anaesthesia is required
- The relaxation associated with anaesthesia may precipitate lower airway obstruction in patients with mediastinal masses

## ☼ **Hypertension**

Treating hypertension aggressively in critical care settings may lead to organ hypoperfusion as autoregulation (particularly cerebral and renal) is often disrupted by acute disease or chronic hypertension. However, accelerated/malignant hypertension requires urgent intravenous treatment to prevent the associated morbidity and mortality.

### Causes
- Primary hypertension
  - No identifiable underlying cause
- Secondary hypertension
  - Drugs
  - Renal/renovascular disease
  - Endocrine (e.g. phaeochromacytoma or Cushing's syndrome)
  - Coarctation
  - Preclampsia/eclampsia
- Reactive hypertension
  - To pain, anxiety, or hypercapnia
  - 'White coat' hypertension

### Presentation and assessment

*Urgent review and treatment*
- Blood pressures >220 mmHg systolic or >120 mmHg diastolic
- Accelerated/malignant hypertension
  - Papilloedema and/or fundal haemorrhages and exudates
  - Acute/impending cardiovascular complications: angina, MI, LVF
  - Acute pulmonary oedema
  - Neurological deficit: encephalopathy, TIA

*Serial blood pressure measurements and consideration of elective anti-hypertensive therapy:*
- Severe (Grade 3) hypertension:
  - Systolic pressure >180 mmHg
  - Diastolic pressure >110 mmHg
- Hypertension with complications
  - Systolic pressure 160–179 mmHg
  - Diastolic pressure >100–109 mmHg
  - Cardiovascular complications/end-organ damage or diabetes

### Investigations
These should be directed by the likely underlying cause; consider
- ABGs
- FBC, coagulation screen, fibrinogen (accelerated hypertension can cause DIC)
- U&Es, LFTs, TFTs, blood glucose
- Urine dipstick looking for haematuria and/or proteinuria
- ECG
- Renal ultrasound
- If end-organ damage suspected consider head CT and cardiac echo

## Immediate management

- Ensure airway, breathing, and circulation are stabilized
- Treat any underlying cause, in particular
  - Ensure adequate analgesia and/or adequate sedation/anaesthesia, particularly where neuromuscular blockade is being used
  - Follow the appropriate treatment protocols for suspected phaeochromocytoma (see p. 250), thyroid storm (see p. 246), or pre-eclampsia (see p. 416)
- If accelerated/malignant hypertension, or if BP >220/120 mmHg, consider immediate IV treatment
  - Aim for a 10–20% reduction in MAP: reductions in blood pressure greater than this can lead to acute complications
  - Insert an arterial line for continuous blood pressure measurement
  - Use short-acting IV drug infusions to achieve initial blood pressure control to allow for titration to desired effect and rapid discontinuation if needed
- Drug choices
  - GTN IV 0.5–12 mg/hour titrated to effect: venodilator (half-life 3 min); side effects include tachycardia, headache, and tolerance
  - Sodium nitroprusside (SNP) 0.25–8 µg/kg/min IV titrated to effect: vasodilator (half-life 2 min), side effects include tachycardia and cyanide toxicity (giving sets need to be protected from sunlight)
  - Esmolol hydrochloride 500 µg/kg/min IV for 1 min, followed by an infusion of 50–300 µg/kg/min IV titrated to effect: β-blocker (half-life 8 min)
  - Labetalol hydrochloride 20 mg IV over 2 min, followed by an infusion at 2 mg/min until a satisfactory response is obtained (maximum dose 300 mg): combined $\alpha_1$ and non-selective β-blocker (half-life 4 h (caution in impaired hepatic function))

Hypertension should not be aggressively treated when it occurs as a response to raised intracranial pressure, i.e. following head injury

## Further management

- Once blood pressure control is achieved consider longer-term anti-hypertensive therapy, e.g. ACE inhibitors, β-blockers, diuretics

## Pitfalls/difficult situations

- Sublingual nifedipine should be avoided for the treatment of severe hypertension as it may cause precipitous drops in blood pressure
- Hypertension as a consequence of acute neurological events may be difficult to manage; in the presence of subarachnoid bleeding hypertension may predispose to re-bleeding whilst hypotension may worsen CPP. It is probably appropriate to treat a raised MAP in a normally normotensive patient in the absence of raised ICP

## Further reading

Santhi R, Worthley LIG (2003). Hypertension in the critically ill patient. *Crit Care Resusc* **5**. 24–42.
OHCC p. 314, OHEA pp. 28, 300.

**Table 4.2** Cardiovascular and haemodynamic variables

| Heart rate and cardiovascular pressures | |
| --- | --- |
| Heart rate | 60–100 beats/min |
| Mean arterial pressure (MAP) | 75–105 mmHg |
| Central venous pressure (CVP) | 0–8 mmHg (0–10 cmH$_2$O) |
| Right atrial pressure (RAP) | 0–8 mmHg |
| Right ventricle pressure, systolic | 14–30 mmHg |
| Right ventricle end-diastolic pressure (RVEDP) | 0–8 mmHg |
| Pulmonary artery pressure (PAP), systolic | 15–30 mmHg |
| Pulmonary artery pressure, diastolic | 5–15 mmHg |
| Pulmonary artery pressure, mean (MPAP) | 10–20 mmHg |
| Pulmonary artery occlusion pressure, mean (PAOP, or PAWP) | 5–15 mmHg |
| Left atrial pressure (LAP) | 4–12 mmHg |
| Left ventricular pressure, systolic | 90–140 mmHg |
| Left ventricular end-diastolic pressure(LVEDP) | 4–12 mmHg |
| **Haemodynamic variables** | |
| Cardiac output (CO) | 4.5–8 L/min |
| Cardiac index (CI) | 2.7–4 L/min/m$^2$ |
| Stroke volume | 60–130 ml/beat |
| Stroke volume index (SVI) | 38–60 ml/beat/m$^2$ |
| Systemic vascular resistance (SVR) | 770–1500 dyn s/cm$^5$ |
| Systemic vascular resistance index (SVRI) | 1860–2500 dyn s/cm$^5$/m$^2$ |
| Pulmonary vascular resistance (PVR) | 100–250 dyn s/cm$^5$ |
| Pulmonary vascular resistance index (PVRI) | 225–315 dyn s/cm$^5$/m$^2$ |
| Left ventricular stroke work index (LVSWI) | 50–62 g.m/m$^2$/beat |
| Rate–pressure product (RPP) | 9600 |
| Ejection fraction (EF) | >60% |
| Oxygen delivery (DO$_2$) | 950–1300 ml/min |
| Systemic oxygen consumption (VO$_2$) | 180–320 ml/min |
| **Haemodynamic variables associated with trans-oesophageal Doppler (TOD)** | |
| Flow time, corrected (FTc) | 330–360 ms |
| Peak velocity at 20 years old | 90–120 cm/s |
| at 50 years old | 70–100 cm/s |
| at 70 years old | 50–80 cm/s |
| at 90 years old | 30–60 cm/s |

**Table 4.2** (*Contd*)

| Haemodynamic variables associated with pulse contour cardiac output analysis | |
| --- | --- |
| Intrathoracic blood volume index (ITBVI) | 850–1000 ml/m$^2$ |
| Extravascular lung water index (EVLWI) | 3–7 ml/kg |
| Stroke volume variation (SVV) | <10% |
| Global end diastolic volume index (GEDVI) | 681–800 ml/m$^2$ |
| Left ventricular contractility | 1200–2000 mmHg/s |
| Cardiac function index (CFI) | 4.5–6.5 L/min |

# Neurology

# :⚙: Decreased consciousness

Decreased consciousness occurs in many diseases requiring admission to intensive care, and is often a cause for admission in its own right. Apart from neurological disease (head injury, space-occupying lesion, subarachnoid haemorrhage), changes in neurological state may be related to worsening respiratory, circulatory, or metabolic disorders.

For intracranial pathology, the primary aim of the immediate management should be to protect airway, ensure adequate breathing and gas exchange, and prevent fluctuations in blood pressure, ensuring adequate oxygen delivery to the brain.

## Causes

*Physiological derangement*
- Hypoxia
- Hypercapnia
- Hypotension
- Hypothermia/hyperthermia

*Intracranial damage*
- Diffuse brain injury
- Extradural haemorrhage
- Subdural haemorrhage
- Intracerebral bleed
- Stroke/ischaemia
- Tumour/other intracerebral mass

*Metabolic and endocrine*
- Hypoglycaemia/hyperglycaemia
- Hyponatraemia/hypernatraemia
- Hyper-osmolar states
- Hypocalcaemia
- Hypermagnesaemia
- Hypothyroidism/hyperthyroidism
- Addison's disease
- Hepatic failure
- Renal failure

*Infections*
- Meningitis
- Encephalitis
- Systemic sepsis

*Drugs and toxins*
- Alcohol
- Sedatives
- Illicit drugs

*Seizures*
- Status epilepticus
- Post-ictal states

**Presentation and assessment**

*Neurological state*

Level of consciousness should be quantified using the Glasgow coma score (GCS) or AVPU systems (rather than poorly defined terms such as unconscious, semi-conscious, obtunded, comatose).

GCS assesses eye, verbal and motor responses and has a maximum score of 15 (fully conscious) and a minimum score of 3 (deeply unconscious/comatose). A GCS <8 equates to 'unconsciousness' (in the AVPU scale P is taken as the cut-off).

---

**Glasgow coma scale**

Best motor response(out of 6)
- Obeys commands        6
- Localizes to pain        5
- Withdraws/normal flexion to pain        4
- Abnormal flexion to pain        3
- Extends to pain        2
- No response to pain        1

Best verbal response (out of 5)
- Appropriate orientated response        5
- Confused speech        4
- Inappropriate/non-conversational speech        3
- Incomprehesible sounds        2
- No speech        1

Best eye response (out of 4)
- Spontaneous eye opening        4
- Eyes open to speech        3
- Eyes open to pain        2
- Eye remain closed        1

     **Minimum score = 3**       **Maximum score = 15**

Painful stimuli should not result in skin damage or marking; alternatives include supra-orbital pressure, jaw thrust manoeuvre, nailbed pressure, and sternal rub

Record each individual component of GCS scores or why they might not be possible (e.g. patient intubated.)

---

**AVPU scale**

An alternative to the GCS, which is particularly useful in children, in which there are four levels of alertness:

**A** – **A**lert
**V** –responds to **V**oice
**P** – responds to **P**ain
**U** – **U**nresponsive

- Transient loss of consciousness, or changes in consciousness are also important, particularly following head injuries
- Obtain a contemporaneous history if possible (e.g. from patient, relatives, or ambulance crew)
  - Mechanism of injury in trauma cases (p. 182) as well as any accompanying amnesia
  - Any history of headaches, limb weakness, seizures, vomiting, slurred speech
  - Any past or current medical history
  - Any medications (especially anti-coagulants) or illicit drug use
  - Previous neurosurgery

Other indicators of altered neurological state may include
- Drowsiness
- Agitation
- Incoherence
- Incontinence
- Headache
- Amnesia
- Vomiting
- Seizures
- Evidence of meningism (painful neck flexion or straight leg raising—often lost if GCS ≤5) may indicate
  - Meningitis
  - Encephalitis
- Evidence of head or neck trauma, especially evidence of vault or base-of-skull fracture (see p. 183)
- Focal neurological signs and symptoms including
  - Loss or change in sensation (anaesthesia or paraesthesia) or power
  - Gait or balance problems
  - Problems speaking or understanding speech
  - Problems reading or writing
  - Abnormal peripheral or central reflexes (including lack of gag/cough reflex)
  - Abnormal plantar responses
  - Visual changes (e.g. blurred or double vision, or loss of visual field)
- Eye examination may reveal
  - Pupil signs: abnormal size, difference in size, reactivity, accommodation, deviation, or movements
  - Fundoscopy (if possible): haemorrhages, papilloedema
- Raised ICP (>25 cmH$_2$O) where monitored

*Other signs and symptoms*
- Airway: grunting, snoring, or complete obstruction may occur (airway obstruction may cause loss of consciousness, or be caused by unconsciousness)
- Respiratory
  - Hypoventilation is a late sign unless associated with narcotic/drug overdose
  - Kussmaul's breathing may indicate a metabolic acidosis (e.g. DKA)

- Cheyne–Stokes breathing is associated with brainstem events or raised ICP
- Tachypnoea causing a respiratory alkalosis may sometimes occur
- Neurogenic pulmonary oedema
- Cardiovascular changes
  - Tachycardia
  - Bradycardia is often a late or pre-terminal sign
  - Hypotension may occur if there is associated trauma (especially spinal)
  - Hypertension may be associated with pain or agitation, or may be associated with severe neurological injury (more likely in patients who are deeply unconscious)
  - Cushing's response of hypertension combined with bradycardia is a late sign indicative of severe intracranial hypertension
  - ECG changes: ischaemic changes can occur in association with subarachnoid or intracerebral bleeding; cardiac ischaemic events or arrhythmias (Stokes–Adams attacks) can cause decreased consciousness; chronic AF is associated with thromboembolic events
- Renal: incontinence, polyurea

## Investigations

- ABGs (for hypoxaemia, hypercarbia, acidaemia)
- FBC, coagulation screen (particularly in anti-coagulated patients, or where acute liver failure is possible)
- U&Es (especially to look for hyponatraemia or ARF)
- LFTs
- Serum glucose, with urinalysis for ketones if indicated (may identify hypo/hyperglycaemia or HONK)
- Plasma osmolality (may help identify ethanol, methanol, or ethylene glycol poisoning)
- Cross-match blood if there is trauma or risk of bleeding
- Blood alcohol levels and/or urine toxicology (for illicit drugs)
- Blood, urine, and sputum cultures where infection is a possible cause
- ECG
- CXR (malignancy or pneumonia may be present)
- Lumbar puncture
- CT scan of head and/or neck (see pp. 162 and 189): good for bony or cerebral lesions, but not brainstem lesions
- MRI scan of head (investigation of choice for suspected brainstem lesions)

In patients with associated trauma also consider
  - C-spine X-rays
  - Other trauma X-rays (e.g. pelvis or long bones)
  - Skull or facial X-rays

**Indications for head CT scan**

*Immediate (once stable)*
- Head injury with any of the following features continuing after resuscitation
  - Diminished consciousness (GCS <13)
  - Deteriorating consciousness
  - Focal neurology
  - Seizures

*Urgent*
- Head injury with confusion, drowsiness, or neurological disturbance lasting >2 hours
- Head injury with persistent severe headache or severe nausea and vomiting
- Suspected or proven skull or base-of-skull fracture; penetrating or open head injury
- New or unexplained seizure activity
- History suggestive of subarachnoid haemorrhage, meningitis, or encephalitis
- Suspected stroke or other central neurological deficit
- Amnesia or loss of consciousness in the elderly or those with a coagulopathy (e.g. patients on warfarin)
- Also consider head CT scan if there is loss of consciousness or severe amnesia associated with a high risk mechanism of injury (see p. 182)

**Immediate management**
- Give 100% $O_2$ and support airway, breathing, and circulation as required
- Care for the cervical spine if trauma is suspected
- Obtain a contemporaneous history if possible (e.g. from relatives or ambulance crew); an 'AMPLE' history (p. 2) should be obtained as a minimum
- Roughly assess neurological state (e.g. conscious and talking, or unconscious) and simultaneously treat neurological complications which may interfere with ABC (e.g. seizures)
- Complete basic ABC primary survey before formerly assessing neurological state

*Airway*
- Airway may be compromised because of impaired conscious level: place patient in recovery position or intubate trachea as appropriate
- If endotracheal intubation is required, a rapid-sequence intubation will be necessary to minimize the risk of aspiration
- Rapid-sequence endotracheal intubation should be considered if
  - GCS ≤8, or rapidly deteriorating
  - There is risk of aspiration of vomit or blood
  - There is a lack of gag reflex

- There is facial or neck trauma putting the airway at risk
- There is evidence of hypoxia ($PaO_2$ <9 kPa on air, <13 kPa on oxygen), hypercarbia ($PaCO_2$ >6 kPa), or marked tachypnoea
- Short-term deliberate hyperventilation is required
- There is ongoing seizure activity
- The patient is unlikely to remain still for investigations (e.g. CT)
- The patient is agitated and combative but requiring treatment
- Any stress response to endotracheal intubation should be avoided if possible

*Breathing*
- Ensure breathing/ventilation is adequate
  - Ventilatory support may be needed to optimize oxygenation; avoid hypoxia
  - Avoid hypercapnia
  - Avoid hyperventilation and hypocapnia unless required for short periods to treat raised ICP
  - If acute pulmonary oedema is present treat with appropriate therapies (see p. 84)

*Circulation*
- Establish IV access
- Avoid hypotension; where possible aim for a blood pressure which would be near normal for the patient
- Resuscitate with fluids and/or inotropes where required

*Neurology*
- Formally assess neurological status, including
  - Glasgow coma score (see p. 159)
  - Eye examination including pupil size and reactivity and fundoscopy if possible
  - Evidence of trauma, especially evidence of vault or base-of-skull fracture
  - Plantar reflexes
- Reassess GCS after stabilizing airway, breathing, and circulation, and continue to reassess consciousness and neurological state at regular intervals

*Others*
- Exclude and treat hypoglycaemia
- Exclude blockage of V–P shunt (if *in situ*)
- Urgent CT scan may be required for diagnosis and appropriate management (prevent hypoxia, hypercapnia, hypotension, and hypertension throughout)
- Raised ICP may be treated with with hypertonic saline or mannitol until more definitive measures can be employed (see p. 190)
- Treat seizures as per protocol (see p. 166)
- Check electrolytes
- Consider the possibility of unexpected overdose (see pp. 428 and 436); trials of naloxone or flumazenil may be appropriate

**Further management**

- Worsening neurological state due to respiratory, cardiac, or metabolic disorders will often respond to successful management of the primary precipitating disorder

*Neurosurgical referral*

- Where decreased level of consciousness is suspected, or proven, to be neurosurgically treatable, referral is indicated.

---

**Indications for neurosurgical referral**

- Fractured skull with impaired consciousness, focal neurology, fits, or other neurology
- Compound skull fractures, depressed skull fractures, or base-of-skull fracture
- Head injury with coma (GCS <9), deteriorating consciousness, neurological disturbance continuing after resuscitation
- Head injury with confusion or neurological disturbance lasting >8 hours
- Evidence of intracranial haemorrhage (subarachnoid, subdural, extradural, or intracerebral) or mass lesion seen on CT

---

*Ventilation*

- Hypoxia should be avoided, as should hypo- or hypercapnia; ideally $PaO_2$ >13 kPa and $PaCO_2$ 4.0–4.5 kPa should be maintained
- Pulmonary oedema may require the addition of PEEP (although caution may be required as high levels of PEEP may increase ICP)
- Aspiration and chest infections are common in patients with decreased consciousness and should be actively investigated/treated
- Head-up positioning may decrease the risk of aspiration and improve cerebral venous drainage

*Cardiovascular*

- Hypotension should be avoided. MAP >90 mmHg should be sufficient initially, MAP may be guided later by ICP (allowing calculation of CPP) or other measurements
- Fluid resuscitation (avoiding hypotonic fluids) is often sufficient, although inotropes may be needed

*Sedation*

- Sedation will be required in most cases where patients are intubated and ventilated
- Sedatives with rapid offset (e.g. propofol) are useful initially as they can be stopped and the level of consciousness rapidly reassessed
- Muscle relaxants may be required initially for endotracheal intubation, or for short periods during transfer or CT scanning, but they run the risk of masking fitting; where they are used consider concurrent sedative infusions with anticonvulsive medications (e.g. propofol or midazolam)

*Metabolic*
- Hyper- or hypoglycaemia should be avoided
- Hyper- or hyponatraemia should be corrected (see pp. 216 and 218)
- Pyrexia should be avoided; the place of mild/moderate hypothermia for severe neurological injuries is unclear, but is practised by some hospitals (mild/moderate hypothermia following cardiac arrest *is* indicated, see guidelines, p. 100)

## Pitfalls/difficult situations

- Drug or alcohol use is frequently associated with other causes of diminished consciousness; a high suspicion of metabolic derangement or head injury/intracranial haemorrhage is essential in these patients
- Diminished consciousness is common in patients sedated in intensive care for prolonged periods, or where there has been renal or hepatic dysfunction leading to a prolonged washout period of sedative medications; a low threshold for suspecting metabolic derangement, intracranial haemorrhage/ischaemia is advisable
- Alcoholic and coagulopathic patients are at increased risk of intracranial haemorrhage even after relatively minor trauma
- Transfer to CT or MRI is hazardous (particularly MRI where monitoring and ventilators need to be 'magnet compatible'); scans should only be attempted once patients are stable
- In some cases, general surgical interventions (e.g. for major internal haemorrhage) may take precedence over investigating or treating neurological problems

## Further reading

Sanap MN, Worthley L:IG (2002). Neurologic complications of critical illness. Part I: Altered states of consciousness and metabolic encephalopathies. *Crit Care Resusc* **4**, 119–32.
Bowie RA, Mahajan RP (2000). Management of head injury. *RCOA Newsl* **51**, 335–7.
National Institute for Clinical Excellence (2003). Head injury. triage, assessment, investigation and early management of head injury in infants, children and adults. Clinical practice algorithms developed by the National Collaborative Centre for Acute Care.
&#x1F4D5; OHEA p. 310, OHEC pp. 27–34.

# ☠ Convulsions and status epilepticus

Epileptic fits warrant intensive care management when they are difficult to control, or when they are associated with underlying disease or physiological disturbance. Prolonged seizure activity carries a significant mortality, especially if there is airway compromise.

Status epilepticus is defined as a tonic–clonic seizure lasting more than 30 minutes or repeated seizure activity without return to full consciousness between the seizures. Ideally, any seizure lasting longer than 5 minutes should be treated as an emergency.

## Causes

*In patients known to have epilepsy the following triggers may be involved*
- Head trauma
- Alcohol
- Intercurrent infection
- Medication failure or sub-therapeutic levels of anti-epileptic medication

*Where there is no history of epilepsy*
- Hypoxia
- Intracranial tumour
- CVA: infarct or haemorrhage
- Traumatic brain injury
- Metabolic disturbances:
  - Electrolyte abnormalities (e.g. sodium, calcium, magnesium)
  - Hypoglycaemia
- Eclampsia (see p. 416)
- Infection: meningitis, encephalitis, brain abscess
- Drug associated:
  - Drug withdrawal, particularly alcohol
  - Drug overdose
  - Illicit drug use, particularly cocaine

## Presentation and assessment

*Seizure activity*
- Loss of consciousness
- Obvious tonic-clonic muscle movements
- Subtle eye movements; sometimes the only sign
- Partial or absence seizures; features may range from episodes of absence, to simple focal twitching with no loss of consciousness, or to complex absences with or without facial tics, autonomic symptoms, and/or hallucinations
- Teeth clenching
- Tongue biting
- Urinary incontinence

*Physiological response to seizure*
- Sweating
- Shallow fast respiration

- Airway obstruction may occur
- Hypoxaemia is associated with airway obstruction and prolonged fits
- Tachycardia
- Hypertension
- Fever

## Investigations

- ABGs: a metabolic lactic acidosis is common
- FBC: raised WCC may indicate meningitis/encephalitis or intercurrent infection leading to reduced seizure threshold in known epileptic
- Serum glucose
- U&Es, LFTs
- Serum magnesium and calcium
- Consider CRP and ESR
- Consider measuring CK following prolonged fits
- Consider urine/blood β-HCG as pregnancy may indicate eclampsia
- Blood and/or urine toxicology screen for alcohol or illicit drugs
- Serum anti-convulsant drug levels in patients with known epilepsy
- CXR to exclude malignancy, infection, or aspiration
- Consider head CT scan/MRI if focal neurology, papilloedema, or signs of head injury are present, or if no obvious precipitant found (urgent CT scanning is indicated in the majority of patients who suffer prolonged seizures but have no previous history of controlled epilepsy)
- Lumbar puncture if infection is possible/likely
- Consider blood, urine, and sputum cultures if infection is likely
- Consider EEG as advised by neurologists

## Differential diagnoses

- Rigors
- Myoclonic jerks
- Pseudosiezures: should be considered in convulsions where consciousness is preserved, or where there is a failure to respond to adequate drug dosing
- Acute withdrawal state without seizure activity
- Acute dystonia
- Syncope from any cause, especially where there are secondary anoxic movements

## Immediate management

- Give 100% $O_2$ initially
- Airway may be compromised because of seizure activity
  - Maintain airway until fit is terminated, adjuncts may be required: consider nasal airways if there is marked jaw clenching
  - Consider placing the patient in recovery position to protect head and airway
  - Where 1st- and 2nd-line anti-epileptic therapies have already failed (or if the patient becomes severely hypoxic, acidotic, or hypotensive during treatment), consider proceeding to endotracheal intubation: employ a rapid-sequence induction technique using thiopental (or propofol) and suxamethonium (see p. 482)
- Ensure breathing/ventilation is adequate
- Assess circulation and obtain IV access
  - Fluid resuscitation may be needed to restore blood pressure

*Seizure assessment and control:*
- Rapidly assess consciousness level and confirm presence of seizure
- Obtain brief history
- Identify any alternative treatable causes:
  - Check blood sugar: if low, or unobtainable/unclear, give 50 ml 50% dextrose IV (the risk of exacerbating cerebral ischaemia is outweighed by the correction of hypoglycaemia)
  - If alcoholism or malnourishment is suspected, give thiamine 250 mg (Pabrinex®, two ampoules) IV over 10 min
  - If eclampsia is suspected follow protocol (see p. 416): magnesium sulphate, loading dose 16 mmol (4g) IV over 5 min, followed by maintenance infusion of 5–10 mmol/hour
- Commence anti-epileptic therapy
  - Lorazepam 4 mg IV (0.025–0.05 mg/kg)—longer-acting with better anti-convulsant activity than diazepam
  - Diazepam 0.1 mg/kg IV (or rectally): alternative to lorazepam
  - Midazolam 10 mg to buccal mucosa, or 200 µg/kg intranasally: an unlicensed alternative to lorazepam
- If seizure activity continues >15 min give 2nd-line anti-epileptics
  - Phenytoin (in 0.9% saline): loading dose 15 mg/kg IV infusion at a rate not exceeding 50 mg/min; ECG monitoring is required
  - Fosphenytoin: 15 mg(PE)/kg IV infusion (max. rate 100–150 mg (PE)/min). Alternative to phenytoin, ECG monitoring required
  - In patients known to be on regular phenytoin avoid loading dose but consider using maintenance dose (see Further management)
- If 1st- and 2nd-line therapies fail to control seizure activity within 45–60 min consider endotracheal intubation (see above), sedation, and 3rd-line therapy (if still required after general anaesthesia initiated)
- If seizure control is achieved reassess airway: sedative effects of treatment may require endotracheal intubation and mechanical ventilation

* Phenytoin equivalents (PE) are used for fosphenytoin: fosphenytoin 1.5 mg = phenytoin 1 mg

**Further management**

- If endotracheal intubation and mechanical ventilation are required
  - Avoid neuromuscular blocking agents if possible (apart from those used for intubation); if they are required, consider using continuous cerebral function monitoring to detect further seizure activity
  - Ventilation should be tailored to avoid secondary brain injury from hypoxaemia or hypercarbia; aim for $PaO_2$ >10 kPa, $PaCO_2$ 3.5–4.5 kPa, pH >7.3 (use a lung protective strategy, see p. 50)
- Perform head CT scan if required (see p. 162)
- Ensure that a full neurological assessment has been carried out and discuss the case with a neurologist
- Consider a third-line anti-convulsant if further treatment is required
  - Phenobarbital 5–12 mg/kg IV (max. rate 100 mg/min)
  - Propofol 1 mg/kg IV followed by 2–10 mg/kg/hour infusion
  - Thiopental 1–5 mg/kg/hour IV
  - Continuous EEG monitoring allows for titration of sedative infusions
  - Infusions should ideally be continued for 24 hour after last seizure activity and weaned slowly
- Phenytoin 300–400 mg/day IV/oral maintenance therapy may be advised (e.g. following head injury)
- Treat complications
  - Where there is evidence of hypotension commence fluid resuscitation with inotropic support if required
  - Hyperpyrexia may extend seizure activity; normothermia should be maintained using surface cooling and antipyretic agents
- Other complications which may require treatment include
  - Cerebral oedema (see p. 190)
  - Neurogenic pulmonary oedema (see p. 86)
  - Aspiration (see p. 64)
  - Lactic acidosis (see p. 212)
  - Electrolyte disturbances (see pp. 211–244)
  - Rhabdomyolysis and acute renal failure (see pp. 272 and 278)
  - DIC (see p. 312)

**Pitfalls/difficult situations**

- Many drugs lower the fit threshold (e.g. flumazenil and antipsychotics)
- Non-convulsive epileptic seizures can also be neurologically damaging: these may present as altered behaviour, absences, or coma, and are diagnosed via EEG changes
- Status epilepticus is not common in epileptics; always consider other causes of convulsions such as infections
- Where tumour or vasculitis are present consider dexamethasone
- Pseudostatus (intentionally simulated status) may be suggested by lack of cyanosis, resistance to passive eye opening, downward plantar reflexes, and the persistence of a positive conjunctival reflex

**Further reading**

Walker M (2005). Status epilepticus: an evidence based guide. *BMJ* **331**, 673–7.
📖 OHCC p. 72, OHEA p. 182.

# :☼: Stroke

A stroke* is defined as an acute focal neurological deficit caused by cerebrovascular disease which lasts more than 24 hours or causes death. If the focal neurological deficit lasts less than 24 hours, the diagnosis is a transient ischaemic attack (TIA)

Strokes cause cerebral infarction either by thromoembolic disorders (85%) or by haemorrhage (10% intracerebral haemorrhage (see p. 176) and 5% subarachnoid haemorrhage (see p. 178); subarachnoid and intra-cerebral haemorrhages may also be caused by trauma/head injury (see p. 182)).

## Causes

The incidence of stroke increases with age
- Previous TIA
- Hypertension
- Smoking
- Heart disease or vascular disease
- Atrial fibrillation
- Diabetes and/or hyperlipidaemia
- Procoagulant disorders such as vasculitis (especially in younger patients)

## Presentation and assessment

Strokes are atraumatic, but *may result in associated trauma* (e.g. by causing falls). They result in rapid focal or global neurological deterioration. Other signs and symptoms may include
- Airway: grunting, snoring, or complete obstruction
- Respiratory: Cheyne–Stokes breathing, tachypnoea, bradypnoea (hypoventilation is a late sign)
  - Neurogenic pulmonary oedema may sometimes occur
- Cardiovascular changes: tachycardia and/or hypertension (hypertension associated with bradycardia is a late or pre-terminal sign)
  - ECG changes: ischaemic changes can occur in association with stroke (especially subarachnoid or intracerebral bleeding); AF is associated with thromboembolic events
- Renal: incontinence
- Neurological: agitation, diminished consciousness, or loss of consciousness
- Common presentations: a commonly used system combining anatomical and clinical systems for classifying strokes is the Oxford acute stroke classification system (see opposite page)
- Atypical presentations: seizures, falls, or personality change

## Investigations

- ABGs
- FBC, coagulation screen
- U&Es, LFTs, serum calcium

---

* The term cerebrovascular accident (CVA) is commonly used in place of stroke; less commonly 'brain attack' is also used

- Serum glucose and lipids
- ECG
- Head CT scan to clarify diagnosis and extent of cerebral damage, to differentiate infarct from haemorrhage, and to exclude hydrocephalus
- Carotid Doppler studies to define if carotid stenosis is >70%
- Echocardiogram (the source of any emboli may be cardiac)
- Consider CRP, ESR, auto-antibodies, thrombophilia screen, plasma electrophoresis, syphilis screen, and blood cultures

**Differential diagnoses**

- Migraine
- Hypoglycaemia
- Partial epileptic seizures, or following siezures (post-ictal states)
- Space-occupying lesions (e.g. tumour, abscess or subdural haematoma)
- Demyelinating disease
- Cerebral venous thrombosis

---

**The Oxford acute stroke classification system**

- TACS[*] (total anterior circulation syndrome): 15% of strokes, mortality ~60%, *all* of
  - Hemiparesis with/without hemisensory loss
  - Homonymous hemianopia
  - Higher cerebral dysfunction (e.g. dysphasia, visuospatial dysfunction, neglect)
- PACS[*] (partial anterior circulation syndrome): 30% of strokes, mortality ~16%, one of
  - Any *two* TACS features (see above)
  - Higher cerebral dysfunction
  - Isolated motor and/or sensory deficit in one limb or the face
- LACS[*] (lacunar syndrome): 20% of strokes, mortality ~11%, any of
  - Pure motor or sensory stroke (involving two of face, arm, or leg)
  - Ataxic hemiparesis
  - Dysarthria or clumsy hand syndrome
- POCS[*] (posterior circulation syndrome): 20% of strokes, mortality ~ 19%, any of
  - Bilateral motor sensory and sensory signs
  - Cerebellar signs, unless accompanied by ipsilateral motor deficit
  - Disorder of conjugate eye movement
  - Ipsilateral cranial nerve palsy with contralateral motor and/or sensory deficit
  - Isolated homonymous visual field deficit

[*] The final letter may be changed to denote the type of stroke: S for syndrome, I for infarct, H for haemorrhage (i.e. TACS, TACI, or TACH)

---

**Immediate and further management**

Immediate and further management of thromboembolic and haemorrhagic stroke, and subarachnoid haenmorrhage, is described on the following pages.

# ① **Thromboembolic stroke**

## Causes

- Thrombosis
  - Rupture of atherosclerotic lesions (risk factors for atherosclerosis include age, male sex, family history, smoking, diabetes, hypertension, and hyperlipidaemia)
  - Vasculitis
  - Cerebral venous thrombosis: caused by hypercoagulable states such as dehydration, polycythaemia, thrombocythaemia, OCP, protein S/C deficiency, factor V Leiden deficiency
- Embolic
  - Platelet aggregates from ruptured atherosclerotic plaques (see above)
  - Infective endocarditis
  - Left atrial thrombus secondary to atrial fibrillation
  - Left ventricular thrombus secondary to poor function or myocardial infarction
  - Paradoxical emboli: venous emboli entering the arterial circulation via patent foramen ovale, ASD, or VSD
  - Prosthetic heart valves
  - Indwelling lines/prosthesis
  - Infective endocarditis
  - Post carotid or cardiac surgery
  - Complication of endovascular coiling of SAH (see p. 178)
- Other
  - Vertebral or carotid dissection (spontaneous or post-traumatic)
  - Vessel occlusion by tumour/abscess
  - Carotid occlusion (post strangulation)
  - Systemic hypotension (e.g. post cardiac arrest)

## Presentation and assessment

Thrombotic stroke often presents with evolving neurology, whilst embolic stroke presents with sudden-onset rapidly developing neurology. For general signs and symptoms, (see p. 170).

Exact presentation varies according to site and extent of lesion. A commonly used system combining anatomical and clinical systems for classifying strokes is the Oxford acute stroke classification system (see p. 171).

## Immediate management

- Give 100% $O_2$ initially, and then titrate to achieve $SpO_2$ >97%
- Airway may be compromised because of impaired conscious level: place patient in recovery position or intubate trachea as appropriate
  - Few stroke patients require invasive ventilatory support but some may if gag reflex is absent, the GCS is <8 and the diagnosis is not convincing before further investigation is undertaken.
- Ensure breathing/ventilation is adequate
- Assess circulation and obtain IV access
  - Commence fluid resuscitation where hypotension is present

- Assess and monitor consciousness level
- Perform a rapid detailed neurological assessment (with fundoscopy)
- Organize an urgent head CT scan if
  - The diagnosis is uncertain or there is evidence of trauma
  - The patient is anti-coagulated or has a known bleeding tendency
  - The patient had a severe headache at the onset of neurology
  - There is rapidly progressive, inconsistent, poorly localized, or fluctuating neurology, or brainstem symptoms
  - The patient has a decreased level of consciousness
  - Papilloedema, fever, or meningism are present
  - Thrombolysis, or early anti-coagulation is being considered
- Aspirin 300 mg (oral or, if dysphagic, rectally or via NGT) should be given once a diagnosis of haemorrhage has been excluded, unless thrombolysis is used when it should be withheld for 24 hours
- Thrombolysis with t-PA may be possible in some centres in confirmed ischaemic strokes with measurable neurological deficit <3 hours old; a head CT scan is required first (see stroke thrombolysis exclusion criteria (p. 175))
- Neurosurgical intervention may be considered in those with cerebellar infarction or a large infarcted area of the middle cerebral artery territory

**Further management**
- Brain imaging should be undertaken within 24 hours where possible
- Ensure adequate hydration and nutrition: often NGT feeding is required until a swallowing assessment can be performed
- Aspirin (50–300 mg) should be continued until an alternative anti-platelet therapy is started
- Anti-coagulation is controversial: heart lesions are the only definite indication for full anti-coagulation
- Lowering blood pressure may extend the infarct, but high blood pressure may increase the risk of haemorrhage: treat if BP is ≥220/110 mmHg (aim to reduce BP slowly; use short-acting agents if required)
- Ensure adequate analgesia and DVT prophylaxis
- Maintaining glycaemic control within the normal range is associated with better outcomes
- Investigate and treat fever aggressively; aspiration is a common cause of infection
- Consider NG feeding
- Aggressive physiotherapy and transfer to a specialist stroke unit are associated with better outcomes
- Consider initiating treatment aimed at modifying cardiovascular risk factors

## Pitfalls/difficult situations

- Strokes in young patients should always raise the suspicion of 'atypical' causes, e.g. procoagulant disorders such as vasculitis
- Up to 5% of patients presenting with stroke have underlying space-occupying lesions (e.g. tumour, abscess, or subdural haematoma)
- Where there is any history of scalp tenderness always consider temporal arteritis and measure ESR
- Careful blood pressure monitoring is important following carotid endarterectomy as strokes associated with hyper/hypotension are common
- Haemorrhagic transformation of ischaemic strokes may occur (with or without thrombolysis)
- Strokes after cardiac surgery or cardiac bypass present diagnostic and therapeutic challenges, especially as these patients are often extensively anti-coagulated

## Further reading

American Heart Association (2005). Adult stroke. *Circulation* **112**, 111–20.
📖 OHCC p. 380, OHEA p. 312.

**Stroke thrombolysis: contraindications**

- Under 18 years old
- Minor or improving symptoms
- Strong suspicion of haemorrhage (even if CT normal), or history of previous intracranial haemorrhage, AVM, or aneurysm
- CT confirmation of haemorrhage, or multilobar infarction (>1/3 of cerebral hemisphere)
- Seizure associated with stroke onset
- Acute pancreatitis
- Pregnancy
- Head trauma, stroke, or neurosurgery in past 3 months
- Active or recent bleeding, or major surgery/trauma in past 14 days
- Recent LP
- Recent non-compressible arterial puncture
- GI bleed or haematuria in past 21 days
- Hypoglycaemia (<3 mmol/L) or hyperglycaemia (>20 mmol/L)
- Systolic BP >185 mmHg or diastolic BP >110 mmHg
- Recent pericarditis following MI
- Anti-coagulation with raised APTT or INR (>1.7)
- Platelet count <100 x $10^9$/L

# ① Intracerebral haemorrhage

Spontaneous intracerebral haemorrhage (SICH) is bleeding into the parenchyma of the brain (bleeding can also extend into the subarachnoid space). Intracerebral haemorrhage may be either supratentorial or infratentorial. The associated mortality is higher than that of either thromboembolic stroke or subarachnoid haemorrhage.

## Causes

*Primary intracerebral haemorrhage (PICH)*
- Chronic hypertension (commonest overall cause)
- Amyloid angiopathy

*Secondary intracerebral haemorrhage*
- Acute hypertension
  - Eclampsia/pre-eclampsia (see p. 416)
  - Drugs: sympathomimetics and recreational drugs such as cocaine
- Coagulopathies, especially following thrombolysis
- Following neurosurgery
- Aneurysms and arteriovenous malformations
- Tumours
- Complicating CNS infections or venous sinus thrombosis
- Haemorrhagic transformation of thromboembolic stroke

## Presentation and assessment

The presentation of intracerebral haemorrhage overlaps with that of stroke (see p. 170)
- Supratentorial haemorrhages cause sensory/motor deficits, aphasia, neglect, gaze deviation, and hemianopia
- Infratentorial haemorrhages cause brainstem dysfunction, cranial nerve defects, ataxia, and nystagmus
- The following are also more common
  - Headache, nausea and vomiting
  - Elevated blood pressure (up to 90% of patients)
  - Seizures (up to 10% of patients)
  - Signs and symptoms of hydrocephalus/raised ICP (see p. 190)

## Investigations (see also p. 170)
- Coagulation studies
- β-HCG (to exclude pregnancy) and serum urate (if pre-eclampsia is suspected)
- Urine toxicology
- Angiography or MRI (especially if no pre-existing hypertension, young patients, or atypical appearance, i.e. tumour or aneurysm, is suspected)

## Immediate management

- Give 100% $O_2$ initially; then titrate to achieve $SpO_2$ >97%
- Airway may be compromised because of impaired conscious level – place patient in recovery position or intubate trachea as appropriate

- Ensure breathing/ventilation is adequate
  - Avoid hypercapnia
  - Avoid hyperventilation and hypocapnia unless required for short periods to treat raised ICP
  - Treat pulmonary oedema appropriately (see p. 86)
- Assess circulation and obtain IV access
  - If there is evidence of hypotension, commence fluid resuscitation
  - Treat severe hypertension only (BP ≥220/110 mmHg), but aim to reduce BP slowly
- Assess and monitor consciousness level
- Perform a rapid detailed neurological assessment with fundoscopy
- Treat seizures as per protocol (see p. 166)
- Consider mannitol 0.5–1 g/kg (~200–400 ml 20% solution) if intracranial mass effect is likely
- Organize urgent head CT scan if haemorrhagic stroke is suspected
- Check for coagulopathies and reverse if possible (specific therapies such as recombinant factor VIIa may be considered)
- Neurosurgical evacuation is more likely to be indicated where
  - A cerebellar clot is present and is >3 cm or has occluded the fourth ventricle
  - A supratentorial haemorrhage of volume 20–80 ml causes an intermediate level of neurological dysfunction (GCS >4 and <13) with midline shift and/or raised ICP, especially if it involves the non-dominant hemisphere
- ICP monitoring may be commenced
- Neurosurgery is unlikely to benefit those patients who have
  - GCS <5
  - Significant comorbidity or are elderly
  - Brainstem haemorrhage
  - Small haemorrhages and are relatively neurologically intact (GCS >12)

## Further management
- Follow the principles outlined for further management of general stroke (see p. 173)
- Avoid hypotonic fluids if possible
- Administer prophylactic anti-epileptic medication if indicated
- Use DVT stockings in preference to heparins in the acute phase
- Maintain CPP >70 mmHg where possible, if appropriate
- Manage intracranial hypertension as appropriate (see p. 190)

## Pitfalls/difficult situations (see p. 174)

## Further reading
Fewel ME, Thompson GB, Hoff JT (2003). Spontaneous intracerebral hemorrhage: a review. *Neurosurg Focus* **15**, E1.

Siddique MS, Mendelow AD (2000). Surgical treatment of intracerebral haemorrhage. *Br Med Bull* **56**, 444–56.

📖 OHCC p. 376.

# :⚙: Subarachnoid haemorrhage

Subarachnoid haemorrhage (SAH) is bleeding into the subarachnoid space and not into the brain parenchyma itself.

## Causes

Risk factors for spontaneous (non-traumatic) SAH include
- Hypertension ( and malignant hypertension)
- Diabetes
- Smoking
- Hyperlipidaemia
- Drug abuse, particularly cocaine and sildenafil (Viagra)
- Family history (up to 20%)
- Females > males, Blacks/Afro-Carribean > Whites/Caucasian
- Associated with Marfan's syndrome, Ehlers–Danlos syndrome, Klinefelter's syndrome
- Associated with polycystic kidney disease and coarctation of the aorta

Saccular (berry) aneurysms account for ~85%(these often occur at the junction of cerebral vessels—the larger the aneurysm, the higher the risk of rupture). Other causes include
- Non-aneurysmal perimesencephalic haemorrhage
- Arterial dissection
- Cerebral or dural arteriovenous malformations
- Mycotic aneurysms
- Vascular lesions of the spinal cord

## Presentation and assessment
- Airway: grunting, snoring, or complete obstruction
- Respiratory: Cheyne–Stokes breathing, tachypnoea, bradypnoea (hypoventilation is a late sign)
  - Neurogenic pulmonary oedema may sometimes occur
- Cardiovascular changes: tachycardia and/or hypertension (hypertension associated with bradycardia is a late or pre-terminal sign)
  - ECG changes: ischaemic changes can occur
- Renal: incontinence

*Neurological signs and symptoms may include*
- Headache (SAH accounts for ~3% of headaches presenting to A&E):
  - Classically a sudden-onset (peaks within minutes) worst-ever 'thunderclap' headache
  - Often occipital, as if the patient has been hit from behind
  - Any severe headache may be suspicious, particularly in patients who do not usually suffer headaches
  - Some patients also describe minor headaches a few days before
- Meningism: nausea and vomiting, photophobia, neck stiffness
- Diminished consciousness, or loss of consciousness
- Seizures
- Focal neurological signs
- Signs of raised ICP may be present (see p. 190)

**World Federation of Neurological Surgeons (WFNS) grading of subarachnoid haemorrhage**

| | | |
|---|---|---|
| I | GCS 15 | Conscious with/without meningism<br>No motor deficit |
| II | GCS 14–13 | Drowsy with no significant neurological deficit<br>No motor deficit |
| III | GCS 14–13 | Drowsy with neurological deficit<br>Motor deficit present or absent |
| IV | GCS 12–7 | Deteriorating patient<br>Major neurological deficit<br>Motor deficit present or absent |
| V | GCS 3–6 | Moribund patient with extensor rigidity<br>Failing vital centres<br>Motor deficit present or absent |

The grade, extent of haemorrhage on CT scan, and patient age, can be used to estimate prognosis The higher the grade, age, and extent of haemorrhage, the worse the prognosis.

Investigations
- ABGs to exclude hypoxia and hypercarbia
- FBC, coagulation studies
- U&Es (salt wasting can be present)
- Serum glucose, serum magnesium (hypomagnesaemia is common)
- LFTs
- ECG (arrhythmias, ischaemia, and infarcts are common)
- CXR may identify pulmonary oedema
- Initial CT scanning to clarify diagnosis, extent of cerebral damage, differentiate infarct from haemorrhage, and exclude hydrocephalus.
- LP, if CT head scan is negative
  - Sequential collection of CSF with RBC count shows no reduction in RBC in any of the 3–4 bottles collected (not always reliable)
  - Xanthochromia may be present (need to wait at least 6–12 hours after episode for blood to lyse in CSF)
  - Opening pressure protein and glucose should also be measured
  - CSF should be examined to exclude meningitis (see p. 208)
- Unenhanced CT scan of brain (within 24 hours): this confirms the diagnosis and can localize the bleeding site

Differential diagnoses
- Meningitis, encephalitis (the major differential diagnosis)
- Migraine, cluster, and thunderclap headaches
- Post dural puncture headache
- Acute hydrocephalus
- Subdural and extradural haemorrhage
- Stroke
- Temporal arteritis

## Immediate management

- Give 100% $O_2$ initially and then titrate to achieve $SpO_2$ >97%
- Airway may be compromised because of impaired conscious level: place patient in recovery position or intubate trachea as appropriate
- Ensure that breathing/ventilation is adequate
  - Avoid hypercapnia
  - Avoid hyperventilation and hypocapnia unless required for short periods to treat raised ICP
  - If acute pulmonary oedema is present, treat with appropriate therapies (see p. 84)
- Assess circulation and obtain IV access
  - If there is evidence of hypotension, commence fluid resuscitation; avoid hypotonic solutions where possible
  - Treat severe hypertension only (BP ≥220/110 mmHg), but aim to reduce BP slowly (use β-blockers or calcium antagonists to avoid effects on cerebral vessel caliber)
- Assess and monitor consciousness level
- Perform rapid detailed neurological assessment with fundoscopy
- Treat seizures as per protocol (see p. 166)
  - Consider prophylactic anticonvulsants
  - Consider CFAM if sedated and ventilated
- Check for and treat raised ICP (see p. 190)
- Ensure adequate pain relief and anti-emesis (provide laxative cover)

## Further management

- Continue regular monitoring for any change in neurological status; any deterioration may warrant a repeat CT scan
- Nurse in quiet darkened environment
- Refer early to a neurological/neurosurgical centre
  - Information should include time from onset of headache, age, comorbidities, GCS, and neurological deficit
  - Transfer to a neurosurgical centre is recommended for effective management and improved outcome
  - Surgical or radiological management may be possible; the aneurysm may be clipped or 'coiled'

*Treatment of neurosurgical complications*

- Re-bleeding: there is a 4% risk of re-bleeding in the first 24 hours and a 1.5% risk every day for the next 4 weeks; each re-bleed may require intubation and ventilation and carries a 60% risk of death
- Seizures: treat aggressively; consider phenytoin 15 mg/kg IV with cardiovascular monitoring
- Where a parenchymal haematoma causes a mass effect surgical evacuation may be required
- Acute hydrocephalus may develop in <24 hours. Signs may include 1 point drop in GCS, sluggish pupils, and bilaterally downward deviating eyes. If hydrocephalus is suspected a CT scan should be done (an extraventricular drain may be inserted, although this may provoke more bleeding)

- Cerebral vasospasm may occur in up to 70% of cases, most commonly between days 4 and 14 post-bleed (not all have symptoms); cerebral ischaemia can cause delayed neurological deficit (diffuse or focal)
  - Oral nimodipine 60 mg 4-hourly used for 21 days has been shown to reduce ischaemic stroke (IV nimodipine may be used instead, but with care to avoid hypotension)
  - If new focal or diffuse neurology is present, and another neuro-logical cause or metabolic disturbance has been excluded, then consider 'triple H' therapy (**h**aemodilution, **h**ypervolaemia and **h**ypertension), and aggressive fluid filling and inotropes/vasopressors to maintain an adequate CPP
  - If neurological symptoms do not resolve consider transluminal angioplasty
- Cerebral salt wasting (may need magnesium or sodium replacement)

*Treatment of medical complications*
40% of patients have medical complications, accounting for 23% of deaths
- LV impairment/cardiogenic shock, arrhythmias, neurogenic pulmonary oedema may occur; treatment of pulmonary oedema with PEEP or vasodilators must be balanced against their detrimental effect on CPP
- Pneumonia and ARDS may occur. A lung protective ventilation strategy is required (see p. 50): chest physiotherapy, careful tracheal toilet, and aggressive treatment of chest infections are advised
- Renal dysfunction and electrolyte imbalance: careful attention to fluid balance is required; the avoidance of hypotonic solutions where possible means that careful monitoring of U&Es is required
- Gut dysfunction: provide early enteral/NG feeding well as stress ulcer prophylaxis
- DVT/PE: DVT prevention with compression stockings or boots is recommended
- Avoid pyrexia (use anti-pyretics if required)
- Avoid hyper/hypoglycaemia

**Pitfalls/difficult situations**
- Diagnosis may often be difficult as less than 50% of patients have the classic headache
- A traumatic SAH may be difficult to differentiate from spontaneous SAH which then causes a fall; assume that other injuries may be present, including cervical spine injuries
- Changes in neurological status may require frequent head CT scans, but maintaining optimal conditions for cerebral protection during transfer to scan may be difficult
- Lumbar puncture is still indicated if the CT scan is negative and SAH is likely (2% of patients with an SAH and a positive history will have a negative CT), or another diagnosis (e.g. meningoencephalitis) is likely

**Further reading**
Al-Shahi R, et al. (2006). Subarachnoid haemorrhage. *BMJ* **333**, 235–40.
Suarez JI, et al. (2006). Aneurysmal subarachnoid haemorrhage. *New Engl J Med* **354**, 387–96.
&#x1F4D6; OHCC p. 378.

# ⊕ Head injury

The vast majority of head injuries are classed as mild. Moderate to severe head injuries involve an element of traumatic brain injury. Head injuries can be classified according to any decrease in consciousness
- GCS 14–15 – mild
- GCS 9–13 – moderate
- GCS 3–8 – severe

The management of traumatic brain injury aims to prevent further neurological damage (secondary brain injury) by
- Rapid removal of intra-cranial haematomas
- Avoidance of hypoxia and hypotension
- Normalization of other physiological parameters
- Minimization of cerebral oedema

Types of cerebral damage associated with head injuries include
- Subdural and extradural haematomas
- Traumatic subarachnoid or intracerebral haemorrhage
- Cerebral contusion

## Causes

A significant head injury should be suspected in cases of
- High-velocity impact (including falls from height)
- Direct head trauma
- Penetrating head trauma
- Other major trauma, especially spinal or chest
- Minor head trauma in an anti-coagulated patient

Head injuries are associated with
- Alcohol and drug use
- Assaults
- Elderly patients

## Presentation and assessment

Identifying the mechanism of injury will help identify high-velocity/high-risk cases, such as
- Pedestrian versus car; car versus car; motor bicycle accident (MBA)
- Ejection from car; turned over car
- Fall >1 m (or five stairs); fall from a horse

Other evidence of a severe head injury includes
- Skull fracture or base-of-skull (BOS) fracture (see p. 183)
- Penetrating head or eye injury
- Sezure following injury
- Diminished consciousness, or loss of consciousness
  - Loss of concsiousness may be delayed when trauma leads to a progressive bleed (especially extradural haemorrhage): the 'transient lucid period'
- Headache
- Amnesia
- Vomiting

- Focal neurology (e.g. problems understanding speech, speaking, reading, or writing, loss of sensation, loss of balance, weakness, problems walking, visual changes, abnormal reflexes)

*General signs and symptoms*
- Airway: grunting, snoring, or complete obstruction
- Respiratory: Cheyne–Stokes breathing, tachypnoea, bradypnoea (hypoventilation is a late sign)
  - Neurogenic pulmonary oedema may sometimes occur
- Cardiovascular changes will depend on the degree of associated trauma and haemorrhage
  - Tachycardia and/or hypotension are likely
  - Hypertension associated with bradycardia is a late or pre-terminal sign
  - ECG changes associated with ischaemia (or myocardial contusion)
- Renal: incontinence
- Trauma injuries, especially
  - Spine and cervical spine fractures
  - Long bone fractures

---

**Signs of base-of-skull fracture**

- CSF rhinorrhoea
- CSF otorrhoea
- 'Raccoon' eyes (bilateral peri-orbital haematoma)
- Mastoid bruising or tenderness (Battle's sign)
- Tympanic blood (on examination with an otoscope)
- Epistaxis
- New unilateral deafness

---

**Investigations**
- ABGs
- Cross-match blood
- FBC, coagulation studies
- Serum glucose
- Serum osmolality (>320 mmol/L is a relative contraindication to mannitol)
- U&Es
- LFTs
- Consider blood alcohol levels and other drug levels where appropriate (e.g. paracetamol and salicylate)
- ECG
- Trauma X-rays (C-spine, CXR, pelvis)
- CT scan (see Indications, p. 162)

**Differential diagnoses**
- Stroke
- Meningitis, encephalitis
- Subarachnoid haemorrhage
- Intoxication (alcohol or drugs), overdose

## Immediate management

- Give 100% $O_2$ and support airway, breathing and circulation as required (see below)
- Use spinal precautions including hard collar, sandbags, and strapping (and in-line manual stabilization for intubation)
- Obtain a contemporaneous history if possible (e.g. from relatives or ambulance crew); an 'AMPLE' history (see p. 2) should be obtained as a minimum
- Roughly assess neurological state (e.g. conscious and talking, or unconscious) and simultaneously treat neurological complications which may interfere with ABC (e.g. seizures)
- Complete basic ABC primary survey before formally assessing neurological state

### Airway

- Airway may be compromised because of impaired conscious level; intubate the trachea as appropriate (placement of the patient in the recovery position is likely to be contraindicated by the need for spinal precautions)
- If endotracheal intubation is needed a rapid-sequence intubation will be required to minimize the risk of aspiration; the hard collar will need to be undone and manual in-line stabilization used in its place
- Rapid-sequence endotracheal intubation should be considered if
  - GCS ≤8 (severe head injury), or rapidly deteriorating
  - There is risk of aspiration of vomit or blood
  - There is facial or neck trauma putting the airway at risk
  - There is evidence of hypoxia ($PaO_2$ <9 kPa on air, <13 kPa on oxygen), hypercarbia ($PaCO_2$ >6 kPa) or marked tachypnoea
  - Short-term deliberate hyperventilation is required
  - There is ongoing seizure activity
  - The patient is unlikely to remain still for investigations (e.g. CT)
  - The patient is agitated and combative but requiring treatment
- Endotracheal intubation may also be required to manage thoracic trauma resulting in respiratory compromise (see pp. 78–82 and 401–2)
- Any stress response to endotracheal intubation should be avoided if possible; IV induction and sedation will help avoid rises in ICP
  - Muscle relaxants may be required for stabilization or transfer, but may mask seizures

### Breathing

- Ensure breathing/ventilation is adequate
  - Ventilatory support may be needed to optimize oxygenation; avoid hypoxia aiming for $PaO_2$ >13 kPa
  - Avoid hypercapnia
  - Avoid hyperventilation and hypocapnia unless required for short periods to treat raised ICP
  - If acute pulmonary oedema is present, treat with appropriate therapies (see p. 86)
- Exclude/treat pneumothorax or haemothorax

*Circulation*
- Establish IV access
- Avoid hypotension; where possible aim for a blood pressure which would be near normal for the patient (or MAP >90 mmHg)
- Resuscitate with fluids and blood as required, avoiding hypotonic fluids; inotropes may be required

*Neurology*
Further useful history may include
- History of significant period of amnesia or loss of consciousness
- Mechanism of injury in trauma cases

Formally assess neurological status, including
- Glasgow coma score (see p. 159)
- Eye examination including pupil size and reactivity and fundoscopy if possible
- Evidence of vault or base-of-skull fracture (otoscopy is required)
- Plantar reflexes
- Reassess GCS once airway, breathing, and circulation have been stabilized, and continue regular reassessment of consciousness and neurological state

*Other*
- Exclude and treat hypoglycaemia
- Urgent CT scan may be required for diagnosis and appropriate management (prevent hypoxia, hypercapnia, hypotension, and hypertension throughout)
  - Patients should be stabilized for transfer prior to CT scan
- Raised ICP may be treated with with mannitol (0.5–1 g/kg IV) or hypertonic saline until more definitive measures are employed (see p. 190)
- Treat seizures as per protocol (see p. 166)
- Aggressively correct any coagulopathy
- Check electrolytes
- Other causes of decreased consciousness, including respiratory or cardiovascular compromise (e.g. intra-abdominal bleeding), should be dealt with

*Isolated head injury*
- Patients with moderate to severe head injuries require CT scans and admission for observation
- Some patients with mild head injuries might also require CT scans (see indications for CT, p. 162), or admission (see p. 188)

In all cases neurosurgical advice should be sought where appropriate (see indications for neurosurgical referral, p. 164)
- Subdural and extradural haematomas should be surgically evacuated
- Head injuries may require active ICP monitoring via an intracranial pressure transducer (a 'bolt')
- A jugular venous probe may be required to measure jugular venous bulb $O_2$ saturations ($SjO_2$)

## Further management

### Ventilation

- Hypoxia should be avoided; ideally, $PaO_2$ >13 kPa and $PaCO_2$ 4.0–4.5 kPa should be achieved
- Pulmonary oedema may require the addition of PEEP (although caution may be required as high levels of PEEP may increase ICP)
  - High intrathoracic pressure should be avoided where possible
- Aspiration events and chest infections are common in patients with decreased consciousness and should be actively investigated/treated
- Head-up positioning may decrease aspiration events and improve cerebral venous drainage

### Cardiovascular

- Hypotension should be avoided
  - An initial MAP >90mmHg should ensure an acceptable CPP
  - Later MAP may be guided by ICP or other measurements
- Fluid resuscitation (avoiding hypotonic fluids where possible) may be sufficient, although inotropes may be needed

### Neurological

- Sedatives with rapid offset such as propofol may initially be advisable as they will allow level of consciousness to be easily reassessed
- Heavy sedation may be required to avoid coughing and gagging on the endotracheal tube (which might otherwise raise ICP)
- Avoid drugs known to cause ICP to rise (e.g. ketamine)
- Muscle relaxants may be required for the initial intubation, stabilization, or transfer, but may mask fitting
  - Where muscle relaxants are used consider concurrent anti-convulsive sedative infusions (such as propofol or midazolam)
- A 30°–45° head-up tilt will aid cerebral venous drainage (where spinal precautions are in place the whole bed may be tilted)
- Where ICP is measured it should be kept ≤20 mmHg (see p. 190)
- Cerebral perfusion pressure (CPP) should be maintained at ≥60 mmHg (CPP = MAP – ICP)
- When measured, aim for jugular venous bulb $O_2$ saturations of 55–75%
  - If $SjO_2$ falls consider treatments for raised ICP (see p. 190)
  - If $SjO_2$ rises consider treatments for hyperperfusion or hyperaemia
- Consider transcranial Doppler (TCD) monitoring for vasospasm
- Consider seizure prophylaxis using phenytoin 300 mg daily IV/NG
- Further head CTs may be indicated if there is any change in GCS, pupils, or neurological signs
- Polyurea may indicate hypothalamic injury causing diabetes insipidus or use of osmotic diuretics

*Trauma*
- A tertiary survey to look for occult traumatic injuries should be done on all head-injured patients with diminished GCS once they are stable
- Spinal precautions (hard collar, sandbags, strapping, supine positioning, and log-rolls) should be in place for all intubated head-injury patients in the initial stages
  - The spine should be cleared as soon as possible according to the Intensive Care Society guidelines to allow better patient management, particularly removal of the hard collar which is likely to impair venous drainage of the head
- Where there is abdominal trauma, intra-abdominal pressures (IAP) should be measured and high pressures avoided in order to avoid rises in CVP and ICP

*General*
- Normoglycaemia should be maintained
- Pyrexia should be avoided; antipyretics may be necessary
- Hypo- and hypernatraemia should be corrected (see pp. 216 and 218)
- Compression stockings should be the first-line DVT prophylaxis where there is a risk of bleeding
- Feeding (via NG if possible) should be instituted in intubated patients as soon as appropriate
- Infections, particularly chest infections, are common following head injuries and should be treated aggressively

## Pitfalls/difficult situations
- There may be a lucid interval between the initial head injury and the development of an intracranial haematoma; close monitoring is advisable for 4–6 hours following serious injuries
- In some cases general surgical interventions (e.g. for major internal haemorrhage) may take precedence over investigating or treating neurological problems

## Further reading

Girling K (2004). Management of head injury in the intensive-care unit. *Contin Educ Anaesth Crit Care Pain* **4**, 52–6.

Morris C, Guha A, Farquhar I (2005). *Evaluation for Spinal Injuries among Unconscious Victims of Blunt Polytrauma: A Management Guideline for Intensive Care.* Intensive Care Society, London.

OHEA p. 176.

**Indications for admission for observation**

- Any head injury requiring CT (see p. 162)
- Moderate to severe headache
- Persistent vomiting
- History of loss of consciousness or amnesia
- Head trauma associated with coagulopathy (e.g. patient on warfarin)
- Alcohol/drug intoxication
- Suspicion of non-accidental injury—patient is likely to remain at risk if discharged
- No companion at home

**Indications for considering ICP measurement**

- Severe head injury (GCS <9 after resuscitation) and an abnormal CT scan (haematomas, contusions, oedema, or compressed basal cisterns)
- Severe head injury (GCS <9 after resuscitation) and a normal CT scan, but two of the following
  - Age >40 years
  - Systolic blood pressure <90 mmHg
  - Decerebrate posturing
- May be considered for moderate or mild head injuries (GCS >8) where sedation or anaesthesia are required for other indications

ICP measurement should be continued until ICP is normal and treatment is not required for 3 days

**Spinal investigations for unconscious patients on ICU where spinal fractures could not be cleared clinically* prior to endotracheal intubation**

- Lateral and AP cervical radiographs
- Multiplane helical (spiral) CT of the entire cervical spine down to and including the T4/T5 disk space **OR** (if no helical CT available) scanning of the cranio-cervical junction and the cervico-thoracic junction (if not seen on plain radiographs) and any suspicious areas of the C-spine
- Thoracolumbar AP and lateral radiographs (unless spinal reconstructions from helical CT of chest/abdomen are available—if so omit)

If **ALL** of the above are satisfied and there are no external signs of injury, the spine may be regarded as stable and uninjured. Close observation during mobilization is essential, but will be limited in this group of patients

* Criteria for clinically clearing the spine are: (1) GCS score 15 and appropriate responses; (2) absence of intoxicants, alcohol, or sedation/opioid analgesics; (3) no midline spinal tenderness, no deformity or steps, and no neurological deficit referable to a spinal injury (e.g. abnormal tone, power or reflexes); (4) no significant distracting injury (e.g. extremity fracture)

Adapted from Morris C, Guha A, Farquhar I (2005). E *Evaluation for Spinal Injuries among Unconscious Victims of Blunt Polytrauma: A Management Guideline for Intensive Care.* Intensive Care Society, London.

# ☠ Raised intracranial pressure

Intracranial pressure (ICP) is the pressure exerted by the brain parenchyma and its contents inside a rigid skull. Normal ICP is 0–10 mmHg.
Raised intracranial pressure is defined as 20 mmHg for >5 minutes.

## Causes
- Space-occupying lesion, including neoplasm, abscess, or haematomas
- Cerebral oedema
  - *Vasogenic* (increasing capillary permeability): traumatic brain injury,
    infection, hepatic encephalopathy, eclampsia, hypertensive
    encephalopathy, sinus thrombosis, altitude cerebral oedema
  - *Cytotoxic* (cell death): post cardiac arrest, acute hyponataemia
  - *Interstitial* (obstruction): hydrocephalus

Certain patients are at higher risk of developing raised ICP
- Following traumatic brain injuries
- Following neurosurgery (especially where haemostasis is poor)
- Younger patients (compared with older patients)

## Presentation and assessment
Raised ICP may be detected within the ICU as a result of ICP monitoring,
via an intraparenchymal transducer or intraventricular drain, showing
- Increased pressures, or
- Abnormal waveforms (normal ICP waves resemble arterial pressure
  waveforms; waveforms affected by raised ICP often have the highest
  peak *after* the dichrotic notch)

Clinical signs and symptoms of raised ICP may include
- Headache (particularly early mornings) and/or vomiting
- Listlessness, irritability, and/or reduced consciousness
- Eyes: unequal, sluggish, or divergent pupils; papilloedema
- Seizures or focal neurological signs
- Hypertension and/or bradycardia
- Cheyne–Stokes respiration

Other signs and symptoms are those associated with decreased consciousness (see p. 158) and any underlying cause, e.g. head injury (see p. 182),
subarachnoid haemorrhage (see p. 178), stroke (see p. 170).

## Investigations
- ABGs
- FBC, coagulation studies
- U&Es, LFTs, serum osmolality and glucose (DM, HONK)
- Core temperature
- Head CT scan is essential if raised ICP is suspected in an unmonitored
  patient; consider if there is an acute rise in monitored ICP

## Differential diagnoses
- Where no monitoring is present: subarachnoid haemorrhage,
  meningitis/encephalitis, migraine, stroke
- Where ICP monitoring is present: incorrect calibration of probe

### Immediate management

- Give 100% $O_2$; support airway, breathing, and circulation as required
- In suspected raised ICP treat any acute cause according to protocol
- Where ICP is shown to be raised in an already intubated ICU patient
  - Check transducers for errors if ICP is monitored
  - Ensure adequate analgesia and sedation
  - Tilt patient up to 30° head up; ensure neck veins not obstructed
  - Check ABGs (and/or end-tidal $CO_2$ monitoring and $SaO_2$); reduce $PaCO_2$ to 4–4.5 kPa and maintain $PaO_2$ ≥10 kPa
  - Aim for CPP ≥70 mmHg using inotropes (once normovolaemia has been achieved) to ensure a MAP ≥80–90 mmHg
  - Avoid treating hypertension unless it becomes severe (e.g. MAP >130 mmHg); use short-acting antihypertensives (e.g. esmolol)
  - Consider giving mannitol 20% 0.5–1 g/kg over 15 minutes (repeat up to every 4 hours; stop if plasma osmolality ≥310 mOsmol/L)

### Further management

- Consider dexamethasone 10 mg IV, then 4–6 mg/4 hours for tumours
- Ensure patient is pain free and well sedated (Ramsey score of 6); consider neuromuscular blockade to prevent coughing on ETT
- Make sure urinary catheter is patent
- Treat pyrexia with surface cooling and paracetamol (avoid core temperature >37°C if possible)
- Treat seizures aggressively with phenytoin 15 mg/kg IV (these can be difficult to diagnosis if paralysed and EEG monitoring may be helpful)
- If ICP continues to increase consider
  - Another bolus of mannitol or a dose of furosemide 20–40 mg
  - Thiopental 50 mg boluses, or a thiopental infusion
  - Inducing moderate hypothermia (34–35°C)
  - Moderate hyperventilation to $PaCO_2$ <4 kPa should only be used as a temporary measure in extreme intracranial hypertension, ideally with accompanying $SjO_2$ monitoring
- Neurosurgical treatment: may include removal of new haematoma, decompressive craniectomy, CSF drainage, or lobectomy
- Consider $SjO_2$ or TCD monitoring

### Pitfalls/difficult situations

- Ventricular drains can block very easily and pressure transducers can become inaccurate; use only as a guide
- Therapy aimed at reducing ICP can reduce CPP
- Fluid overload from volume resuscitation to maintain MAP can 'leak' across a more permeable BBB and increase cerebral oedema
- Electrolyte abnormalities are common and should be corrected

### Further reading

Mayer S, Chong J (2002). Critical care management of increased intracranial pressure. *J Intensive Care Med* **17**, 55–67.
 OHCC pp. 134, 382, OHEA p. 174.

# ☢ Meningitis and encephalitis

(See also p. 340)

Meningitis is a life-threatening inflammation of the meninges and CSF surrounding the brain and spinal cord. Encephalitis is inflammation of the brain parenchyma. Both carry a significant risk in terms of both mortality and morbidity. Rapid diagnosis and aggressive treatment are essential.

Meningitis is diagnosed following identification of pathogens and white cells in cerebrospinal fluid (CSF) obtained by lumbar puncture.

## Causes

- Risk factors for infectious meningitis include
  - Head injury
  - Ear and/or sinus infection
  - Immunocompromised patients, including those with diabetes, chronic renal failure, or on immunosuppressant drugs (particularly steroids)
- Infectious causes
  - Common bacteria: *Streptococcus pneumoniae* (common, especially in asplenic patients), *Haemophilus influenzae*, *Neisseria meningitides*, *Listeria monocytogenes*
  - Common viruses: herpes simplex virus, Coxsackie virus
  - Nosocomial bacteria: *Escherichia coli*, *Pseudomonas*, *Klebsiella*, *Acinetobacter*
  - In the immunocompromised: TB, fungal infections (e.g. Cryptococcus)
  - Following neurosurgery: *Staphylococcus aureus*, *Staphylococcus epidermidis*

Non-infectious causes include subarachnoid haemorrhage, malignant infiltration (lymphoma/leukaemic involvement), and autoimmune processes.

## Presentation and assessment

A high index of suspicion is the key to quick and effective management.
- Neurological/meningeal signs and symptoms
  - Headache and/or neck stiffness (not always found with encephalitis)
  - Altered mental state or decreased consciousness
  - Photophobia
  - Vomiting
  - Cranial nerve lesions and/or focal neurological signs
  - Seizures
  - Papilloedema*
- Signs of infection
  - Tachycardia
  - Tachpnoea
  - Pyrexia and/or rigors
  - Evidence of severe sepsis: hypotension, cardiovascular collapse, DIC, ARDS
  - Rash
- Airway and cardiorespiratory signs and symptoms associated with decreased consciousness (see p. 158) may also be present

---

* Papilloedema is an unreliable sign which can be difficult to detect and may be absent or present late

Often the classical symptoms and signs are not present, especially in immunosuppressed or elderly patients where behavioural changes and/or low-grade fever may be the only signs.

**Viral meningitis** should be considered in cases of reduced consciousness
- Diagnosis should be suspected on history and CT appearances
- Personality/behavioural changes are associated with HSV infection
- May be associated with a history of exotic travel
- Viral meningitis is often self-limiting
- Rash may be vesicular in nature

**Meningococcal septicaemia** may occur with meningococcal meningitis (~70% of cases) (see p. 350)
- Meningococcus tends to occur in clusters, especially where there is close contact (e.g. new university students, pilgrimages)
- Prodromal symptoms are non-specific and influenza like
- Rash is a characteristic purpuric non-blanching rash, which may initially appear erythematous

**Intracerebral abscess** may be associated with meningitis (see p. 342)

Investigations
- ABGs
- FBC, coagulation screen
- G&S
- U&Es, LFTs, serum osmolality
- Serum glucose
- Serial CT scan may be required according to neurological status
- Blood cultures, LP, throat swabs, and skin scrapings
- Serial blood cultures or microbiological samples may be required
- Blood serology may be indicated for HIV, HSV, or mumps
- Other investigations may be required depending upon severity of complications

Differential diagnoses
Differential diagnoses for meningitis include causes of severe headache and/or decreased consciousness
- Migraine
- Subarachnoid haemorrhage (exclude with CT scan)
- Causes of raised ICP (see p. 190)

Causes of aseptic meningitis (i.e. no organism found in LP samples)
- Viral meningitis (HSV, EBV, varicella-zoster, CMV, geographically limited viruses, e.g. Murray Valley encephalitis)
- Partly treated bacterial meningitis

- Bacterial meningitis due to tuberculosis, syphilis, Lyme disease, rickettsiae
- Fungal meningitis (Candida, Cryptococcus, Histoplasma, Coccidioides)
- Protozoal meningitis (cerebral malaria, Toxoplasma)
- Non-infective meningitis (lymphoma/leukaemia, vasculitis)

## Immediate management

- Give 100% $O_2$ initially, and then titrate to achieve $SpO_2$ >97%
- Airway may be compromised because of impaired conscious level: place patient in recovery position or intubate trachea as appropriate
  - Keep patients nil by mouth initially as they are at risk of requiring intubation and ventilation
- Ensure breathing/ventilation is adequate
- Indications for intubation and ventilation include
  - GCS <10 or airway compromise
  - Respiratory insufficiency ($PaO_2$ <8 kPa or $PaCO_2$ >6.5 kPa)
  - Marked seizure activity
- Assess circulation
  - Obtain IV access
  - Commence fluid resuscitation with inotropic support as required
- Assess and monitor consciousness level
- Perform a rapid detailed neurological assessment
- Treat seizures as per protocol (see p. 166)

**If you suspect bacterial meningitis do not delay treatment.** Antibiotic therapy should be commenced immediately. If meningococcal disease is suspected, benzylpenicillin may have already been given by the GP or the admitting physicians.

*Meningitis treatment:*
- Give third-generation cephalosporin (e.g. ceftriaxone 2 g IV 12-hourly): local guidelines vary according to patterns of resistance*
- Start dexamethasone 10 mg IV 6-hourly for 4 days with first dose of antibiotic
- Perform a CT scan prior to lumbar puncture to exclude raised ICP and other causes of meningitis
- Perform lumbar puncture (see p. 510)
  - Measure opening pressure (often elevated),
  - Take three 0.5 ml CSF samples for urgent Gram stain, microscopy, and culture, PCR and protein
  - Take 0.5 ml in glucose bottle for CSF glucose (and send a corresponding plasma sample)
  - See p. 208 for interpretation of results
- Perform blood cultures (at least two) and throat swab
- If there are vasculitic lesions send scrapings (if skin pustules are present send aspirations) for culture/PCR

* If the patient is known to have severe penicillin allergy consider chloramphenicol 1 g IV 6-hourly

**Further management**

- Admission to a critical care facility may be required for further monitoring of neurological state and treatment of complications including:
  - Seizure activity resistant to anticonvulsants
  - Decreased level of consciousness, especially where airway is at risk
  - Sepsis or SIRS requiring vasopressors or mechanical ventilation (meningococcal meningitis)
- If bacterial meningitis is present discuss with microbiology regarding the need to inform public health and provide prophylaxis for staff, especially if there is close contact with secretions or blood (oral ciprofloxacin 500 mg, single dose)
- Reconsider antibiotic treatment after advice from microbiologist once the Gram stain result is available. Common treatment variations include the following
  - If a Gram-negative bacillus is identified consider adding gentamicin
  - Where Listeria is identified (or the patient is immunosuppressed and at risk) consider switching to amoxicillin and gentamicin
  - Where *Staph. aureus* is present consider switching to flucloxacillin
  - Where viral meningitis is suspected treatment should be targeted at HSV treatment (the most destructive virus); if there is any suspicion start aciclovir 10 mg/kg 8-hourly (over 1 hour via CVP line)
  - Where Cryptococcus or Toxoplasma are identified consider checking HIV status
- Consider re-culturing the CSF if clinical improvement is slow
- If aseptic meningitis is found obtain a travel history to help identify unusual organisms (rickettsiae, viral causes, Histoplasma, Coccidioides, cerebral malaria)
- Treat complications as required
  - Meningococcal septicaemia: shock (likely to require inotropes), coagulopathy, renal failure, ARDS, adrenal insufficiency
  - Raised ICP: treat aggressively with 30° head up, mannitol, and other treatments as required (see p. 190)
  - Seizures: treat aggressively according to protocol (see p. 166); use of muscle relaxants may prevent the identification of fits
  - SIADH or cerebral salt wasting may occur; check fluid balance and electrolytes regularly
  - Infections: concurrent pneumonia is common, requiring aggressive treatment; skin vesicles are likely to become infected
- Other complications include
  - Venous sinus thrombosis
  - Cerebral infarcts
  - Intracranial collections (subdural effusions, intracerebral abscess formation)

### Pitfalls/difficult situations

- Administration of antibiotic therapy prior to admission and lumbar puncture may prevent the identification of a causative organism.
- CSF analysis does not always add clarity to the diagnosis, as a CSF pleocytosis has a number of causes including partially treated bacterial meningitis, TB, Lyme disease, sarcoidosis, and Behçet's syndrome.
- If SAH has been excluded the next most common cause, and the most life threatening, is an infectious cause which should be treated aggressively
- The development of new focal neurology warrants a further CT scan to exclude subdural empyema formation

### Further reading

Van de Beek D (2006). Community acquired bacterial meningitis in adults. *New Engl Med J* **354**, 44–53.

📖 OHCC p. 374.

# ☼ Agitation, confusion, and aggression

Agitation and confusion are commonly found in the critically ill, and may lead to difficulty in treating or investigating the patient's illness, or result in aggression directed towards staff or the patient's relatives.

## Causes

Most critical care agitation or aggression stems from delirium. Causes and risk factors of delirium include:

* **H**ypoxia
* **E**lderly patients
* **A**cidaemia
* **D**rug interactions and/or side effects
* **W**ithdrawal states (especially alcohol)
* **A**nalgesia (either inadequate, or as a drug side effect)
* **T**ired/sleep deprivation
* **C**erebral illnesses (e.g. Alzheimer's disease, post-ictal states, stroke)
* **H**ypotension
* **E**ndocrine or metabolic derangement
* **R**are causes (e.g. heavy metal poisoning)
* **S**epsis/infections

Metabolic abnormalities may include hypo- or hyperglycaemia, uraemia, liver failure (hepatic encephalopathy), hyper- or hyponatraemia, hypercalcaemia

Drugs related to agitation and delirium include alcohol (acute intoxication or acute withdrawal), illicit drugs (e.g. opioids or hallucinogens), benzodiazepines, antidepressants, steroids, dopamine, anticholinergics.

Inadequate analgesia may be caused by urinary retention or constipation.

## Presentation and assessment

Levels of agitation or aggression commonly fluctuate over the course of the day (often worse at night) and may present in a variety of ways.

* Fidgeting and interfering with invasive lines or monitoring
* Shouting or calling out
* Disorientation in time, place, or (less commonly) person
* Paranoia
* Inability to follow complex commands
* Overfocusing on certain subjects (pain may be exaggerated)

Cardiorespiratory signs and symptoms may be present, especially where agitation is associated with physiological compromise (i.e. hypoxia), including hyperventilation, tachycardia, and hypertension

## Investigations

* ABGs
* FBC
* U&Es, LFTs, serum glucose, calcium, magnesium
* Consider CRP and blood alcohol level
* Consider CXR (if chest infection likely)
* Consider head CT if there are associated neurological abnormalities

**Immediate management**

- Give 100% $O_2$ first, and then titrate to achieve $SpO_2$ >97%
- Support airway, breathing, and circulation as required
- Perform a brief neurological assessment
- Diagnose and treat any underlying cause
  - Check $SaO_2$, electrolytes, blood sugar, catheter patency
- Reassure confused patients of their surroundings and who you are
- Avoid confrontation with aggressive patients
- Antipsychotic or sedative medication should only be used if the patient is a risk to themselves or others
  - Haloperidol 1–2 mg IV/IM every 2–4 hours (decrease dose in the elderly; in extreme agitation up to 15 mg may be required)
  - Alternatively olanzapine 2.5–5mg PO/SL/IM once daily may be used (if dementia is present risk of stroke may be increased)
  - Chlorpromazine 12.5 mg IV (slow) may be used as an alternative
  - Monitor airway and ECG if high doses are used
- Avoid benzodiazepines in delirium unless required to treat specific states (e.g. alcohol withdrawal) or for rescue therapy
  - Lorazepam 1–2 mg IV/IM or midazolam 2.5–5 mg IV/IM
  - Where patients refuse treatment make an early assessment of mental capacity. Questions should include
  - Are they oriented in time, place, and person?
  - Are they suffering from any delusions?
  - Do they understand the treatment proposed and the potential consequences of refusal of treatment?

**Further management**

- Attentive medical/nursing care may alleviate the need for medication
  - Avoid too many changes in nursing staff if possible
  - Involve family and relatives where possible; have familiar objects from the patient's home in the room
  - Remind patients of the day, time, location; provide a clock/calendar
  - Create a day–night cycle; minimize excess noise at night
  - Provide patients with their glasses, hearing aid, and dentures
  - Provide an interpreter if required

**Pitfalls/difficult situations**

- In some critical care units physical restraints may be used in place of, or in combination with, chemical treatments. Do not use these unless you are familiar with indications, technique, and complications
- Delirium may present with agitated behaviour or with hypoactive (e.g. withdrawn, quiet, paranoid) behaviour
- Overt aggression or violence from mentally capable patients is unacceptable; consider involving security or police

**Further reading**

Borthwick M, Bourne R, Craig M, *et al.* (2006). *Detection, Prevention and Treatment of Delirium in Critically Ill Patients* (UK Clinical Pharmacy Association, South Wigston, Leics).
📖 OHCC p. 370, OHEA p. 308.

# :◯: **Alcohol withdrawal**

Withdrawal from alcohol (or other drugs) is common in the hospital setting, and often goes unnoticed in the early stages. Responses can range from cravings with mild physical symptoms to overt psychosis and life-threatening autonomic dysfunction.

## Causes

Patients may suffer from alcohol withdrawal if they have previously had a high alcohol intake and have
- Voluntarily stopped or reduced their alcohol intake
- Become incapacitated or otherwise unable to ingest alcohol

Identifying patients with a history of high alcohol intake will allow the use of anti-withdrawal prophylaxis.

## Presentation and assessment

Symptoms commonly occur 24–72 hours after cessation of alcohol and last for 5–7 days. Peak intensity occurs 24 hours after onset.

Signs and symptoms may include
- Anxiety, agitation, insomnia, anorexia
- Confusions, disorientation, hallucinations, delusions
- Gross tremor
- Seizures occur in 2% of withdrawing patients and are more likely if
  - There is a past history of epilepsy
  - Hypoglycaemia, hypomagnesaemia, or hypokalaemia are present
- Autonomic disturbance
  - Sweating and flushing
  - Fever
  - Tachycardia and hypertension
  - Mydriasis

Moderate to severe withdrawal (delirium tremens (DTs)) is associated with increasing degree of confusion, hallucinations, and autonomic disturbance.

## Investigations
- FBC, coagulation studies
- U&Es, LFTs
- Serum glucose, magnesium, and calcium
- Consider sepsis screen (blood, urine, and sputum samples)
- Consider CRP
- ECG
- Consider head CT scan and LP (if meningitis likely)

## Differential diagnoses
- Meningitis/encephalitis
- Hypoglycaemia
- Sepsis
- Hyperthyroidism
- Schizophrenia

Immediate management

- Give 100% $O_2$ first and then titrate to achieve $SpO_2$ >97%
- Support airway, breathing, and circulation as required
- Airway may become compromised because of seizure activity or sedatives given as treatment
  - Keep patients nil by mouth initially as they are at risk of requiring intubation and ventilation
- Ensure breathing/ventilation is adequate
- Commence fluid resuscitation with inotropic support as required
- If autonomic instability is severe consider IV sedation with propofol
  - Consider adding agents such as clonidine or β-blockers
- Perform a rapid detailed neurological assessment
- Treat seizures as per protocol (see p. 166)

*Withdrawal treatment:*
- Chlordiazepoxide 20 mg 6-hourly PO (reduce by 25% every 2 days over 8 days); extra doses up to 200 mg/day may be required (reduce doses in the elderly or patients with severe liver impairment)
- Alternatively IV lorazepam or diazepam may be used
- Consider infusions with propofol, benzodiazepines, or barbiturates
- Avoid antipsychotics where possible because of the risk of lowering the seizure threshold
- Where withdrawal is unintentional and/or complicating other critical illness consider giving alcohol; 10% ethanol infusions have been used

Further management

- Supplemental vitamin therapy (may be given orally unless coma, delirium, or Wernicke–Korsakoff syndrome is likely)
  - Thiamine 300 mg PO daily, ascorbic acid 100 mg PO daily
  - Pabrinex® 1–2 pairs IV 12-hourly for up to 7 days should be used (contains ascorbic acid 500 mg, glucose 1 g, nicotinamide 160 mg, pyridoxine 50 mg, riboflavin 4 mg, thiamine 250 mg)
- Avoid dextrose-containing solutions until after thiamine administration
- Consider treatment with vitamin K if PT is prolonged
- Phosphate and magnesium electrolyte replacement may be required

Pitfalls/difficult situations

- Chlordiazepoxide has a long half-life and may accumulate in liver failure, causing prolonged sedation
- Wernicke–Korsakoff syndrome may occur, causing ocular abnormalities (diplopia, nystagmus, VI nerve palsy, and conjugate gaze defects), confusion, amnesia, confabulation, hypotension, hypothermia, and coma; this may be prevented by vitamin supplementation

Further reading

DeBellis R, Smith B, Choi S, *et al.* (2005). Management of delirium tremens. *J Intensive Care Med* **20**, 164–73.

# ① Neuromuscular weakness and paralysis

There are many causes of weakness or paralysis in patients on the intensive care unit. A systematic approach is required.

Causes
- **Central problems**
  - CVA
  - Space-occupying lesions in brain or spinal cord
  - Trauma to brain or spinal cord
  - Multiple sclerosis
- **Anterior horn cell disease**
  - Motor neuron disease
  - Poliomyelitis
- **Peripheral nerve conduction**
  - Guillian–Barré syndrome
  - Critical illness neuropathy
  - Autoimmune diseases
  - Metabolic disorders (diabetes, porphyria, thyroid, liver or renal failure)
  - Nutritional deficiencies
  - Toxins/poisons (including alcohol) or drugs (isoniazid, vincristine)
  - Sarcoid
  - Malignancy
- **Neuromuscular junction**
  - Myasthenia gravis
  - Eaton–Lambert syndrome
  - Botulism
  - Muscle relaxant effects (including suxamethonium apnoea)
  - Venoms
- **Muscle problems**
  - Endocrine myopathies
  - Electrolytes disturbances (including periodic paralysis)
  - Polymyositis
  - Acute rhabdomyolysis
  - Congenital abnormalities (including the muscular dystrophies)
  - Critical illness myopathy

Critical illness myopathy is associated with high-dose steroids (including asthma therapy), muscle relaxants, and aminoglycoside antibiotics.

Presentation and assessment
- The exact presentation will depend on the cause.
- A full history and examination is of paramount importance.
- Difficulty weaning from the ventilator is often the first sign of impending problems

Investigations
- ABGs
- FBC, U&Es, LFTs

- Serum CK, magnesium, phosphate, and calcium
- Serum B12, folate, and iron
- Autoimmune screen
- Nerve conduction studies and/or muscle biopsy
- Lumbar puncture
- Imaging of brain and spinal cord (MRI may be more useful than CT)
- Pulmonary function tests (PFTs)

### Differential diagnoses

The patient may be receiving heavy doses of sedation or muscle relaxants

### Immediate management

- Give 100% $O_2$ initially and then titrate to achieve $SpO_2$ >97%
- Support airway, breathing, and circulation as required
- If the protective reflexes of the upper airway become obtunded, early intubation must be considered
- Assess adequacy of ventilation by measuring FVC and $FEV_1$
  - Support ventilation if FVC <15 ml/kg, or FVC less than predicted TV, or aspiration occurs; repeat PFTs 4-hourly
- Endotracheal intubation and mechanical ventilation are likely to be more appropriate than non-invasive ventilation because of the lack of airway protective reflexes and the likely length of treatment
- Fluid resuscitation or inotropes may be required, particularly in trauma or spinal shock
- Correct calcium, magnesium, potassium, and phosphate

### Further management

- Prolonged mechanical ventilation may require a tracheostomy
- Autonomic disruption causing cardiovascular instability, gastric stasis, and urinary retention can occur with many causes
- Impaired swallowing may be present, requiring NG or PEG feeding
- Treatments aimed at reducing complications of neuromuscular weakness or paralysis include
  - Respiratory infections: regular physiotherapy and tracheal toilet
  - DVT/PE: compression stockings or LMWH
  - Skin damage, joint contractures: pressure area care, physiotherapy
  - Bowel care may be needed

### Pitfalls/difficult situations

- Recovery of function may take months
- The use of suxamethonium may cause hyperkalaemia in patients
- suffering from prolonged immobility

### Further reading

Maramattom BV, Wijdicks FM (2006). Acute neuromuscular weakness in the intensive care unit. *Crit Care Med* **34**, 2835–41.
Sanap MN, Worthley LIG (2002). Neurologic complications of critical illness. Part II: Polyneuropathies and myopathies. *Crit Care Resusc* **4**, 133–40.
&#x1F4D5; OHCC pp. 368, 388, OHEA pp.188, 314.

# ① **Guillain–Barré syndrome**

Guillain–Barré syndrome (GBS, also far less commonly known as Landry–Strohl syndrome) is an acute ascending inflammatory demyelinating polyradiculoneuropathy. Remyelination occurs in most patients, although about 25% of patients require intensive care and 5% die.

## Causes

GBS is more common in women, and although its aetiology is not known it is assumed to be autoimmune mediated. Two-thirds of cases are associated with the following risk factors

- Infection
  - Viral: influenza, parainfluenza, varicella, EBV, measles, HIV, CMV, HBV
  - Bacterial: Camplyobacter, mycoplasma pneumonia
- Immunization (especially tetanus and typhoid)
- Surgery
- Bone marrow transplant

## Presentation and assessment

GBS typically occurs 7–10 days after a precipitating event and develops over 2–3 weeks. Signs and symptoms include
- Ascending symmetrical motor weakness/paralysis
- Absent or reduced reflexes
- Minimal sensory loss, although paraesthesia or pain may occur

Variants of GBS exist including a pure sensory form, a cranial form (ataxia, ophthalmoplegia (Miller–Fisher variant)), and a unilateral form

Autonomic dysfunction may occur
- Arrhythmias (tachycardias and bradycardias; asystole may even occur)
- Blood pressure instability (hyper/hypotension)
- Gut and bladder paralysis

## Investigations (see also p. 202)

Consider
- Lumbar puncture (CSF protein >0.5 g/L, cell count normal—changes present by the second week)
- Nerve conduction studies (decreased conduction velocities)
- Nerve biopsy

## Differential diagnoses (see also p. 202)
- Spinal cord injury (especially epidural abscess or haematoma)
- Botulism
- Periodic paralysis
- Tick paralysis
- AIDS, CMV polyradiculoneuropathy
- Acute porphyria
- Critical illness polyneuropathy
- Arsenic exposure
- Suxamethonium apnoea

## Immediate management

- Give 100% $O_2$ initially and then titrate to achieve $SpO_2$ >97%
- Support airway, breathing, and circulation as required
- If the protective reflexes of the upper airway become obtunded early intubation must be considered
- Assess adequacy of ventilation by measuring FVC and $FEV_1$
  - Support ventilation if FVC <15 ml/kg, or FVC is less than predicted TV, or aspiration occurs; repeat PFTs 4-hourly
- Cardiovascular monitoring may be required if autonomic disturbance is noted
  - Tachycardias or bradycardias may need treatment with short-acting agents; expect exaggerated responses to vasoactive medications

*Guillain-Barré syndrome treatment*

Treatment may decrease the need for ventilation; mortality is unaffected
- Human immunoglobulin (gammaglobulin, IVIG) 0.4 g/kg/day IV for 5 days
- Alternatively, plasmapheresis (or plasma exchange) may be used: four to six exchanges over 8–10 days (total exchange of 250 ml/kg)

## Further management (see also p. 203)

- Supportive care and treatment of the complication's paralysis will be required
- Ventilation is likely to be prolonged
- SIADH may occur (monitoring of U&Es is advisable)
- Analgesics are likely to be required for muscle, joint, and soft tissue pain

## Pitfalls/difficult situations

- Steroids may make outcome worse
- Suxamethonium may provoke dysrhythmias
- About 10% of patients develop a chronic relapsing form of GBS whilst 15% are left with residual neurological disability

## Further reading

OHCC p. 384.

# ℹ **Myasthenia gravis**

Myasthenia gravis is an autoimmune disease. Ninety per cent of patients have antibodies to post-synaptic acetylcholine receptors in the neuro-muscular junction. Critical care is most likely to be required in myasthenia gravis for myasthenic or cholinergic crises.

## Causes

Myasthenia gravis affects mostly women in their twenties and thirties or men over 50 (often associated with thymoma).
- Myasthenic crises may be precipitated by
  - Trauma
  - Infections
  - Drugs, especially muscle relaxants, sedatives, aminoglycosides, antiarrhythmics (lidocaine, procainamide, quinidine), antihistamines, lithium, and phenytoin
- Cholinergic crises
  - Typically occur following excess anticholinergic administration

## Presentation and assessment

Myasethenia gravis presents with gradual-onset muscle weakness which worsens with exercise and prdominantly affects proximal muscles. The most commonly affected sites include the extra-ocular (ptosis, diplopia), bulbar (dysphagia, aspiration), neck, and shoulder muscles.

There is no sensory loss or pain, and reflexes are normal. Ask the patient to perform repetitive shoulder or upward gaze eye movements and look for fatigue
- Myasthenic crises (may be the first presentation of myasthenia gravis)
  - Severe weakness with respiratory insufficiency
  - Inability to swallow oral secretions
  - Pyrexia and tachycardia may be present if infection is the precipitant
- Cholinergic crises
  - Cholinergic crises may present with profound muscle weakness causing respiratory failure and bulbar palsy, and associated with hyper-salivation, lacrimation, vomiting, miosis, and sweating

## Investigations (see also p. 202)
- Edrophonium test (also known as a Tensilon test)
- Electromyography
- ACh receptor antibodies (present in 80% of cases)
- TFTs (for both hyper- and hypothyroidism)
- FBC, CRP, septic screen—if infection is likely to be a precipitant
- CXR (looking for aspiration, or if considering Eaton–Lambert syndrome for bronchial carcinoma)
- Chest CT may be considered at a later point (to identify thymoma)

## Differential diagnoses (see also p. 202)
- Eaton–Lambert syndrome (muscle weakness improves with exercise)
- Suxamethonium apnoea
- Organophosphate or nerve-agent poisoning

**Immediate management**

- Give 100% $O_2$ initially and then titrate to achieve $SpO_2$ >97%
- Support airway, breathing, and circulation as required
- If the protective reflexes of the upper airway become obtunded, early intubation must be considered
- Assess adequacy of ventilation by measuring FVC and $FEV_1$
  - Support ventilation if FVC < 15 ml/kg, or FVC is less than predicted TV, or failure to expectorate secretions occurs
  - Repeat PFTs 4-hourly
- Cardiovascular monitoring should be applied
- Perform edrophonium test
  - Give edrophonium 2 mg IV and wait for 30–60 seconds
  - Observe for cholinergic symptoms (have atropine available)
  - Give further 8 mg IV edrophonium
  - Improvement in muscle function should occur within 5–10 min
  - Stop if cholinergic symptoms occur/worsen

*Myasthenic crisis (responds to edrophonium)*

- Discontinue possible medication triggers and treat infections
- Commence acetylcholinesterase inhibitor treatment (e.g. pyridostigmine or neostigmine)
- Where respiratory failure is present, consider human immunoglobulin or plasmapheresis treatment
- In severe cases immunosuppressants may be required (e.g. methotrexate or azathioprine)
- Steroids may be required, but may exacerbate the illness in the acute stages (use as directed by a neurologist)

*Cholinergic crisis (does not respond to edrophonium)*

- Withdraw anticholinesterase medication
- Control cholinergic symptoms with atropine 1 mg IV every 30 min (up to 8 mg)
- Re-introduce anticholinesterase treatment when edrophonium test becomes positive

**Further management** (see also p. 203)
Supportive care and treatment of the complications paralysis

**Pitfalls/difficult situations**

- Where possible avoid muscle relaxants
- Respiratory infections caused by pulmonary aspiration and/or atelectasis are common
- Thymectomy may reduce symptoms of myasthenia, but careful post-operative management within critical care may be required
- Where patients with severe myasthenia gravis require mechanical ventilation for other reasons, plasma exchange or immunosuppressive therapy may be considered to aid weaning

**Further reading**
📖 OHCC p. 386.

# Cerebrospinal fluid and other neurological variables

**Table 5.1** Normal CSF values

| | | |
|---|---|---|
| Pressure | 7–18 cmH$_2$O | |
| Specific gravity | 1.0062–1.0082 | |
| Protein | 0.15–0.45 g/L | |
| Chloride | 120–130 mmol/L | |
| Glucose | 2.8–4.2 mmol/L | 75% of blood glucose |
| Cell count | | |
|    Lymphocytes | ≤5/mm$^3$ | |
|    Neutrophils | Nil | |
| Xanthachromia index | <0.015 | |

**Table 5.2** CSF findings associated with disease

| | Pressure | Cell count/mm$^3$ | Protein | Glucose |
|---|---|---|---|---|
| Bacterial meningitis | ↑ | 1000–60 000 Neutrophils | ↑ | ↓ (<60%) |
| TB meningitis | ↑ | <1500 Neutrophils initially Lymphocytes later | ↑ | ↓ (<60%) |
| Viral meningitis | Normal or ↑ | Normal or ↑ (<500) Mononuclear cells may be seen | Mildly ↑ (<2 g/L) | Normal (>60%) |
| HSV meningitis | ↑ | ↑ Lymphocyte count | ↑ | Normal (>60%) |
| Fungal meningitis | ↑ | <500 Mostly lymphocytes | ↑ | ↓ (<60%) |
| Abscess | ↑ | Variable | ↑ | Normal (>60%) |
| Tumour | ↑ | Mononuclear or blast cells may be seen | Sometimes >5 g/L | Normal or ↓ |

**Table 5.3** Neurological variables

| | | |
|---|---|---|
| Jugular venous bulb saturations ($SjO_2$) | 55–75% | |
| Intracranial pressure (ICP) | 0–10 mmHg | 0–14 cmH$_2$O |
| Transcranial Doppler (TCD) temporal windows | | |
|    MCA, mean flow velocity | 55 ± 12 cm/s | |
|    ACA, mean flow velocity | 50 ± 11 cm/s | |
|    PCA, mean flow velocity | 40 ± 10 cm/s | |
|    TICA, mean flow velocity | 39 ± 9 cm/s | |
| Electroencephalogram (EEG) | | |
| Cerebrofunction monitor (CFM) | Abrupt spikes in epilepsy | Up to 50 µV |
| Bispectral index (BIS) | Indicates anaesthesia | <50 |

# Metabolic and endocrine

# :O: Metabolic acidaemia

Metabolic acidosis is defined as pH <7.36 associated with low bicarbonate (<23 mmol/L). $PaCO_2$ is usually decreased (respiratory compensation). Increased $PaCO_2$ along with reduced levels of bicarbonate would suggest mixed, metabolic, and respiratory acidosis (see p. 52).

Base excess (BE), or base deficit, is commonly used as a means of isolating the metabolic component of an acidosis or alkalosis where there is a mixed respiratory/metabolic picture.

Commonly measured cations ($Na^+$ and $K^+$) exceed the measurable anions ($Cl^-$ and $HCO_3^-$); this is known as the anion gap (normal 7–12 mmol/L). When the anion gap is increased, this can indicate the accumulation of unmeasurable acid. BE is measured by gauging the amount of acid or base that is required to correct blood pH to 7.4, given a $PCO_2$ level of 40 mmHg at 37°C. The normal range is is +2 to –2; a BE more negative than –5 indicates a significant metabolic acidosis.

## Causes (see p. 214)

## Presentation and assessment

The main presentation will be of the presenting illness or precipitating cause of metabolic acidosis (i.e. heart failure); in addition the following may also be present

- Respiratory signs and symptoms: tachypnoea, dyspnoea, gasping or sighing breathing (Kussmaul's breathing)
  - $PaCO_2$ is often <3.5 kPa because of compensatory hyperventilation
  - Bradypnoea is often a late or pre-terminal sign
- Cardiovascular changes: decreased myocardial contractility, vasodilatation, haemodynamic instability, decreased responsiveness to inotropes
  - ECG: increased incidence of dysrhythmias
  - Bradycardia is often a late or pre-terminal sign
- Neurological symptoms: agitation, confusion, coma
- Gastrointestinal: impaired perfusion of gut, poor gut motility
- Renal: where hypoperfusion or renal failure are present oliguria or anuria may be present

## Investigations

- ABGs and serum lactate
  - Venous gases may be used where metabolic acidosis alone (i.e. no hypoxia or hypercapnia) is suspected; venous pH is slightly lower than arterial pH
- Serum osmolality and osmolar gap
- FBC and coagulation screen
- U&Es and anion gap (indication of dehydration, renal failure; electrolyte imbalance)
- Serum magnesium, phosphate, and calcium
- Serum glucose
- LFTs and amylase
- Septic screen: blood, urine, and sputum cultures
- Urine sample/dipstick for ketones, protein, or myoglobinurea

- Consider testing for serum ketones as some dipstick tests do not detect β-HBA, the predominant ketone body in DKA
- ECG, CXR
- Further imaging (e.g. abdominal ultrasound or CT scan) and investigations may be indicated by history and examination

**Differential diagnoses**
- Diabetic ketoacidosis
- Drug poisoning: salicylates, metformin

**Immediate management**
- Give $O_2$ and support airway, breathing, and circulation as required
- Primary concern should be to treat the cause
- Provide organ system support as indicated
  - Ventilation support may be required (see directions below)
  - Inotropic support may be required
  - Treat arrhythmias if these cause haemodynamic compromise
- Control of acidaemia
  - Maintain respiratory compensation; avoid sedatives in awake patients
  - If mechanical ventilation is required temporarily maintain a supra-normal minute volume
  - Consider 50–100 mmol of $NaHCO_3$ IV if pH <7.1 and haemodynamic instability is present (mild acidaemia of pH ~7.2 may be protective)
  - 50–100 mmol of $NaHCO_3$ IV may be the drug of choice in acidaemia complicated by hyperkalaemia
  - Resistant or profound cases of metabolic acidaemia may require haemofiltration (see renal replacement indications, p. 277), a degree of cardiovascular stability will be required for successful haemofiltration to be performed

**Further management**
- Continue full invasive monitoring
- Continue to monitor for ABG and electrolytes
- Correct any electrolyte abnormalities
- Sepsis screen and antibiotics
- Specific treatment for poisoning (see pp. 427–461) or diabetic ketoacidosis (insulin therapy)

## Causes of metabolic acidosis

| Normal anion gap (<12 mmol/L) | Raised anion gap (>12 mmol/L) | |
|---|---|---|
| | Normal serum osmolality (osmolal gap < 10 mOsm/kg $H_2O$) | Raised serum osmolality (osmolal gap > 10 mOsm/kg $H_2O$) |
| • Renal tubular acidosis | • Diabetic ketoacidosis | • Any form of alcohol ingestion |
| • Carbonic anhydrase inhibition, acetazolamide | • Drugs and poisons | • Ethanol |
| • Gastrointestinal loss | • Salicylates | • Methanol |
| • Diarrhoea | • Tricyclic antidepressants | • Ethylene glycol |
| • Small bowel/biliary fistula | • Toluene exposure (glue sniffing) | • Isopropyl alcohol |
| • Ureteroentrostomy | • Renal failure | • Paraldehyde |
| • Hyperchloraemic acidosis (commonly following aggressive saline resuscitation) | • Rhabdomyolysis | |
| | • Lactic acidosis with tissue hypoperfusion | |
| | • Shock/prolonged hypotension | |
| | • Hypoxia | |
| | • Anaemia/blood loss | |
| | • Sepsis | |
| | • Hypo-, hyperthermia, | |
| | • Lactic acidosis without tissue hypoperfusion | |
| | • Metformin and phenformin | |
| | • Hepatic or renal failure | |
| | • Pancreatitis | |
| | • Malignancy | |
| | • Glucose-6-phosphate deficiency | |

### Anion gap

- The calculation of anion gap involves four measured ions, and so the error is much higher than that of a single electrolyte determination; laboratory errors often result in a low anion gap
- Albumin is the major unmeasured anion and contributes almost the whole of the value of the anion gap; every 1 g decrease in albumin will decrease the anion gap by 2.5–3 mmol
  - Low albumin is common in ICU patients and will lower the anion gap so that what should give rise to a raised anion gap (i.e. lactic acidosis) may result in a normal anion gap.

### Pitfalls/difficult situations

- Cause may not be immediately apparent, especially in poisoning
- Suspect gut ischaemia in patients with severe unexplained lactic acidosis
- Inotropes and anti-arrhythmic drugs may not be effective if pH is <7.15
- Hyperkalaemia often accompanies metabolic acidosis; hypokalaemia may develop on treating acidosis
- Be prepared to treat severe arrhythmias

### Further reading

Sirker AA, Rhodes A, Grounds RM, Bennett ED (2002). Acid-base physiology: the 'traditional' and the 'modern' approaches. *Anaesthesia* **57**, 348–56.

http://www.anaesthesiamcq.com/AcidBaseBook/ABindex.php

OHCC pp. 98, 432, 434.

# :☼: Hypernatraemia

Sodium is the major extracellular cation, and so hypernatraemia is always accompanied by hyperosmolality.
- Mild          145–150 mmol/L
- Moderate      151–160 mmol/L
- Severe        >160 mmol/L

## Causes
- Hypovolaemic, associated with low extracellular volume
  Water loss > sodium loss
  - Extrarenal losses (especially if water only is replaced): diarrhoea, vomiting, fistulas, significant burns
  - Renal losses: osmotic diuretics, diuretics, post-obstructive diuresis, intrinsic renal disease, uncontrolled diabetes mellitus
  - Adipsic: this is secondary to decreased thirst; may be behavioural or secondary to head injury and hypothalamic damage.
- Hypervolaemic, associated with high extracellular volume
  Sodium gains > water gains
  - Administration of high-concentration sodium bicarbonate
  - Hypertonic saline
  - Conn's syndrome: hypertension, hypokalaemia, alkalosis
  - Cushing's syndrome
- Euvolaemic, associated with normal extracellular volume
  - Diabetes insipidus (nephrogenic or cranial): intracellular and interstitial water loss predominates; <10% is intravascular
  - Any increase in insensible losses: hyperventilation, fever

## Presentation and assessment
Patients may be asymptomatic, or signs and symptoms may include
- General signs and symptoms: weakness, malaise, decreased skin turgor
- Neurological: irritability, confusion, delirium, brisk tendon reflexes, muscle twitches, spasticity, seizures, coma, intracranial haemorrhage
- Cardiovascular
  - Hypovolaemic: resting or postural hypotension
  - Hypervolaemic: S3 heart sound, oedema
- Gastrointestinal: diarrhoea, vomiting, excessive drain/fistula output
- Renal: polyuria, polydypsia, massive diuresis

## Investigations
- U&Es and plasma glucose (to exclude hyperglycaemic osmotic diuresis)
- Urinary sodium, coupled urinary and plasma osmolality
- Consider head MRI/CT scan, looking for intracranial haemorrhage, dural sinus thrombosis, or pathological cause of central hypernatraemia
- Consider water-deprivation test (urine osmolality does not increase in line with serum hyperosmolality in either type of DI)
- ADH stimulation (if nephrogenic DI is present, urine osmolality does not increase after ADH or desmopressin administration)

## Differential diagnoses
- HONK

## Immediate management

- Give $O_2$ and support airway, breathing, and circulation as required

**Sodium correction: depends on rate of onset of symptoms**
- If hyperacute (<12 h) rapid correction can be attempted
- Chronic hypernatraemia: correction should be attempted over 24–72 hours to minimize the risk of cerebral oedema; aim to lower plasma sodium at a rate of <0.8 mmol/hour

**Guide treatment according to cause**
- Hypovolaemic
  - If possible, encourage oral fluids/NG water
  - If hypotensive consider giving colloid initially, or 0.9% saline to correct hypovolaemia (0.9% saline will be hypotonic compared with plasma sodium)
  - Follow this with 0.45% saline or 5% dextrose IV
- Hypervolaemic:
  - Stop any high-sodium-containing infusions/feed
  - Start 5% dextrose and add NG water
  - Consider furosemide 20 mg IV
  - Haemofiltration with low-sodium dialysate may be considered if patient is severely fluid overloaded or already on CVVH
- Euvolaemic
  - Encourage oral intake/NG water
  - 0.45% saline or 5% dextrose IV (may need >5 L/day)
  - Where DI is present replace urinary losses and give desmopressin IV/SC/IM 1–2 µg 12-hourly; or via intranasal spray 10 µg 12-hourly

## Further management

- Investigate any causes and treat appropriately
- Minimize sodium intake, e.g. from colloids, feed, or sodium bicarbonate
- Maintain a strict input–output chart, including all drain losses
- Monitor electrolytes frequently, 1–2-hourly initially, then ~4-hourly

## Pitfalls/difficult situations

- In liver failure keep sodium >145 mmol/L to avoid cerebral oedema

---

**Urine osmolality states**

| Osmolality | Likely cause |
|------------|--------------|
| High | Extrarenal hypotonic fluid losses, salt overload |
| Low | Diabetes insipidus |
| Normal | Diuretics or salt wasting |

---

## Further reading

Adrogue HJ, Madias NE (2000). Hypernatraemia. *N Engl J Med* **342**, 1493–9.
Reynolds RM, Padfield PL, Seckl JR (2006). Disorders of sodium balance. *BMJ* **332**, 702–5.
OHCC p. 416, OHEA p. 280.

# ☼ Hyponatraemia

Mild                125–134 mmol/L
Moderate            120–124 mmol/L
Severe              <120 mmol/L

## Causes

Hypovolaemic (associated with loss of sodium *and* water)
- Renal losses (urinary sodium >20 mmol/L): diuretics, DKA, Addison's disease, sodium-losing nephropathies, diuretic phase of ARF
- Extra-renal (urinary sodium <20 mmol/L): diarrhoea, vomiting, fistula/drain losses, burns, small bowel obstruction, pancreatitis

Hypervolaemic (urinary sodium usually >20 mmol/L), associated with total body water rise *greater than* sodium rise: oedema is present
- Iatrogenic: TUR syndrome (see p. 390), excess water administration
- Cardiovascular: CCF (urinary sodium <20 mmol/L)
- Respiratory: pneumonia, TB, lung abscess, cystic fibrosis, vasculitis
- Neurological: trauma, CVA, SAH, malignancy, vasculitis, infection
- Gastrointestinal: cirrhosis with ascites
- Renal: severe renal failure, nephritic syndrome
- Drugs: opiates, haloperidol, amitriptyline, vasopressin, carbamazepine, oxytocin, chlorpropamide, thiazides, ecstasy overdose
- Endocrine: severe myxoedema, psychogenic polydipsia
- Malignancy: lung (small-cell), pancreatic, lymphoma, prostatic

Euvolaemic causes a slight increase in total body water, minimal oedema (urinary sodium >20 mmol/L, urine osmolality >100 mosmol/kg, serum osmolality <270 mosmol/kg)
- General: following surgical stress response, HIV
- Endocrine: glucocorticoid deficiency, hypothyroidism, SIADH

## Presentation and assessment

Signs and symptoms depend on rate and magnitude of the decrease
- General: change in skin turgor, weakness, incontinence
- Neurological
  - (sodium ~120 mmol/L): headache, confusion, restlessness, irritability
  - (sodium ~110 mmol/L): ataxia, hallucinations, seizures, coma, fixed unilateral dilated pupil, decorticate or decerebrate posturing
- Cardiovascular: hypertension, CCF, elevated CVP/JVP, S3 heart sound, oedema, bradycardia
- Respiratory: hypoventilation or respiratory arrest associated with coma
- Gastrointestinal: anorexia, nausea and vomiting

## Investigations
- U&Es, TFTs
- Random serum cortisol, ACTH stimulation test
- Urinary sodium level, coupled urinary and plasma osmolality
- Imaging: CXR, consider head CT

## Differential diagnoses
- Sampling error: tourniquet used on sample arm
- Artificially low sodium due to hyperlipidaemia or hyperglycaemia

## Immediate management

- Give $O_2$ and support airway, breathing, and circulation as required

**Sodium correction depends on rate of onset of symptoms**
- Chronic hyponatraemia: correction should not exceed 0.5 mmol/L/hour in first 24 hours and 0.3 mmol/L/hour thereafter
- Acute hyponatraemia: allows faster correction, but no greater than 20 mmol/L/day is advised
- In hypovolaemia
  - If symptomatic, give hypertonic saline
  - If asymptomatic, give isotonic saline
- In hypervolaemia with no oedema
  - If symptomatic (seizures, muscle twitching) give 0.9% saline
  - Consider cautious hypertonic (1.8%) saline in 100 mL aliquots
  - Check plasma sodium levels every 2 hours if using hypertonic solutions
- In hypervolaemia with oedema
  - If symptomatic give furosemide (20 mg IV PRN) and mannitol (100–500 mL 20% over 20 minutes)
  - Replace urinary sodium losses with hypertonic saline as above
- If asymptomatic, fluid restrict to 1–1.5 L/day. Persistent hyponatraemia in this circumstance points to SIADH
  - If SIADH is present give isotonic saline and demeclocycline
- If in established renal failure, dialysis may be necessary
- Monitor plasma potassium and magnesium concentrations as they may alter dramatically

## Further management

- Accept a plasma sodium level of 125–130 mmol/L
- Use isotonic solutions for drug reconstitution and TPN
- Correct other electrolyte abnormalities (hyponatraemia may intensify the cardiac effects of hyperkalaemia)
- Correct adrenal insufficiency or hypothyroidism

## Pitfalls/difficult situations

- Rapid large corrections risk central pontine myelinolysis
- Where possible perform frequent plasma sodium checks rather than using equations to calculate excess water
- If the patient has LVF consider giving furosemide (20 mg IV PRN) and replacing urinary sodium with hypertonic saline aliquots
- Hyponatraemia can occur with a normal osmolality if abnormal solutes (e.g. ethanol, ethylene glycol) have been ingested
- Urine osmolality and electrolytes will be affected by diuretics; these should be stopped for >24 hours) before urine osmolality and electrolyte measurement if a cause other than diuretics is considered likely

## Further reading

Arieff AI, Ayus JC (2000). Hyponatremia. *N Engl J Med* **343**, 886–8.
📖 OHCC p. 418, OHEA p. 282.

## ☠ Hyperkalaemia

Hyperkalaemia is relatively common and can have severe side effects unless corrected rapidly.

- Mild        5.5–6.0 mmol/L
- Moderate    6.1–7.0 mmol/L
- Severe      >7.0 mmol/L

### Causes

- Acute or chronic oliguric renal failure
- Potassium-sparing diuretics, NSAIDs, β-blockers
- Suxamethonium given to patients with the following conditions
  - Major burns
  - Spinal trauma
  - Prolonged immobility
  - Mild serum elevation of potassium
- Cell injury from rhabdomyolysis, crush injury, tumour lysis, or burns
- Metabolic acidosis
- Excess intake of potassium (e.g. via infusions, medications, or diet)
- Addison's disease
- Massive blood transfusion
- Malignant hyperthermia

### Presentation and assessment

Hyperkalaemia is often an incidental laboratory finding; signs and symptoms when present may include

- Neuromuscular symptoms: muscle cramps, fatigue, weakness, paraesthesia, paralysis (this may even present as failure to wean)
- Cardiovascular changes
  - ECG changes: tall tented T waves, slurring of ST segments into T waves, small P waves, prolonged PR interval, widened QRS, complete heart block, asystole or VF
- Gastrointestinal: nausea, vomiting, or diarrhoea
- General effects: hyperkalaemia may potentiate the effects of 'lows': low calcium, low sodium, low pH, and low temperature

Hyperkalaemia should be suspected in patients who have

- Pre-existing renal failure, especially if dialysis has been missed
- Dehydration and acidaemia (e.g. DKA)

### Investigations

- ABGs (or venous blood gases)
- FBC
- U&Es and serum calcium
- ECG ( it is not essential to perform an ECG prior to treatment)

### Differential diagnoses

- Sampling error: tourniquet used on sample arm
- Thrombocytosis: platelets leak $K^+$ in clotted sample
- Severe leucocytosis: for the same reason as above
- Blood sample left to rest for a long time before testing
- Tight tourniquet leading to crushed RBCs/haemolysis

Immediate management

- Give $O_2$ and support airway, breathing, and circulation as required
- If the patient is mechanically ventilated consider temporarily increasing the ventilation rate to 'buy time' by decreasing acidosis/inducing alkalosis and so lowering $K^+$ levels
- Obtain IV access
- Commence continuous ECG monitoring
- If hyperkalaemia is moderate or severe, or if the patient is symptomatic (or has ECG changes), consider
  - Calcium chloride 3–5 ml of 10% solution IV over 3 min: has a cardioprotective effect only; will not lower potassium
  - Calcium gluconate 10 ml 10% IV over 2 min: alternative to calcium chloride
  - The cardioprotective effect of calcium lasts ~1 hour; if ECG changes are present these often resolve after calcium
  - The calcium dose may need to be repeated if hyperkalaemia persists
  - Insulin 15–20 units soluble insulin in 50 ml 50% dextrose IV over 30–60 min
  - Salbutamol 5 mg nebulized; other β-agonists may be considered as alternatives
  - Sodium bicarbonate 8.4% 25–50 ml IV may be considered if there is accompanying profound acidosis

Further management
- Re-check $K^+$ level regularly to guide therapy: ABG analysers which allow $K^+$ analysis may be quicker than sending formal laboratory samples
- Consider polystyrene sulfonate resin (calcium resonium) 15 g PO 8-hourly, or as a 30 g enema (this requires colonic irrigation after 9 hours to remove $K^+$ from colon)
- Treat the cause (e.g. steroids for Addison's disease)
- Avoid suxamethonium
- If hyperkalaemia does not respond to treatment proceed to dialysis

Pitfalls/difficult situations
- It is important to note that insulin and salbutamol only move $K^+$ into cells; excess $K^+$ must eventually be removed from the body either in the urine or via the bowels.
- If the patient is anuric haemofiltration or dialysis is usually required to remove $K^+$
- Hyperkalaemia can prolong neuromuscular blockade
- If a rapid-sequence intubation is required, consider using a modified technique with rocuronium rather than suxamethonium
- The rate of rise of $K^+$ governs arrhythmia potential: some patients with chronic renal failure and marked hyperkalaemia are quite stable

Further reading
Kuvin JT (1998). Electrocardiographic changes of hyperkalaemia. *N Engl J Med* **338**, 662.
Evans KJ, Greenberg A (2002). Hyperkalaemia: a review. *J Intensive Care Med* **20**, 272–90.
OHCC p. 420, OHEA p. 276.

# ☼ Hypokalaemia

- Mild      2.5–3.0 mmol/L
- Severe    <2.5 mmol/L

## Causes

- Decreased intake: malnutrition, omission from IV fluid, TPN
- Renal losses: RTA, leukaemia (unknown mechanism), magnesium depletion, haemofiltration losses
- Endocrine: SIADH, Cushing's syndrome, Conn's syndrome (Conn's syndrome should be suspected where there is a hypertensive hypokalaemic alkalosis in a patient not taking diuretics)
- Gastrointestinal losses: diarrhoea, enemas or laxative abuse, vomiting or NG suctioning, intestinal fistula, rectal villous adenoma, pyloric stenosis, refeeding syndrome
- Drugs: diuretics (especially metolazone in the elderly), β-agonists, steroids, theophylline, and aminoglycosides
- Purgative or liquorice abuse
- Alcoholism
- Trans-cellular shifts: insulin usage, alkalosis, hypothermia, familial periodic paralysis
- Rare syndromes: Gitelman's syndrome, Liddle's syndrome, Bartter's syndrome, Fanconi's syndrome

## Presentation and assessment

Hypokalaemia is often an incidental laboratory finding; signs and symptoms, when present, may include:

- Neurological symptoms: psychosis, delirium, hallucinations
- Neuromuscular: muscle weakness, decreased tendon reflexes, paralysis, paraesthesia, cramps, hypotonia (this may present as respiratory failure, or difficulty weaning from ventilator)
- Cardiovascular: palpitations
  - ECG changes: prolonged PR interval, ST depression, small/inverted T waves, visible U wave (after T), dysrhythmias (SVT, VT, torsade de pointes)
- Gastrointestinal: abdominal cramps, constipation, nausea and vomiting
- Renal: polyuria, nocturia, polydypsia

## Investigations

- ABGs
- U&Es, serum magnesium, calcium, and phosphate
- Glucose
- Digoxin level (if on digoxin, as hypokalaemia can potentate arrhythmias)
- ECG

## Differential diagnoses

- Sampling error: tourniquet used on sample arm
- Cushing's disease/syndrome
- Conn's syndrome
- Hypomagnesaemia
- Hypocalcaemia

## Immediate management

- Give $O_2$ and support airway, breathing, and circulation as required
- Obtain IV access
- Commence continuous ECG monitoring
- Where possible stop causative drugs
- If symptoms or arrhythmias are life threatening:
  - Give KCl replacement neat at 20 mmol/30 min via central line only (do not give replacement any more concentrated than 40 mmol/L via a peripheral line)
- If symptoms are moderate:
  - Give 40 mmol KCl in 1 L of fluid, this may be infused peripherally over 4–6 hours
  - Alternatively 40 mmol KCl in 100 ml of fluid may be infused via a central line over 4–6 hours
- If symptoms are mild and without arrhythmias
- Give oral therapy if possible using Sando-K®, 2–4 tablets 6–8-hourly

## Further management

- Monitor $K^+$ level hourly via ABG initially and treat underlying causes
  - Discontinue laxatives and add $H_2$ receptor antagonists and/or motility agents to decrease NG losses
- Correct any hypomagnesaemia which will antagonize attempts at potassium correction
- If diuretics are essential, consider switching to potassium-sparing drugs (e.g. spironolactone or amiloride)

## Pitfalls/difficult situations

- Potassium replacement in patients with renal insufficiency may result in hyperkalaemia
- Chronic hypokalaemia is better tolerated than acute hypokalaemia
- Where patients have an associated acidaemia consider correcting hypokalaemia before or alongside acidaemia correction in order to avoid alkali-induced shift of $K^+$ into cells
- If bicarbonate is high, then any hypokalaemia is likely to have been long-standing and may take up to 2 days to replace adequately
- Take care to avoid hypokalaemia when treating DKA
- Oral $K^+$ replacement may be limited by patient tolerance; some patients develop nausea or even GI ulceration
- Some causes of hypokalaemia are amenable to surgical correction: renal artery stenosis, adrenal adenoma, intestinal obstruction, villous adenoma
- Hypokalaemia increases the risk of digoxin toxicity
- Maintaining $K^+$ levels of 4–4.5 mmol/L following myocardial injury or infarction may decrease the incidence of dysrhythmias

## Further reading

Lederer E, Lerbeck K. Hypokalaemia. Available online at: www.emedicine.com/med/topic1124.htm
Gennari FJ (1998). Hypokalemia. *N Engl J Med* **339**, 451–8.
📖 OHCC p. 422, OHEA p. 278.

# ! Hypercalcaemia

| Normal | 2.2–2.5 mmol/L (ionized 0.9–1.1 mmol/L) |
| --- | --- |
| Mild | 2.6–3.0 mmol/L |
| Moderate | 3.0–3.4 mmol/L |
| Severe | >3.4 mmol/L |

Corrected calcium (mmol/L) = measured calcium + 0.02 × (40 − plasma albumin g/L)

## Causes

- Most commonly secondary to malignancy, especially squamous cell lung carcinoma, myeloma, breast carcinoma, or any other carcinoma with bone metastases
- Primary or tertiary hyperparathyroidism
- Hyperparathyroidism, hyperthyroidism, phaeochromocytoma (MEN II), Addison's disease
- Vitamin D intoxication, milk alkali syndrome, excess antacid ingestion
- Granulomatous disease: sarcoidosis, TB
- Familial benign hypocalciuric hypercalcaemia
- Renal failure (initiation of chronic haemodialysis), post renal transplantation
- Drugs: thiazide diuretics, lithium, theophylline
- Hypophosphataemia (<1.4 mmol/L)
- Immobilization, Paget's disease, AIDS, advanced chronic liver disease

## Presentation and assessment

Often identified as a result of blood tests, rather than clinically. Urgent treatment is required for calcium >3 mmol/L. Symptoms are classically described as 'bones, stones, abdominal groans, and psychic moans'.

- General symptoms: polyuria, polydypsia, dehydration, corneal calcification
- Cardiovascular: raised BP, bradycardia, dysrhythmias, cardiac arrest
  - ECG changes: shortened QT
- Neurological: confusion, lethargy, depression, coma, hyper-reflexia, tongue fasciculations
- Gastrointestinal: abdominal pain, anorexia, weight loss, peptic ulceration, nausea, vomiting, constipation, pancreatitis
- Renal: kidney stones, renal failure

## Differential diagnoses

- Falsely elevated levels: elevated serum protein levels, high paracetamol level, alcohol or hydralazine, and with haemolysis

## Investigations

- FBC
- U&Es, calcium, magnesium, phosphate, LFTs
- PTH levels
- Amylase
- ECG
- CXR
- Urinary calcium, creatinine, and sodium
- 24 hour urinary calcium, urinary cAMP

Immediate management

• Give $O_2$ and support airway, breathing, and circulation as required
• Rehydrate with IV fluids (normally 0.9% saline); volumes of 4–6 L/24 hours may be required
• Give a loop diuretic, e.g. furosemide (40 mg IV repeated as necessary)
**Do not use a thiazide diuretics**
• Consider dialysis if renal failure is present (use low-calcium dialysate)
• If calcium >3.4 mmol/L, give sodium pamidronate 30–90 mg in 1 L 0.9% saline IV over 4 hours (works over 2–3 days with maximum effect in 1 week)

Further management

• Aim to decrease serum calcium by 0.5 mmol/L over 1–2 days
• Endocrinology or oncology referral may be required
• Continued bisphosphonate treatment may be required: sodium clodronate (300 mg/day for 7–10 days), or etidronate sodium (7.5 mg/kg/day over 4 hours for 3 days)
• Consider glucocorticoids in haematological malignancy, granulomatous disease, or vitamin D toxicity (prednisolone 120 mg/day)
• Calcitonin (8 U/kg over 8 hours), an osteoclast inhibitor, is rarely used as serum calcium fall is minimal and tachyphylaxis develops within 2–3 days
• Consider slow IV phosphate infusion(<10 mmol/12 hours) which increases bone reuptake, decreases gut absorption, and inhibits osteoclasts
• Oral phosphate therapy (5 g 8-hourly) may also be used (causes diarrhoea)
• Chemotherapy may decrease calcium in malignancy

Pitfalls/difficult situations

• It is ionized calcium which is physiologically active; therefore use corrected calcium level which eliminates the influence of serum albumin
• Severe elevations in calcium levels may cause coma
• Elderly patients may manifest symptoms from moderate elevations
• The symptoms of hypercalcaemia may overlap with the symptoms of the patient's malignancy
• Hypercalcaemia associated with renal calculi, joint complaints, and ulcer disease is more likely to be due to hyperparathyroidism
• No imaging studies definitively diagnose hypercalcaemia
• Always consider malignancy, particularly if cachexia or bone pain are present
• Always consider hypercalcaemia in patients with multiple non-specific complaints and associated lung mass
• In moderate to severe hypercalcaemia anaesthetic agents may potentiate the risk of serious arrhythmias
• Rebound hypercalcaemia can occur after stopping calcitonin therapy

Further reading

Bilezikian JP (1992). Management of acute hypercalcaemia. *N Engl J Med* **326**, 1196–1203.
 OHCC p. 426, OHEA p. 284.

## ☼ **Hypocalcaemia**

- Hypocalcaemia    <2.2 mmol/L (ionized <0.9 mmol/L)

Corrected calcium (mmol/L) = measured calcium + 0.02 × (40 − plasma albumin g/L)

### Causes
- Transfusion of large quantities of citrated blood products
- Alkalosis or hyperventilation, causing reduction of ionized calcium fraction
- Hypomagnesaemia exacerbates hypocalcaemia and causes end-organ resistance to PTH
- Hypovitaminosis D: dietary deficiency, chronic renal failure
- Hyperphosphataemia (binds calcium): chronic renal failure, rhabdomyolysis, parathyroidectomy
- Following surgery: small bowel syndrome, parathyroidectomy
- Acute pancreatitis causing saponification of calcium by free fatty acids in peritoneum
- Sepsis (especially toxic shock syndrome), burns, or critical illness causing low albumin
- Drug administration: protamine, glucagon, heparin
  - Bisphosphosonates may cause rebound hypocalcaemia after being used to treat hypercalcaemia
- Over-hydration
- Osteomalacia
- Malignancy: osteoblastic metastases and tumour lysis syndrome

### Presentation and assessment
- Neurological: neuromuscular symptoms
  - carpopedal spasm, cramp, tetany, convulsions, confusion
  - Chvostek's sign (tapping over the facial nerve, anterior to tragus of ear, stimulates facial twitching: positive in 10% of normocalcaemic individuals)
  - Trousseau's sign (inflating a BP cuff above systolic pressure causes local ulnar and median nerve ischaemia resulting in carpal spasm)
- Respiratory: wheeze, stridor, rales
- Cardiovascular: dysrhythmias, reduced cardiac output, hypotension, heart failure, angina
  - ECG changes: prolonged PR interval, prolonged QT interval
- Gastrointestinal: dysphagia, diarrhoea, colic

### Investigations
- ABGs
- Clotting profile
- U&Es, calcium, magnesium, phosphate
- LFTs, including albumin
- CK and urine myoglobin
- Amylase
- Plasma PTH level
- 12-lead ECG
- Consider skull X-ray

**Differential diagnoses**

- Sampling error: tourniquet used on sample arm
- Falsely depressed levels seen with iron dextran, heparin, oxalate, citrate, or hyperbilirubinaemia

**Immediate management**

- Give $O_2$ and support airway, breathing, and circulation as required
- Inotropic support may be required
- Calcium supplementation
  - Central administration is preferable as vasoconstriction and ischaemia can occur around tissues at injection site
  - 10 ml 10% calcium chloride IV (2.25 mmol) over 10 min
  - Alternatively, 10 ml 10% calcium gluconate IV over 10 min (slower onset)
  - Calcium infusion may be needed: 10% calcium chloride at 5–10 mmol/hour (2.25 mmol/hour)

**Further management**

- If respiratory alkalosis is present consider adjusting ventilator settings
- Where spontaneous over-breathing is present in intubated patients consider deepening sedation to inhibit it
- Correct any coexisting hypokalaemia and hypomagnesaemia
- Consider enteral supplementation of calcium or vitamin D analogues

**Pitfalls/difficult situations**

- Watch for an increase in cardiac output or BP during calcium administration

**Further reading**

Marx SJ (2000). Hyperparathyroid and hypoparathyroid disorders. *N Engl J Med* **343**, 1863–75. OHCC. 428, OHEA p. 286.

# ⓘ Hyperphosphataemia

- Normal    0.8–1.4 mmol/L
- Severe    2.0–4.0 mmol/L

## Causes

- Renal failure (acute or chronic)
- Malignant disease: leukaemia, lymphoma, chemotherapy treatment
- Trauma or burns (white phosphorus in particular)
- Excessive exercise: release from muscle stores
- Any cause of acidosis
- Ischaemic bowel
- Malignant hyperpyrexia
- Hypothermia
- Haemolysis, outdated blood transfusion
- Prolonged immobilization
- Excessive intake or potassium phosphate treatment
- Hypoparathyroidism, acromegaly, thyrotoxicosis, glucocorticoid withdrawal
- Syndrome of familial intermittent hyperphosphataemia

## Presentation and assessment

Signs and symptoms are secondary to the hypocalcaemia which occurs alongside hyperphosphataemia

- General: cataracts, muscle cramps, Chvostek's sign, Trosseau's sign, perioral paraesthesia
- Neurological: altered sensorium, delirium, decreased consciousness, seizures, coma
- Cardiovascular: hypotension, cardiac failure
  - ECG changes: prolonged PR interval, prolonged QT interval

## Investigations

- ABGs
- FBC
- U&Es, calcium, magnesium, phosphate
- Serum glucose
- LFTs
- Serum PTH level
- Urinary myoglobin level
- ECG: prolonged QTc may occur

## Differential diagnoses

- Hypermagnesaemia
- Hyper- or hypocalcaemia

## Immediate management

- Give $O_2$ and support airway, breathing, and circulation as required
Treatment of the hypocalcaemia, which occurs as symptoms arise, takes precedence (see p. 226).
- Administration of insulin can hasten intracellular passage of phosphate as a temporizing measure
- Oral phosphate binders may be given (some can cause hypercalcaemia); avoid aluminium-containing binders as these may exacerbate renal failure
- Where toxic ingestion has occurred, gastric lavage and oral phosphate binders may be appropriate
- Consider using saline 0.9% with acetazolamide to increase urinary excretion
- Consider haemodialysis/haemofiltration for severe refractory cases or those with established renal failure

## Further management

- Continue to treat the underlying cause

## Further reading

Bugg NC, Jones JA (1998). Hypophosphataemia pathophysiology, effects and management on the intensive care unit. *Anaesthesia* **53**, 895–902.

Malluche HH, Mawad H (2002). Management of hyperphosphataemia of chronic kidney disease: lessons from the past and future directions. *Nephrol Dial Transplant* **17**, 1170–5.

# :Ö: Hypophosphataemia

- Normal     0.8–1.4 mmol/L
- Moderate   0.4–0.6 mmol/L
- Severe     &lt;0.4 mmol/L

## Causes

- Critical illness
- Re-feeding syndrome, post starvation, or during hyperalimentation
- Inadequate dietary intake: secondary to vitamin D deficiency and phosphate deficiency
- Ingestion of phosphate binding antacids
- Chronic liver disease or alcoholism
- Diuretic therapy, especially loop diuretics
- Hyperparathyroidism
- Lymphoma or leukaemia
- Hyperaldosteronism
- Steroid therapy
- Respiratory acidosis
- After high-dose glucose and insulin therapy
- Neurolept malignant syndrome

## Presentation and assessment

Hypophosphataemia is most commonly an incidental finding in the ICU. Where signs and symptoms are present they may include

- General symptoms: metabolic acidosis, myopathy, rhabdomyolysis
- Cardiovascular: cardiomyopathy, decreased cardiac output, VE
- Respiratory: failure to wean, respiratory failure, left shift of ODC secondary to decreased 2,3-diphosphoglycerate levels
- Neurological: encephalopathy, irritability, paraesthesia, seizures, coma
- Haematological: leucocyte and erythrocyte dysfunction, reduced platelet half-life, haemolytic anaemia

## Investigations

- ABGs
- FBC
- U&Es, calcium, magnesium, phosphate
- Serum glucose
- LFTs
- Serum PTH level
- Urinary myoglobin level

## Differential diagnoses

- Sampling error: tourniquet used on sample arm
- Alcoholic ketoacidosis
- DKA
- Guillain–Barré syndrome
- Hyperventilation syndrome

## Immediate management

- Give $O_2$ and support airway, breathing, and circulation as required
- Treatment is normally reserved for those with severe or sustained hypophosphataemia
  - IV therapy (usually reserved for phosphate <0.6 mmol/L): potassium acid phosphate 30 mmol over 4–6 hours in 100 ml saline if given centrally, or in 1000 ml saline if given peripherally
  - Oral therapy: Phosphate-Sandoz® two tablets 8-hourly

## Further management

- Continue to treat the underlying cause

## Pitfalls/difficult situations

- Replacing phosphate too rapidly may cause hypocalcaemia and metastatic calcification

## Further reading

Neligan P (2001). Phosphate. Available online at: www.ccmtutorials.com/misc/phosphate.
Mailhot T (2006). Hypophosphatemia. Available online at: www.emedicine.com/emerg/topic278.htm
OHCC p. 430.

# :⚙: **Hypermagnesaemia**

- Normal   0.7–1.0 mmol/L
- High   >2.5 mmol/L

## Causes

- Excessive intake or administration, most commonly due to
  - Magnesium-containing antacids, vitamins, or cathartics in patients with renal failure
  - Purgative abuse in anorexia nervosa
  - Inadvertent IV magnesium overdose, i.e. when treating PIH or dysrhythmias
- Intestinal hypomotility: decreased GI elimination and increased absorption
- Tumour lysis syndrome and rhabdomyolysis
- Adrenal insufficiency
- Hypothyroidism, hypoparathyroidism
- Lithium toxicity (also see below)
- Extracellular volume contraction in DKA or severe dehydration

## Presentation and assessment

- General symptoms: skin flushing, light-headedness
- Neurological: sedation, stupor, coma
- Neuromuscular: weakness, disappearance of tendon reflexes
  - Prolongation of neuromuscular blockade if muscle relaxants used
- Cardiovascular: hypotension, vasodilatation, bradycardia, arrhythmias (asystole, AF, intraventricular conduction delay), cardiac arrest
  - ECG changes: prolonged PR interval, broad QRS complexes, heart block
- Respiratory: bronchodilatation, respiratory depression, failure to wean
- Gastrointestinal: diarrhoea, nausea, vomiting
- Haematological: impaired coagulation due to platelet clumping and delayed thrombin formation

## Investigations

- ABGs
- U&Es, magnesium, calcium, phosphate
- Blood glucose
- TFTs
- PTH level
- Serum CK
- Urinary myoglobin level
- ECG

## Differential diagnoses

- Hypercalcaemia
- Hyperkalaemia
- Hypoparathyroidism
- Hypothyroidism and myxoedema coma
- Acute or chronic renal failure
- Rhabdomyolysis
- Lithium toxicity

### Signs of hypermagnesaemia

| Visible sign | Magnesium level (mmol/L) |
| --- | --- |
| Abolition of knee jerk | 3.0–5.5 |
| Risk of respiratory arrest | 5.0–7.5 |
| All deep tendon reflex abolition | >10 |
| Cardiac arrest | >15 |

### Immediate management

- Give $O_2$ and support airway, breathing, and circulation as required
- Give 10 ml 10% calcium gluconate IV over 10 min; repeat dose if necessary
- Give 50 ml 50% dextrose and 10 IU human soluble insulin over 1 hour
- Infuse saline 0.9% at 1 L/hour initially, inducing a diuresis using furosemide 20–40 mg IV; this may be repeated as necessary
- Dialysis with magnesium-free dialysate may be indicated in life-threatening situations

### Further management
- Treat any precipitating cause

### Pitfalls/difficult situations
- Elevation of magnesium is not commonly an isolated entity
- Magnesium potentiates the effects of muscle relaxants
- Avoid magnesium in patients with muscular dystrophies or myasthenia gravis

### Target plasma magnesium levels for therapies

| Treatment description | Target level (mmol/L) |
| --- | --- |
| General therapeutic level | 1.25–2.5 |
| Severe asthma | >1 |
| Pregnancy induced hypertension | 2–4 |

1 g magnesium = 4 mmol magnesium

### Further reading
Noronha JL, Matuschak GM (2002). Magnesium in critical illness: metabolism, assessment and treatment. *Intensive Care Med* **28**, 667–79.
📖 OHEA p. 288.

# ① Hypomagnesaemia

Hypomagnesaemia complicates >20% of critical care episodes. Serum ionized magnesium concentration is affected by many factors, including albumin concentration, and is a poor indicator of total body stores. Magnesium supplementation may required be in patients at risk of hypomagnesaemia, or symptomatic patients, even in the absence of low levels.

- Normal      0.7–1.0 mmol/L
- Low          <0.7 mmol/L

## Causes

- Elderly, malnourished, chronic alcohol abuse
- Metabolic acidosis, especially DKA with insulin administration
- Inadequate magnesium replacement with IV fluid therapy or TPN
- Diarrhoea, prolonged NG suction or drainage, bowel fistulae
- Malabsorption: colitis, radiation injury, short bowel syndrome
- Pancreatitis
- Excess renal losses: diuretic phase of ATN, interstitial nephritis, osmotic diuretics
- Drugs: loop diuretics, digoxin, gentamicin, amphotericin, cisplatin, cyclosporin
- Hyperaldosteronism
- Massive blood transfusion or volume overload
- 'Hungry bone syndrome' following surgery for hyperparathyroidism

## Presentation and assessment

Hypomagnesaemia is most commonly found as an incidental finding in ICU. Where signs and symptoms are present they may include

- General symptoms: anxiety, confusion, depression, psychosis
- Neurological and neuromuscular symptoms: coma, seizures, ataxia, vertigo, nystagmus, dysarthria, dysphagia, myoclonus, Trousseau's sign, Chvostek's sign, hyper-reflexia, weakness, muscle cramps
- Cardiovascular symptoms: palpitations, hypertension and angina, arrhythmias (most commonly SVT or AF; less commonly VT/VF or torsade de pointes)
  - ECG changes include prolonged PR and QT intervals, broadened QRS, inverted or peaked T waves, ST depression, U waves
  - Increased risk of digoxin toxicity
- Respiratory symptoms: stridor
- Biochemical: hypomagnesaemia may potentiate hypokalaemia and hypocalcaemia

## Investigations

- ABGs
- U&Es, magnesium, calcium, phosphate
- Serum glucose
- ECG

## Differential diagnoses

- Sampling error: tourniquet used on sample arm
- Hypocalcaemia
- Hypokalaemia

## Immediate management

- Give $O_2$ and support airway, breathing, and circulation as required
- Life-threatening complications such as stridor (see p. 16), coma (see p. 158), seizures (see p. 166), and tachycardia (see p. 140) should be treated according to the appropriate protocols alongside magnesium replacement
- Consider magnesium supplementation in patients at risk even in the absence of low levels

### Magnesium replacement/treatment regimens

- Asymptomatic, or minor symptoms
  - Replacement infusion: 20 mmol (5 g) over 1–2 hours (in 100 ml 5% dextrose) via central line; may need to be repeated; aim for symptom control with a plasma concentration >0.8 mmol/L
- PIH/eclampsia
  - Magnesium sulphate 16 mmol (4 g) IV in 100 ml* over 30 min
  - Followed by 4 mmol/hour (1 g/hour) over the the 24 hours following last seizure
  - If another seizure recurs in this time, give 8–16 mmol (2–4 g) over 5 min; aim for therapeutic level of 2–4 mmol/L
- Acute severe asthma
  - Magnesium sulphate 8–10 mmol (2.5 g) IV in 100 ml* over 5–10 min
  - Followed by 50–100 mmol (12–25 g) over the next 24 hours
- Dysrhythmias
  - AF or atrial flutter: consider a bolus of magnesium sulphate 8–10 mmol (2.5 g) IV in 100 ml* over 5–30 min depending upon severity, followed by a replacement infusion if required, aiming for plasma concentration of 1.4–1.8 mmol/L
  - In torsade de pointes give as per the severe asthma protocol
- Acute MI: routine magnesium treatment is no longer recommended
- Stroke and neurological injury: some centres use magnesium therapy; there is no commonly accepted protocol

* Low concentrations of magnesium may be given via peripheral IV access and are compatible with either 0.9% saline or 5% dextrose

## Further management

- Continue to treat precipitants
- Keep magnesium level >0.8 mmol/L

## Pitfalls/difficult situations

- Rapid administration of magnesium can lead to hypotension and/or flushing and muscle weakness. Where rapid replacement is required it may be advisable to simultaneously volume resuscitate or provide vasopressor/inotropic support to those with initial compromise
- Alcohol withdrawal can be exacerbated by hypomagnesaemia

## Further reading

Tong GM, Rude RK (2005). Magnesium deficiency in critical illness. *J Intensive Care Med* **20**, 3–17.
📖 OHCC p. 424, OHEA p. 290.

# :❂: **Diabetic ketoacidosis**

Diabetic ketoacidosis (DKA) occurs almost exclusively in type I diabetes and is a state of absolute or relative insulin deficiency aggravated by ensuing hyperglycaemia, dehydration, ketonaemia, and acidosis.

## Causes

One way of remembering the causes of DKA is to consider the "five I's"
- Infection (30%): commonly UTI, URTI, LRTI, or skin
- Incidental new diabetes (25%)
- Insufficient insulin (20%)
- Infarction: MI, CVA, GI tract, peripheral vasculature
- Intercurrent illness: almost any underlying condition can precipitate DKA, but diarrhoea and/or vomiting are particularly common catalysts

## Presentation and assessment

- General signs and symptoms
  - 2–3 day history of gradual deterioration and ensuing dehydration, associated with polydipsia, polyuria
  - Ill appearance, dry skin and mucous membranes, decreased skin turgor
  - Hypothermia or fever if infection present
- Neurological and neuromuscular symptoms: decreased reflexes, drowsiness, coma (resulting from the fall in pH)
- Cardiovascular symptoms: tachycardia, hypotension
- Respiratory symptoms: hyperventilation or breathlessness; characteristic Kussmaul's respiration with subjective dyspnoea
  - Smell of acetone on the breath (described as similar to pear-drops/nail-varnish remover)
- Gastrointestinal: abdominal pain, nausea, and vomiting
- Biochemical: triad of hyperglycaemia (blood glucose >10 mmol/L), ketonaemia (urinary ketones), and acidaemia (pH <7.3, serum bicarbonate <15 mmol/L)

Diagnosis requires positive serum ketones and arterial pH <7.30 and/or serum bicarbonate <15 mmol/L

## Investigations

- ABGs (to assess pH and bicarbonate/base excess, but see Pitfalls)
  - Venous blood gases may be used as an alternative
- FBC, as WCC often elevated.
- U&Es, LFTs, serum phosphate, magnesium, calcium
- Serum glucose, normally >10.0 mmol/L, although acidosis can still exist at lower levels if insulin has only recently been used
- CRP
- Cardiac enzymes/troponins
- Septic screen: blood, sputum, and urine cultures
- Urinalysis: strongly positive for ketones (captopril can give a false-positive test for urinary acetone); may also suggest UTI
- CXR, looking specifically for any infective foci
- ECG, to eliminate MI

**Differential diagnoses**

Any conditions causing acidosis without elevation of plasma glucose including

- Sepsis
- Renal failure
- Salicylate overdose
- Inborn errors of metabolism
- Alcoholic ketoacidosis
- Hyperosmolar non-ketotic coma

**Immediate management**

- Give $O_2$ and support airway, breathing, and circulation as required

The priority is to correct hypovolaemia

- Site large-bore IV cannula; central access may be needed in patients with major cardiac disease or autonomic nephropathy or the elderly
- If hypotensive and oliguric give IV colloids or saline to restore BP
- Rehydrate with
  - 1 L saline 0.9% over 30 min
  - 1 L saline 0.9% with $K^+$ 2-hourly for 8 hours
  - 1 L saline 0.9% with $K^+$ 4-hourly until rehydrated
  - The above should be followed with caution in the elderly or those with cardiac disease by careful titration with CVP and clinical status, aiming to restore hydration status within 12–24 hours
- In unstable or severely acidotic patients insert arterial line to monitor replacement adequacy via ABGs
- Catheterize if patient is oliguric or has a high serum creatinine

  Commence glycaemic correction once fluid resuscitation is underway
  - Give insulin (0.1 unit/kg IV bolus, then infusion at 0.1 unit/kg/hour)
  - Titrate insulin according to an accepted regime (see p. 239)
  - Aim for fall of 5 mmol/L/hour with correction of bicarbonate and acidosis
  - Replace potassium according to an accepted protocol (see p. 239) as insulin shifts $K^+$ into the cells causing life-threatening hypokalaemia
  - Avoid bicarbonate, even if the acidosis is severe pH<7. It can cause severe sodium overload and intracellular acidosis. Relative CSF alkalosis will depress respiration which compromises respiratory compensation

Give 5000 units heparin SC as DVT prophylaxis

**Further management**

- Initially monitor $K^+$, glucose, creatinine, and bicarbonate hourly
- Watch for dysrhythmias due to changes in $K^+$ level
- Once glucose <11 mmol/L, change fluids to 5% dextrose or dextrose 4%–saline 0.18%
- Gastroparesis is common; consider placing an NGT
- Continue to investigate the cause of the disturbance that initiated the episode

**Pitfalls/difficult situations**

- Plasma glucose is not always high, especially if the patient has been vomiting
- High WCC may be seen, even in the absence of infection
- Ketonaemia may result in falsely high creatinine levels
- Hyponatraemia is common
- Ketonuria does not mean ketoacidosis; alcohol may be the cause if glucose is normal
- Amylase is often raised (by up to 10×) along with non-specific abdominal pain, even in the absence of pancreatitis
- If the patient requires mechanical ventilation, hyperventilate to maintain physiological compensation for acidosis and monitor ABGs
- Bicarbonate therapy may be indicated in those with ketoacidosis and a normal anion gap as they have fewer ketones available to regenerate bicarbonate during insulin administration
- Hyperchloraemic acidosis caused by aggressive fluid resuscitation may complicate the recovery stage 12–24 hours later; clinical indices of recovery are usually reassuring by this stage
- Repeated arterial blood sampling is painful, and some diabetic patients become reluctant to present to hospital as a result; in most cases ABGs are not required or venous gases may be used instead
- Amylase (amylase may be high and abdominal pain or vomiting present, even in the absence of pancreatitis); if pancreatitis is suspected consider US or CT imaging
- In some cases as the insulin rate is reduced ketogenesis increases; it may be necessary to keep the insulin infusion rate high and maintain blood glucose with 10% dextrose

**Further reading**

BSPED recommended DKA guidelines (2001). Available online at: www.bsped.org.uk/dka.htm
DiNubile MJ (1983). Plasma acid–base patterns in ketoacidosis. *N Engl J Med* **308**, 1165.
OHCC pp. 440, 442, OHEA p. 246.

**Suggested insulin sliding scale for diabetic ketoacidosis**

| Hourly blood glucose (mmol/L) | Insulin infusion (units/h)[*] |
|---|---|
| 0.0–2.0 | 0.5 (give IV glucose)[†] |
| 2.1–5.0 | 0.5 |
| 5.1–7.0 | 1 |
| 7.1–10.0 | 2 |
| 10.1–15.0 | 3 |
| 15.1–20.0 | 4 |
| 20.1–28.0 | 6 |
| >28.1 | Call doctor |

[*] Add 50 units Actrapid insulin to 50 ml saline 0.9%
[†] If hypoglycaemia is refractory to treatment stop insulin and seek senior advice

**Potassium replacement during resuscitation of diabetic ketoacidosis**

| Plasma potassium | Amount of $K^+$ added to each litre |
|---|---|
| <3.0 mmol/L | 40 mmol |
| <4.0 mmol/L | 30 mmol |
| <5.0 mmol/L | 20 mmol |

# ✺ Hyperosmolar non-ketotic crisis

Hyperosmolar non-ketotic crisis (HONK) typically occurs in elderly type II diabetic patients who present following a longer history. Compared with DKA the blood sugar is often very high (>35 mmol/L) and severe dehydration with no acidosis is present.

## Presentation and assessment

- Respiration is usually normal
- Neurological symptoms predominate
  - Confusion, agitation, or drowsiness are common
  - Coma is more frequent and mortality is much higher than in DKA
  - Presentation occasionally includes focal neurology, CVA, seizures
- Thrombotic events may occur: DVT or MI
- Biochemistry
  - Acidosis is not usually present as there is sufficient insulin to prevent lipolysis and ketogenesis
  - Serum osmolality >340 mosmol/kg

## Investigations

The same investigations as those required in DKA are suggested (see p. 236). The following findings may be apparent:

- ABGs (typically there is no acidaemia, coexistent lactic acidaemia considerably worsens the prognosis)
- Serum glucose (usually >35 mmol/L)
- Plasma osmolality (>350 mosmol/L)
- U&Es: severe dehydration causes a greater rise in urea than creatinine, and significant hypernatraemia may be hidden by the high glucose

## Immediate management

As for DKA (see p. 237) with slight differences:

- Give $O_2$ and support airway, breathing, and circulation as required
- Fluid replacement
  - Treat as for DKA but give 0.45% saline if plasma Na >150 mmol/L
  - Replace fluids at half rate of DKA regime over 48 hours as there is a risk of cerebral oedema; the suggested rate is 100–200 mL/hour
- Insulin treatment
  - Wait 1 hour before giving insulin as it may not be needed
  - Patients are often hypersensitive to insulin
- Correct serum phosphate and magnesium which often fall rapidly

Risk of DVT is higher; therefore full anticoagulation is advised

## Further reading

www.diabetesindia.com/diabetes/hyperglycaemic_honk.htm
📖 OHCC p. 444.

## ☠ Hypoglycaemia

Hypoglycaemia most commonly occurs in insulin-dependent diabetic patients, but can also occur in other conditions. Rapid recognition and correction is essential to avoid fitting or other complications. Prolonged hypoglycaemia can cause irreversible brain damage.

- Normal              3.5–5.5 mmol/L (fasting)
- Hypoglycaemia       <2.8 mmol/L[*]

Causes

- Insulin
    - Deliberate/accidental insulin overdose
    - Inappropriate insulin (e.g. given when unable to eat)
    - Insulinoma
- Oral hypoglycaemics: sulphonylureas
- Other drugs: aspirin, β-blockers, quinine, septrin, pentamidine
- Endocrine: Addison's disease, hypopituitarism, hypothyroidism
- Hepatic failure
- Starvation
- Alcohol
- Severe sepsis
- Sarcomas

Presentation and assessment

Hypoglycaemia is more common in the elderly

- Adrenergic symptoms
    - Hunger, or nausea and vomiting
    - Pallor, sweating, palpitations, tremor
    - Tachycardia and tachypnoea
- Neuroglycopenic symptoms
    - Confusion, agitation, aggression
    - Focal neurological signs, blurred vision
    - Fatigue, drowsiness
    - Seizures, coma

In sedated patients signs and symptoms may be missed. Regular blood sugar monitoring is essential, especially in those at high risk

- Patients on tight glycaemic control regimes
- Liver failure
- Extremes of age
- Patients on quinine therapy for malaria

Investigations

- Bedside blood sugar monitoring (BM sticks) is adequate in most cases
    - Where BM is persistently low confirm the reading with a formal blood glucose reading

---

[*] Symptoms of hypoglycaemia can occur at normal blood sugar levels in diabetic patients, particularly those with poor blood sugar control

Other investigations may be indicated:
- FBC, coagulation screen
- U&Es, LFTs
- TFTs, cortisol
- Blood alcohol level, paracetamol and salicylate levels
- C-peptide if an endogenous source of insulin is suspected
- Septic screen: blood, sputum, and urine cultures
- CXR
- CT head, lumbar puncture

**Differential diagnoses**
- Hypothyroidism
- Psychosis
- Neurological disorder: stroke, CVA, epilepsy, meningitis
- Inadvertent sympathomimetic overdose

**Immediate management**

- Give $O_2$ and support airway, breathing, and circulation as required
- Treat any seizures (see p. 166) and simultaneously correct glucose
- Glucose replacement
  - Oral sugary fluids or snacks
  - Glucagon 1 mg IM if unable to take oral glucose
  - 25% glucose 25 ml IV
  - A continuous infusion of high-dose glucose (i.e. 50% glucose at 10–50 ml/hour, ideally given via a central line) may be required
- Regularly monitor BM

**Further management**
- Monitor potassium levels: replacement will be required for those patients who have been given large amounts of glucose and have a functioning pancreas, or who have also taken large quantities of insulin
- If on an insulin sliding scale consider adjusting the regime to avoid further episodes
- If no cause for hypoglycaemia is found consider giving hydrocortisone 200 mg IV to exclude Addison's disease
- Octreotide may help in cases of insulinoma
- Give thiamine if alcoholism or malnutrition is suspected

**Pitfalls/difficult situations**
- Hypoglycaemia occurring with long-acting sulphonylureas such as chlorpropamide or glibenclamide may be prolonged
- Deliberate insulin overdose can result in prolonged intractable hypoglycaemia, which may recur after treatment; prolonged BM monitoring will be required
- Surgical excision of the insulin injection site has been attempted for large overdoses of long-acting insulin
- Check blood sugar in patients when confronted with seizures or coma
- In the elderly the effects of hypoglycaemia can mimic a stroke

**Further reading**
📖 OHCC p. 438, OHEA p. 262.

## ☢ Addison's disease

Addison's disease is an endocrine disorder caused by failure of the adrenal glands to produce enough of the hormone cortisol and, in some cases, the hormone aldosterone. The disease is also called adrenal insufficiency or hypocortisolism. Addisonian crisis occurs when there is a severe phase of the attack, usually due to a precipitating cause.

### Causes
- Autoimmune adrenalitis (80%)
- Tuberculosis or malignant secondaries of the adrenal glands
- Adrenal haemorrhage (Waterhouse–Friedrichsen syndrome)
- Hypopituitarism
- Drugs: metyrapone, aminoglutethamide, ketoconazole, etomidate (especially given via infusion), rifampicin, phenytoin, phenobarbitone
- Physiological stressors (these can also be crisis precipitants): infection, trauma, surgery, sepsis, burns
- Cessation of steroid therapy

### Presentation and assessment
- General signs and symptoms
  - Weight loss, fatigue, weakness, myalgia, anorexia dehydration
  - Precipitant symptoms: fever, night sweats (infection), flank pain (infarction)
  - Hyperpigmentation may occur in chronic disease
- Cardiovascular
  - Postural hypotension
  - Shock, tachycardia, peripheral vasoconstriction, oliguria
  - Life-threatening arrhythmias
- Gastrointestinal
  - Nausea and vomiting
  - Diarrhoea and abdominal pain are present in 20% of cases
- Psychiatric features: asthenia, depression, apathy and confusion

### Investigations
- ABG, showing a metabolic acidosis, respiratory failure, low bicarbonate
- FBC, anaemia with normal MCV, moderate neutropenia, relative eosinophilia/lymphocytosis
- U&Es: likely to reveal hyponatraemia/hyperkalaemia with Na:K ratio <21:1; dehydration
- Serum glucose: may show hypoglycaemia
- Serum calcium: may be high but when corrected usually normal
- Serum cortisol/ACTH: prior to hydrocortisone administration (baseline cortisol <400 nmol/L and should be >1000 nmol/L in sick patients)
- Short synacthen test: no response expected (250 µg tetracosactide given, cortisol measured at 0 and 30 min: if second cortisol >500 nmol/L and 200 nmol/L greater than baseline, Addison's disease is excluded)
- Septic screen: blood, urine, and sputum cultures
- ECG to exclude MI, PR/QTc prolongation
- CXR: previous TB or bronchial carcinoma
- AXR: adrenal calcification

**Differential diagnoses**
- Acute abdomen
- Septic shock

**Immediate management**

- Give $O_2$ and support airway, breathing, and circulation as required
Do not delay treatment whilst awaiting urgent laboratory tests
- Take blood for cortisol (10 mL heparin or clotted) and ACTH (10 mL heparin)
- Give hydrocortisone 200 mg IV stat followed by 100 mg 6-hourly
- Resuscitate with colloid first; then maintenance saline 0.9%
- Inotropes/vasopressors may be required, but are likely to be ineffective unless cortisol replaced
- Serum glucose should be monitored as there is a danger of hypoglycaemia
  - If hypoglycaemic give 50 ml 50% dextrose

**Further management**
- Treat primary cause
- Guide fluid therapy using more invasive monitoring if necessary so as to avoid extreme fluid overload
- If response is poor suspect other autoimmune diseases: check TFTs, do coeliac serology
- Consider fludrocortisone PO 50 µg every second day up to 0.15 mg daily
- Hypoadrenalism related to sepsis can be treated with hydrocortisone 50 mg IV 6-hourly for 7 days; a reducing dose is then given over 7 days
- Dexamethasone can be used for steroid replacement for 48 hours before the synacthen test as it does not interfere with cortisol assays

**Pitfalls/difficult situations**
- Unexplained abdominal symptoms could herald the disease
- Do not be afraid to perform a synacthen test if at all suspicious

| Equivalent doses of glucocorticoids | |
| --- | --- |
| Dexamethasone | 0.75 mg |
| Methylprednisolone | 4 mg |
| Triamcinolone | 4 mg |
| Prednisolone | 5 mg |
| Hydrocortisone | 20 mg |
| Cortisone acetate | 25 mg |

**Further reading**
Cooper MS, Stewart PM (2003). Current concepts: corticosteroid insufficiency in acutely ill patients. *N Engl J Med* **348**, 727–34.
Masterson GR, Mostafa SM (1998). Adrenocortical function in critical illness *Br J Anaesth* **81**, 308–10.
OHCC p. 448, OHEA p. 260.

# :O: **Thyroid storm**

Thyroid storm is a clinical syndrome marked by exaggerated manifestations of thyrotoxicosis. It represents the most serious complication of hyperthyroidism and carries a high mortality.

## Causes
- Graves disease, hyperfunctioning thyroid multinodular goitre, TSH-secreting tumour, radio-iodine therapy, excess thyroxine intake
- Excess handling of thyroid gland intra-operatively
- Various conditions or treatments may trigger thyroid storm in susceptible individuals
  - Surgery or trauma
  - Sepsis, DKA, PE, MI
  - Labour
  - Drugs: ephedrine, atropine, radiocontrast

## Presentation and assessment
- General signs and symptoms:
  - Fever (>38.5°C), often hyperpyrexia
  - Sweating, fatigue, other signs associated with of hyperthyroidism
- Cardiovascular: angina, sinus tachycardia >140 beats/min (disproportionate to fever), AF, multifocal ventricular ectopics, hypertension followed by hypotension, cardiac failure (30% of cases)
- Respiratory: tachypnoea, failure to wean, 'fighting' the ventilator
- Neurological: agitation, delirium, aggression, seizures, coma
- Gastrointestinal: anorexia, weight loss, abdominal pain, nausea, vomiting, diarrhoea, hepatic failure
- Renal failure (secondary to rhabdomyolysis)
- Multi-organ failure

## Investigations
Diagnosis is clinically based; no laboratory tests are diagnostic. Do not delay treatment whilst awaiting laboratory results.
- TFTs (T3, free T4 and TSH): elevated T4/T3, suppressed TSH
- ABGs
- FBC
- U&Es, LFTs, calcium, magnesium, serum glucose
- Blood and urine cultures
- Urinary myoglobin
- ECG
- CXR

## Differential diagnoses
- MH
- Phaeochromocytoma
- Infection/sepsis
- Anticholinergic or adrenergic drug intoxication
- CCF
- Essential hypertension
- Hyperthyroidism

Immediate management

- Give $O_2$ and support airway, breathing, and circulation as required
Symptom control is the priority, rather than correcting thyroid status
- Do not await laboratory test confirmation of suspected diagnosis
- Protect and support airway and breathing as required
- Circulatory support with IV saline may be required in view of large insensible losses
- Replace glucose as required
- Hyperpyrexia (also see p. 252) cooling measures; consider
  - Tepid sponging, femoral ice packs, cooling blankets
  - Peritoneal or NG lavage with ice-cold fluid
  - Haemofiltration or endovascular temperature therapy catheter
  - Antipyretics: IV paracetamol 1 g 6-hourly; **do not use NSAIDs or other drugs which displace thyroid hormone from binding sites**
  - Consider dantrolene as $T_4$ causes calcium release from SR, similar to MH (see p. 258)
- Hyperadrenergic state
  - Propranolol 1–5 mg IV up to 10 mg (can precipitate CCF); aim for pulse rate <100 beats/min
  - Alternatively consider esmolol 250–500 μg/kg loading, then 50–100 μg/kg/min (but see comments below)
  - Reserpine 2.5–5 mg 6-hourly may be given.
  - Consider deepening sedation to obtund any exaggerated sympathetic responses
  - Adrenal insufficiency: give IV hydrocortisone 200 mg 6-hourly or dexamethasone 2 mg IV 6-hourly
- Excess $T_4/T_3$ treatment
  - Propranolol and steroid (as above) in combination reduce organification of iodine, inhibit iodide transport, reduce peripheral conversion of $T_4$ to $T_3$ and reduces $T_4$ release (**only propranolol has this effect**)

Further management
- Following IV loading, commence oral propranolol 20–40 mg 6-hourly
- Start oral propylthiouracil 1 g loading, then 200–300 mg 6-hourly

**It is important to give propylthiouracil first, as iodine can cause increased release of thyroid hormone.**
- Following propylthiouracil, give oral Lugol's iodine 5–10 drops 6-hourly
  - Alternatively: sodium iodide 500 mg 8-hourly IV , or
  - Potassium iodide 200–600 mg IV over 2 hours then 2 g/day PO
- Consider carbimazole 60–120 mg/day PO (beware of agranulocytosis)
- Treat the precipitating condition

Pitfalls/difficult situations
- Cardioversion of dysrhythmias is unlikely to be successful until the patient is biochemically euthyroid
- β-Blockade with propanolol may still be the drug of choice even where cardiac failure is present

- Thyroid hormone has a half-life of 3–6 days; amelioration of symptoms cannot occur until this vascular pool has been depleted; peritoneal dialysis and plasmaphoresis may speed up vascular depletion
- Oral cholestyramine resin PO can bind thyroid hormone entering the gut via the enterohepatic circulation, resulting in resin–hormone complex excretion

### Further reading

Migneco A, Ojetti V, Testa A, De Lorenzo A, Gentiloni Silveri N (2005). Management of thyrotoxic crisis. *Eur Rev Med Pharmacol Sci* **9**, 69–74.

Singhal A, Campbell DE (2004). Thyroid storm. Available online at: www.emedicine.com/ped/topic2247.htm

OHCC p. 446, OHEA p. 256.

# ☼ Phaeochromacytoma

Phaeochromocytomas are catecholamine-producing tumours, 90% of which derive from the adrenal medulla. They occasionally present acutely, or coincidentally with another condition.

## Causes

Phaeochromocytomas may present in isolation (10% malignant, 10% bilateral, 10% familial, 10% extra-adrenal) or as part of a syndrome

- von Recklinghausen's disease (phaeochromocytoma, neurofibromata, café au lait spots, Lisch nodules, axillary freckling)
- von Hippel–Lindau disease (phaeochromocytoma, cerebellar haemangioblastomas, retinal haemangiomas, other neoplasms)
- MEN 2a (phaeochromocytoma, hyperparathyroidism, and medullary carcinoma thyroid).
- MEN 2b (phaeochromocytoma, Marfanoid appearance, thyroid carcinoma, bowel ganglioneuromatosis, hypertrophied corneal nerves)

## Presentation and assessment

Symptoms and signs are more likely to manifest after painful procedures, endotracheal intubation, or direct tumour manipulation.

- General signs and symptoms
  - Anxiety, tremor, weakness, faintness, paraesthesia
  - Cold extremities, pallor, drenching perspiration
- Cardiovascular
  - Myocardial ischaemia, palpitations, tachycardia, AF or VF
  - Hypertension: sustained or paroxysmal
- Metabolic: unexplained lactic acidosis

## Investigations

- ABGs (to exclude tissue acidosis)
- U&Es (hypokalaemia and hyperuricaemia may be present)
- Serum glucose (hyperglycaemia may be present)
- 24 hour urine collection for VMA level (a catecholamine metabolite; false-positive results occur in 15% of essential hypertensives)
- 24 hour collection for catecholamines and metanephrine
- Plasma catecholamines (sample must be heparinized and kept on ice during rapid transfer for analysis; test may not be available)
- Pentolinium suppression test (plasma catecholamine samples taken 10 and 30 min after 2.5–5 mg pentolinium IV should be suppressed)
- CT/MRI scan to localize any tumour
- MIBG scan (to localize tumour or seek secondaries)
- Serial ECG/troponins/echocardiography

## Differential diagnoses

- Inadequate sedation, analgesia, or anaesthesia
- Pre-existing uncontrolled hypertension exacerbated by invasive procedures or poor sedation
- Pre-eclampsia
- Raised intracranial pressure

- Thyroid storm or hyperthyroidism
- Carcinoid
- Insulinoma
- Inadvertent bolus of vasopressors
- Administration of indirect acting vasopressors (e.g. ephedrine, pseudo-ephedrine) to patients taking monoamine oxidase inhibitors

### Immediate management

- Give $O_2$ and support airway, breathing, and circulation as required
- Stop any avoidable stimulus
  - Deepen any anaesthesia/sedation whilst administering IV opioids
- Insert invasive monitoring
  - An arterial line will be needed to monitor BP closely
  - Commence adequate fluid replacement with CVP monitoring, as most patients are volume depleted
- Adrenergic control
  - Sole β-blockade may precipitate a hypertensive crisis due to unopposed α-receptor stimulation
  - Give phentolamine (non-selective α-blocker) 2–5 mg IV bolus and repeat as necessary to control hypertension
  - Alternatively doxazosin 2–4 mg/day (selective $α_1$ blocker; therefore less need for β-blockade)
  - If further hypertensive control is required, consider adding magnesium sulphate 5 g (20 mmol) loading, then 2 g/hour (8 mmol)aiming for a therapeutic level of 1.5 mmol/L, or sodium nitroprusside 0.5–1.5 µg/kg/min
  - After α-blockade, if HR >100 beats/min or frequent VEs, give labetalol 5–10 mg IV increments (β-blocker with weak $α_1$ blockade)
  - For further tachyarrhythmias consider esmolol 1.5 mg/kg bolus IV

### Further management

- Stabilize on anti-hypertensive regime
- The definitive treatment is excision of the primary tumour

### Pitfalls/difficult situations

- MI can develop rapidly, particularly in elderly patients or those with pre-existing stable or unstable cardiac disease
- If undiagnosed, peri-operatively phaeochromacytoma has a 50% mortality
- Sole β-blockade can lead to severe hypertension and congestive cardiac failure; do not institute β-blockade until α-blockade is established.
- IV labetalol should not be given as the sole anti-hypertensive as it has a β:α blockade ratio of 7:1
- Phaeochromocytoma causes patients to have volume depletion masked by hypertension

### Further reading

Nguyen-Martin MA, Hammer GD (2006). Phaeochromocytoma: an update on risk groups, diagnosis and management. *Hosp Physician* **42**, 17–24.
📖 OHEA p. 258.

# :Ö: Hyperpyrexia

Hyperthermia is defined as core body temperature above normal (>38°C). Severe hyperthermia is core body temperature >40.5°C sustained for over 1 hour.

At >42°C cellular enzymes cease to function, proteins are denatured, and there is extensive damage to vital organs, particularly endothelium, nervous tissue, and liver.

## Causes

Hyperthermia is caused by increased production of body heat, decreased dissipation, or a combination of both. The common causes of hyperthermia in critical care are

- Infection, sepsis
- Burns (probably due to resetting of central thermostat)
- Acute liver failure
- Mismatched blood transfusion (release of pyrogens)
- Post-traumatic
- Endocrine disorders: hyperthyroidism, phaeochromocytoma
- CNS disorders: head injury, SAH, meningitis, encephalitis, seizures
- Specific syndromes: toxic epidermal necrolysis, neurolept malignant syndrome, malignant hyperthermia
- Toxicity: amphetamines, salicylates, cocaine, phencyclidine, lysergic acid diethylamide (LSD)

A number of factors can predispose to developing hyperthermia
- Behavioural factors: inappropriate over-clothing, poor fluid intake/ dehydration, hyperactivity/over-exertion
- Drugs: anticholinergics and phenothiazines (lack of sweating), salicylates (uncouple oxidative phosphorylation), diuretics (dehydration), ketamine (vasoconstriction), tricyclic antidepressants (increased muscle rigidity, depressed sweating), MAO inhibitors (increased muscle rigidity), sympathetic (α- and β-receptor) blockers (decreased heat loss), sympathomimetics (increased heat production), hallucinogens (ecstacy: depressed sweating, increased muscle activity, increased metabolism)
- Illnesses: Parkinsonism, delirium tremens, psychosis, cardiovascular disease (inability to increase CO for heat dissipation), autonomic dysfunction, endocrine dysfunction

## Presentation and assessment

*In a non-sedated patient the following may be present*
- Mild hyperthermia (37–39°C)
  - Apathy, malaise
  - Headache
  - Dizziness
  - Tachycardia/wide pulse pressure
  - Hyperventilation
  - Metabolic acidosis
  - Nausea and vomiting

- Severe hyperthermia (>40.5°C)
  - Confusion
  - Ataxia
  - Muscle rigidity/dystonia
  - Syncope
  - Focal neurological signs
  - Seizures
  - Coma
  - Metabolic acidosis
  - Tachycardia and hypotension
  - Hyperventilation/respiratory exhaustion/hypercapnia

*In a sedated and ventilated patient, the following may be present*
- Arrhythmias, tachycardia, and/or cardiovascular failure
- Metabolic acidosis
- Hypercapnia
- Muscle rigidity

*Prolonged untreated hyperthermia can lead to*
- Muscle damage/rhabdomyolysis
- Cardiovascular failure
- ARDS
- DIC (denatured clotting factors, endothelial damage)
- Renal failure (due to dehydration, hypotension, rhabdomyolysis)
- Liver dysfunction
- Lactic acidosis
- Electrolyte imbalance (hypernatraemia, hypo/hyperkalaemia, hypocalcaemia)

Investigations
- ABGs
- FBC and coagulation screen
- U&Es (to look for dehydration, renal failure; electrolyte imbalance)
- CK (to look for rhabdomyolysis)
- Serum magnesium, phosphate and calcium
- LFTs and amylase
- TFTs, serum cortisol
- Septic screen: blood, urine, and sputum cultures
- Urine for toxicology
- Urine myoglobinurea
- ECG
- CXR
- Consider CT scan or lumbar puncture (for evidence of infection)

Differential diagnoses
- Malignant hyperpyrexia: more likely to present during anaesthesia and surgery after exposure to a triggering agent (see p. 258)
- Neurolept malignant syndrome: associated with history of intake of neuroleptic drugs (phenothiazines, butyrophenones) or tranquillizers. Can also be seen after withdrawl of anti-parkinsonian drugs and metaclopramide

## Immediate management

- Give $O_2$ and support airway, breathing, and circulation as required
- Start cooling as soon as possible
- Sedation and ventilation along with neuromuscular block may be required to reduce heat production
- Give IV fluids ideally guided by CVP and other invasive
- haemodynamic monitoring
- For cooling consider
  - Antipyretics (paracetamol and/or NSAIDs)
  - Peripheral cooling using exposure, sponging, and fan
  - Cooling blankets and mattresses
  - Cold IV fluids
  - Cold irrigation of the stomach
  - Use of central venous systems (Coolguard™)
  - Haemofilteration using cold fluids
- Avoid rapid changes in pH; severe metabolic acidosis (pH <7.1) may be corrected using bicarbonate infusion

## Further management

- Active cooling should continue until core temperature reaches <38°C
- Continue full invasive monitoring
- Continue to monitor for DIC, metabolic acidosis, and electrolyte imbalance during and after cooling
- Correct any electrolyte changes
- Treat arrhythmias if these cause haemodynamic compromise
- Consider supportive measures for rhabdomyolysis (see p. 278)
- Seizures prevention or treatment may be required with phenytoin or diazepam (see p. 166)
- Inotropic support may be required
- Ventilation support may be required
- Drug therapy with paracetamol or NSAIDs may be effective in patients with hyperthermia due to proven infection
- α-Antagonists have been used to vasodilate to improve heat loss

## Pitfalls/difficult situations

- Peripheral temperature in a vasoconstricted patient may not reflect central temperature
- Be prepared to treat severe arrhythmias
- Peripheral cooling may cause vasoconstriction preventing further heat loss

## Further reading

📖 OHCC p. 518.

# ✪ Neuroleptic malignant syndrome

This is potentially a fatal idiosyncratic response to neuroleptic drugs and tranquillizers. These drugs include phenothiazines, butyrophenones, thioxanthines, and lithium; more common in males and at <40 years of age.

## Causes
- Drugs as above
- Often triggered by: exercise, exhaustion, dehydration

## Presentation and assessment
- Muscle rigidity and akinesia
- Sweating
- Rapid rise in core body temperature
- Labile blood pressure (autonomic impairment)
- Tachycardia and other dysrhythmias
- Metabolic acidosis
- Complications as in hyperpyrexia (see p. 253)

## Investigations
As for hyperpyrexia (see p.252)

## Differential diagnoses
- MH
- Sepsis
- Tetanus
- Heat stroke
- Parkinson's disease

## Immediate management
- Stop causative agents
- Supportive management as in hyperpyrexia (see p. 254)
- Cooling as in hyperpyrexia (see p.254)
- Consider the following drug therapy
  - Dantrolene (see MH for dosage p.258)
  - Diazepam
  - Levodopa (orally)
  - Bromocriptine
  - Amantidine

## Further management
- Repeat drug therapy if required
- Continue monitoring and support therapy for at least 72 hours
- Otherwise follow management plan for hyperpyrexia

## Further reading
Adnet P, Lestavel P, Krivosec-Horber R (2000). Neuroleptic malignant syndrome *Br J Anaesth* **85**, 129–35.

# ☠ Malignant hyperpyrexia

This is an inherited disorder which in susceptible individuals exposed to triggering agents causes intense muscle activity and a hypermetabolic state. MH is unlikely to occur in critical care as most triggering agents are used during anaesthesia; however, these patients will be admitted to critical care for management.

## Guidelines for the management of a malignant hyperthermia crisis

*Know where dantrolene is stored*

**Diagnosis, consider MH if**
1. Masseter muscle spasm after suxamethonium
2. Unexplained unexpected tachycardia together with
3. Unexplained unexpected increase in end-tidal $CO_2$

**Early management**
1. Withdraw all trigger agents (i.e. all anaesthetic vapours)
2. Install clean anaesthetic breathing system and hyperventilate
3. Abandon surgery if feasible
4. Give dantrolene IV 1 mg/kg initially and repeat PRN up to 10 mg/kg
5. Measure ABGs, $K^+$, and CK
6. Measure core temperature
7. Surface cooling avoiding vasoconstriction

**Intermediate management**
1. Control serious arrhythmias (e.g. with β-blockers)
2. Control hyperkalaemia and metabolic acidosis

**Later management**
1. Clotting screen to detect DIC
2. Take first voided urine sample for myoglobin estimation
3. Observe urine output for developing renal failure
4. Promote diuresis with fluid/mannitol (20 mg dantrolene contains 3 mg mannitol)
5. Repeat CK at 24 hours

**Late management**
1. Consider other diagnoses and do appropriate investigations, e.g. VMA, thyroid function tests, WCC, CXR
2. Consider possibility of myopathy, neurological opinion, EMG
3. Consider possibility of recreational drug abuse (ecstasy)
4. Consider possibility of neurolept malignant syndrome
5. Counsel patient and/or their family regarding implications of MH
6. Refer patient to MH unit

Adapted from guidelines of the same name supported by the Association of Anaesthetists of Great Britain and Ireland and the British MH Association. 1998

## Further reading

Hopkins PM (2000). Malignant hyperthermia: advances in clinical management and diagnosis. *Br J Anaesth* **85**, 118–128

📖 OHEA p. 248.

# ☼ Hypothermia

Hypothermia is defined as core temperature (and not peripheral temperature) of <35°C. Mild hypothermia is between 32 and 35°C, moderate between 28 and 32°C, and severe <28°C.

Temperature measured at peripheral sites (skin) may be up to 2°C lower than that measured at central sites (close to the core). In states of poor circulation, this difference may increase. Temperature measured in the rectum, oesophagus, nasopharynx, and tympanic membrane approximates core temperature.

## Causes

The common causes of hypothermia in critical care are:
- Post-operative patient after prolonged extensive surgery
- Post-operative patient after cardiac surgery
- Massive blood/fluid transfusion
- Exposed body surfaces (burns)
- Extracorporeal procedures: haemodialysis/haemofiltration, ECMO
- Irrigation of body cavities: peritoneal, bladder
- Hypometabolic states: hypothyroid, hypoglycaemia, hypopituitarism, adrenal insufficiency
- Toxicity: alcohol, barbiturates, central depressants, antidepressants

A number of factors can predispose to developing hypothermia
- Immobility
- Impaired consciousness
- Extremes of age
- Autonomic neuropathy
- Malnutrition
- Renal failure

## Presentation and assessment

Mild hypothermia
- General: shivering, with resultant increased oxygen demand
- Respiratory: dyspnoea, increased rate/depth of breathing
- Cardiovascular: vasoconstriction, tachycardia, increased cardiac output
- Neurological: confusion/lethargy, dizziness, ataxia, dysarthria,
- Renal: increased renal blood flow with resultant diuresis
- Other: <35°C platelet function and clotting factor function is progressively impaired

Moderate/severe hypothermia
Progressive depression of organ function occurs
- General: shivering stops at very low temperature (i.e. <32°C)
- Respiratory: reduced respiratory rate and depth, depression of cough reflex, apnoea (<24°C)
- Cardiovascular: bradycardia, progressive cardiovascular depression
  - ECG changes include bradycardia, prolonged PR and QT intervals, J wave (<33°C), AF, VF (<28°C)
- Neurological: coma, loss of reflexes and dilated pupils
- Renal: oliguria will develop associated with ATN and ARF

- Haematology: neutropenia or thrombocytopenia (splenic sequestration)
- Other: hyperglycaemia (secondary to reduced insulin secretion and peripheral insulin resistance); hypoglycaemia may occur with prolonged hypothermia
  - Mixed respiratory and metabolic acidosis

*In a sedated patient/post-operative patient, the following may be present*
- At mild/moderate hypothermia
  - Inappropriately excessive sedation
  - Lack of post-operative recovery
  - Bradycardia or arrhythmias
  - Loss of reflexes
  - Metabolic acidosis

*Prolonged untreated hypothermia can lead to*
- Infections, pneumonia
- ARDS
- Renal failure
- Bowel ischaemia
- Pancreatitis
- Rhabdomyolysis
- DIC

### Investigations

- ABGs (allow for temperature correction, partial pressure of oxygen may be increased during hypothermia; approximate correction factor for oxygen is 7%/°C.)
- FBC (WCC may be raised if infection present)
- U&Es (indication of dehydration, renal failure; K may be increased)
- Serum glucose (to exclude hypoglycaemia, but it may be high)
- Serum magnesium, phosphate, and calcium ($Mg^{2+}$ and $PO^{4-}$ may be decreased)
- CK (to look for rhabdomyolysis)
- Amylase (indicates pancreatitis)
- Urine for toxicology
- TFTs
- Serum cortisol
- Septic screen: blood, urine, and sputum cultures
- Urine: for protein or myoglobinurea
- ECG, CXR

### Immediate management

- Give 100% $O_2$ (shivering increases oxygen demand by 200–500%)
- Support airway, breathing, and circulation as required
- Confirm hypothermia using a suitable low-reading thermometer (oesophageal, rectal, or bladder)

- If resuscitation is required, the ALS protocol should be adjusted for hypothermia
  - At <30°C, resuscitative drugs will not be effective; hence they should be withheld until the temperature is corrected to >30°C
  - At <30°C, three DC shocks can be tried; if unsuccessful, no further shocks should be given until the temperature is >30°C
  - Start active rewarming and continue CPR and ventilation
  - At 30°C the lowest recommended dose of the drugs can be given at twice the recommended interval in the ALS protocol
- Central access is extremely important because of sluggish peripheral circulation
- Invasive haemodynamic monitoring is mandatory
- For rewarming consider following

Mild hypothermia
- Rewarm gradually using passive means
  - Remove any wet clothing, and replace with dry garments
  - Keep in a warm environment
  - Apply blankets; consider using foil or 'space' blankets

Moderate hypothermia (<32°C): include
  - Warmed humidified oxygen
  - Warmed IV fluids: avoid fluids containing lactate (hypothermic liver has reduced capacity to metabolize lactate)
  - Heat lamps
  - Heated forced-air air blankets
  - Warmed fluid mattresses
- Careful cardiovascular monitoring for dysrhythmias and hypotension

Severe hypothermia (<28°C)
- Consider rewarming using gastric, bladder, colonic, or peritoneal lavage with warmed fluids in patients with stable cardiac rhythms
- If significant cardiac dysrhythmias are present consider
  - Pleural/thoracic lavage
  - AV heating using modified bypass technique with a Level One fluid warmer
  - Haemodialysis/haemofiltration
  - Cardiac bypass (spontaneous cardiac output is not required)
- Rewarming at rates >2°C/hour has been shown to reduce mortality in cases of severe hypothermia
- Volume expansion will be required during rewarming; use CVP as a guide
- Avoid rapid changes in pH; severe metabolic acidosis (pH <7.1) may be corrected using bicarbonate infusion
- Monitor blood glucose levels (early moderate hyperglycaemia should be tolerated; later hypoglycaemia can occur with rewarming)
- Active resuscitation should continue until core temperature ≥35°C

## Further management

- When not associated with immersion hypothermia is commonly associated with sepsis; consider starting antibiotics
- Continue active rewarming: aim for up to 1°C/hour increase in core temperature
- Continue full invasive monitoring
- Continue to monitor for DIC, metabolic acidosis, and electrolyte imbalance during and after rewarming
- Avoid hyperventilation
- Correct any electrolyte changes
- Treat arrhythmias if these cause haemodynamic compromise
- Give thiamine 250 mg IV if there is history of alcohol intake
- If temperature is slow to correct, suspect hypothyroid or Addisonian crisis; treat with liothyronine 20 µg IV and hydrocortisone 200 mg IV repeated as necessary
- Infection commonly occurs with hypothermia; antibiotic treatment may be indicated
- Treat any frostbite/gangrene

## Pitfalls/difficult situations

- Profound bradycardia or bradypnoea may be present in hypothermic patients; allow as much as 1 minute to confirm their presence/absence
- Rough handling/inappropriate CPR may precipitate arrhythmias
- The possibility of secondary hypothermia should be considered and causes looked for
- Many drugs are ineffective at hypothermic temperatures and may cause rebound/unwanted side effects as the patient is rewarmed
- Core temperature may drop during rewarming; this 'after-drop' is probably due to temperature equilibration between core and periphery rather than return of cold blood from the peripheries
- In endocrine disorders and sepsis the cause of hypothermia may be difficult to diagnose in the first instance
- Be prepared to treat severe arrhythmias during hypothermia and rewarming
- Death cannot be diagnosed in a hypothermic patient; CPR along with rewarming and active management should continue until core temperature is >35°C
- Assessment of neurological status is also impaired during hypothermia
- MOF is common after profound and prolonged hypothermia

## Further reading

Epstein E, Anna K (2006). Accidental hypothermia. *BMJ* **332**, 706–9.
American Heart Association (2005). Hypothermia. *Circulation* **112**, IV136–8.
📖 OHCC p. 518, OHEA p. 272.

# Renal

# ① /⚙ **Fluid-balance disorders**

Fluid-balance disorders include hypovolaemia (oligaemia), dehydration/acute fluid depletion, and hypervolaemia/fluid overload.

Careful attention to fluid-balance is essential in ICU. Patients will require 'maintenance' fluids in addition to any fluid resuscitation.

## Causes

Hypovolaemia (see also shock, p. 106) occurs when there is a decrease in the volume of circulating blood. It can be accompanied by a decrease in total body water (dehydration/acute fluid depletion); but can also occur in patients who have an overall increase in total body water caused by fluid leaking out of the intravascular space (e.g. in sepsis). Causes include
- Haemorrhage (see p. 114)
- Third-space losses (e.g. fluid leaking into the interstitial compartment/oedema caused by diseases such as sepsis or pancreatitis)
  - This may occur rapidly, especially where surgical/radiological drainage of large amounts of ascites or pleural fluid (especially transudate) promotes rapid re-accumulation of fluid
- Severe dehydration
- Aggressive negative balance with CVVH/HD

Dehydration/acute fluid depletion
- Inadequate intake or inadequate fluid resuscitation
- Increased losses
  - GI: diarrhoea, vomiting
  - Renal: polyuria/diuresis (diuretic therapy, DKA, DI)
  - Other: severe burn injury, hyperpyrexia/heat exhaustion
  - Aggressive negative balance with CVVH/HD

Hypervolaemia/fluid overload
- Iatrogenic
- Acute renal failure
- Polydipsia
- Chronic heart failure
- Cirrhosis
- Nephrotic syndrome

## Presentation and assessment

Fluid-balance/volume status assessment will include
- The patient's fluid charts (and anaesthetic charts)
- Any history of diarrhoea, vomiting, diuresis

Hypovolaemia may present as shock (see shock, p. 106, and haemorrhage, p. 114). Signs and symptoms of fluid depletion may include
- General: thirst, skin turgor, dry mucous membranes, sunken eyes
  - Pyrexia may be present if it is associated with the cause of fluid loss
- Neurological: altered mental state, decreased consciousness, syncope
- Cardiovascular: tachycardia, normotension or hypotension
  - Increased capillary refill time
  - Decreased JVP/CVP

- Renal: oliguria, raised urea and creatinine
  - Polyurea may be present if it is associated with the cause (i.e. DKA)
  - Metabolic acidosis
- GI: vomiting or diarrhoea may be present
- Haematology: raised Hct and Hb (haemoconcentration)
- Other: hypernatraemia, raised serum osmolality

Acute fluid overload signs and symptoms may include
- General: peripheral/dependent oedema, enlarged and tender liver; ascites may be present **if** there is acute-on-chronic overload
- Neurological: altered mental state and decreased consciousness may occur
- Respiratory: pulmonary oedema may occur
- Cardiovascular: tachycardia, raised JVP (>4 cm from sternal angle), CVP (>15 cmH$_2$O), or PAOP (>18 mmHg)
  - Gallop rhythm, S3 may be present
  - Hypotension may be present if there is coexisting cardiogenic shock
- Renal: pre-existing renal failure or oligura may be present; polyurea may also be present
- Haematology: lowered Hct and Hb (haemodilution)
- Other: hyponatraemia, decreased serum osmolality

**Investigations**
- ABGs
- FBC, coagulation screen
- U&Es, LFTs
- Serum magnesium, calcium, and phosphate
- Serum glucose
- Serum osmolality
- Consider a full septic screen (blood, urine, sputum cultures)
- Stool culture, if diarrhoea present
- Consider cardiac enzymes
- 12-lead ECG (if cardiogenic shock suspected)
- CXR
- CVP measurement
- Urinalysis
- Consider echocardiography and/or cardiac output measurement

**Differential diagnoses**
Dehydation/acute fluid depletion
- HONK
- Meningitis
- Adrenal insufficiency
- Hypothyroidism

Acute fluid overload
- Cardiac failure
- TUR syndrome

## Immediate management

- Give $O_2$ as required; support airway, breathing, and circulation
- Manage shock/hypotension as per protocol (see p. 106)
- Manage haemorrhage as per protocol (see p. 114)

*Dehydation/acute fluid depletion*

- Prescribe maintenance fluids (usually crystalloids) and resuscitation fluids (crystalloids or colloids) separately
- Assess patient fully, including age, weight, working diagnosis, comorbidities, and volume status (CRT, HR, BP, C/JVP, UOP)
  - Urinary catheterization is likely to be required
- Prescribe appropriate fluid challenge
  - 250–500 ml IV gelatin colloid (e.g. Gelofusine®) over 15–60 min
  - In patients who are very small, elderly with IHD, or known to have poor LV function consider reducing fluid challenge to 200 ml over 30–60 minutes
  - In fit healthy severely dehydrated patients (e.g. patients with severe DKA) consider speeding initial fluid challenges up to 1000 ml over 15–30 minutes
- Review patient following fluid challenge, noting changes in haemodynamic and urinary variables
- Prescribe further fluid challenges as appropriate, and review again

*Acute fluid overload*

- Treat pulmonary oedema as per protocol (see p. 86)
- Consider monitoring degree of overload using CVP measurement
- Consider therapies such as
  - Diuresis (furosemide IV 20–40 mg, relies upon having functioning kidneys)
  - Vasodilatation using GTN IV infusion if patient is normo- or hypertensive (1 mg/ml at 0–15 ml/hour) and/or morphine IV 2–10 mg (repeated doses may accumulate in renal failure)
  - If *in extremis* consider venesecting 200–400 ml of blood whilst preparing other treatments
  - CVVH/HD

## Further management

- Common electrolyte abnormalities associated with acute fluid-balance problems may occur:
  - Hyponatraemia/hypernatraemia
  - Hypokalaemia/hyperkalaemia
- Other electrolytes which may be clinically relevant in certain situations include
  - Calcium: hypocalcaemia in massive blood transfusion, pancreatitis
  - Phosphate: hyperphosphataemia in acute renal failure secondary to tubular obstruction (i.e. tumor lysis syndrome, rhabdomyolysis)
  - Magnesium: hypomagnesaemia secondary to marked diuresis
- Acid–base abnormalities associated with acute fluid-balance problems include
  - Hyperchloraemic metabolic acidosis secondary to excessive replacement with 0.9% saline

- Hypochloraemic hypokalaemic metabolic alkalosis secondary to HCl loss with persistent vomiting, or excess NG aspirates
- Metabolic acidosis secondary to excess bicarbonate loss from small bowel fistula, or urethroenterostomy
- Metabolic acidosis secondary to diabetic ketoacidosis

## Pitfalls/difficult situations

- Glucose-containing fluids such as 5% dextrose spread into interstitial and intracellular fluid spaces, whilst the oncotic pressure generated by colloids forces fluid to remain in the intravascular space for longer; as an approximate rule of thumb regarding intravascular fluid replacement 1 L of colloid is equivalent to 2–3 L of saline 0.9% is equivalent to 8–9 L of 5% dextrose
- Hypotonic fluids may exacerbate cerebral oedema and increase ICP in head-injured patients
- Salt loading should be avoided in heptic failure

---

### Prescribing maintenance fluids

- Daily fluid requirements
  - ~40 ml/kg/day or 1.5 ml/kg/hour
  - Increase if there are large losses from urine, diarrhoea, vomiting, or skin (e.g. burns losses)
- Daily electrolyte requirements
  - Sodium ~1–2 mmol/kg/day[*]
  - Potassium ~0.5–1mmol/kg/day[†]

[*] Larger daily amounts of sodium are regularly given to critically ill patients, especially during acute resuscitation. Hyponatraemic/hypo-osmolar fluids should be avoided in head injuries; sodium- containing fluids should be avoided if possible in liver failure

[†] Potassium requirements may be increased by certain diseases or medications, or decreased by renal failure or tissue destruction

A sample daily fluid regimen for an 70 kg patient would contain 2800 ml (i.e. 120 ml/hour) of saline 0.9% or dextrose 4%–saline 0.18% (each litre containing ~20 mmol KCl)

In practice U&Es should be regularly checked and potassium supplementation given as required. Maintenance fluids may be adjusted according to plasma sodium, e.g.

- $Na^+$ <135 mmol/L          0.9% saline
- $Na^+$ 135–145 mmol/L    Hartmann's solution or dextrose 4%–saline 0.18%
- $Na^+$ >145 mmol/L        5% glucose

Maintenance fluids may also be provided in the form of enteral feed or TPN

---

## Further reading

Nolan J (1999). Fluid replacement. *Br Med Bull* **55**, 821–43.
📖 OHCC pp. 274, 414.

Commonly available IV fluids

| Fluid | Other names/similar solutions | Contents (mmol/L) | | | | pH |
|---|---|---|---|---|---|---|
| | | Na$^+$ | K$^+$ | Cl$^-$ | Other | |
| Saline 0.9% | Saline; 'normal' saline | 154 | 0 | 154 | | 5 |
| Dextrose 4%–saline 0.18%saline | Dextrose saline; 4% and a fifth | 30 | 0 | 30 | | 4 |
| Hartmann's solution | Compund sodium lactate; Ringer's lactate | 131 | 5 | 111 | Ca$^{2+}$ 2 Lactate ~30 | 6.5 |
| 5% Dextrose | | 0 | 0 | | | 4 |
| Sodium bicarbonate 8.4% | | 1000 | | | | 8 |
| Colloids | Gelofusine$^®$ Haemaccel$^®$ Starch solutions Human albumin solution 4.5% (HAS) | ~150 Haemaccel$^®$ ~5 | Haemaccel$^®$ ~5 | 125–145 | Haemaccel$^®$ Ca$^{2+}$ ~6 | ~7.4 |

Commonly available IV colloids

| Fluid | General information | Indictaions | Complications |
|---|---|---|---|
| Albumin | Available as 4.5% and 20% preparations<br>MW ~68 kDa | Unclear: shown to be as safe as crystalloids for acute resuscitation<br>Provides plasma expansion for ~4 hours | Theoretical risk of transmission of vCJD<br>Prepared from pooled donors<br>Expensive |
| Blood (packed red cells) | Expands intravascular compartment only<br>Increases oxygen carriage | Haemorrhage, anaemia | Immune reaction, infection, immunosuppresssion |
| Dextrans | Polysaccharide products of sucrose<br>Classified by their molecular weights<br>Dextran 70: MW 70 000 kDa | Provides volume expansion for ~12 hours | Alter platelet function<br>Incidence of allergic reactions<br>Rouleaux formation affects cross-matching |
| Gelatins | Widely variable molecular size<br>Excreted by unchanged kidney<br>Long shelf life | Provides plasma expansion for ~4 hours | Anaphylaxis |
| Starches | Polymerized cornstarch<br>Hespan: 450 000 kDa<br>Haes-steril: 200 000 kDa<br>Voluven: 130 000 kDa | Provides volume expansion for ~24 hours | May impair coagulation: Factors VII and vWF<br>May accumulate in RES – if large volumes given (>33 ml/kg/24 hour) – long-erm pruritus |

# ① **Acute renal failure**

Acute renal failure (ARF) is a rapid decrease in renal function/glomerular filtration (GFR). In critical care ARF commonly presents with oliguria or anuria.

Causes

Pre-renal causes
- Dehydration
  - GI losses: diarrhoea, vomiting
  - Renal losses: polyuria/diuresis (diuretic therapy, DKA, DI)
  - Other losses: severe burn injury, hyperpyrexia/heat exhaustion
  - Inadequate intake
- Hypotension
  - Haemorrhage
  - Shock (e.g. septic, cardiogenic)

Intra-renal causes
- Drug toxicity: NSAIDs and ACE inhibitors (particularly in combination with pre-renal failure); radiocontrast agents
- Rhabdomyolysis
- Renal artery obstruction (stenosis, emboli, or aortic surgery)
- Venous obstruction: intra-abdominal compartment syndrome
- Vasculitis: SLE, PAN
- Thrombotic disease: TTP, DIC
- Infection (particularly streptococcal and TB)
- Glomerulonephritis
- Carcinoma: myeloma

Post-renal causes
- Ureteric obstruction: calculi, carcinoma, retroperitoneal fibrosis, surgical disruption (e.g. after emergency hysterectomy)
- Bladder outflow obstruction: clot, tumour, neurogenic bladder, catheter obstruction

ARF is more likely to develop in patients with pre-existing renal impairment. Up to 10% of the population have mild to moderate renal impairment (grades 1–3), and 0.4% have severe renal impairment or renal failure (grades 4–5). Individuals at risk include patients with
- Diabetes
- Hypertension
- Cardiac failure
- Vasculitis
- Previous renal or aortic surgery

Presentation and assessment
Features of ARF include
- Oliguria (<0.5 ml/kg/hour), or anuria, is the most common presenting feature
- Features of fluid overload (e.g. pulmonary oedema) may occur
- Hyperkalaemia may develop
- Metabolic acidosis
- Increasing urea and creatinine will develop over time

Other signs and symptoms may include
- General: thirst, skin turgor if fluid depletion is present
  - Pyrexia may be present if there is associated infection
- Neurological: altered mental state, decreased consciousness
- Respiratory signs and symptoms: tachypnoea, dyspnoea, gasping or sighing breathing (Kussmaul's breathing)
  - $PaCO_2$ is often <3.5 kPa because of compensatory hyperventilation
- Cardiovascular
  - Tachycardia, hypotension, increased capillary refill time, and decreased JVP/CVP in shock
  - Tachycardia, raised JVP (>4 cm from sternal angle), CVP (>15 $cmH_2O$), or PAOP (>18 mmHg) in fluid overload
  - ECG changes associated with hyperkalaemia: tall tented T waves, slurring of ST segments into T waves, small P waves, prolonged PR interval, widened QRS, complete heart block, asystole or VF
- GI: nausea and vomiting, diarrhoea
  - Intra-abdominal pressure (IAP) may be raised
- Other: evidence of trauma or compartment syndrome may be present

## Investigations
- ABGs (metabolic acidosis will occur, with/without respiratory compensation)
- FBC, coagulation studies
- U&Es (serial measurements are required to monitor potassium levels, as well as rises in urea and creatinine)
- LFTs
- Serum CK (raised in rhabdomyolysis), serum CRP
- Serum magnesium, calcium, and phosphate
- Serum glucose, serum osmolality
- Consider a full septic screen (blood, urine, sputum cultures)
- Stool culture, if diarrhoea present
- 12-lead ECG (if cardiogenic shock or hyperkalaemia suspected)
- Consider renal ultrasound (or abdominal CT), or rarely IVU
- Urine dipstick
- Urine U&Es, osmolality, and microscopy (for cells, casts, crystals)
- Consider testing urine for myoglobin or Bence-Jones protein
- Consider autoantibody screen, complement concentrations, serum immunoglobulins, and electrophoresis
- Consider renal biopsy for certain conditions

## Differential diagnoses
- Traumatic renal rupture (urine collecting in abdomen)
- LVF/pulmonary oedema
- Catheter obstruction
- Shock/hypotension

## Immediate management

- Give $O_2$ as required; support airway, breathing, and circulation

*Treatment of complications*

- Treat pulmonary oedema as per protocol (see p. 86)
- Hyperkalaemia may be temporarily controlled by insulin IV
  15–20 units soluble insulin in 50 ml 50% dextrose over 30–60 minutes
  - If signs of potassium toxicity are present give calcium chloride IV
    3–5 ml of 10% solution over 3 minutes for cardioprotecton
- Severe acidosis can be transiently controlled with boluses of sodium
  bicarbonate 8.4% IV 25–50 ml

*Renal support*

- Stop any nephrotoxins (e.g. NSAIDs)
- Insert a urinary catheter and monitor urine output and fluid balance
- Consider outflow obstruction
  - Wash out the bladder to ensure the urinary catheter is patent
  - Consider renal tract imaging (renal US or CT of abdomen)
    if ureteric obstruction/hydronephrosis is a possibility
  - If ureteric or bladder obstruction is present obtain urological
    advice; a suprapubic catheter or nephrostomy may be required
- Optimize renal perfusion
  - Insert a CVC and give fluid challenges, aiming for a CVP of
    12–14 mmHg
  - Avoid hypotension, using vasopressors or inotropes if required,
    aiming for MAP ≥70 mmH
  - Monitor and treat raised IAP (see p. 294)
- Low-dose dopamine or furosemide boluses/infusions have not been
  shown to prevent the onset of ARF

*Renal replacement therapy (RRT)*

- Indications for RRT (see p. 277)
- Within ICU/HDU this is usually haemodialysis (HD) or continuous
  veno-venous haemofiltration (CVVH); HF and HD are considered
  equivalent
- Insert a dialysis line for RRT; correct clotting abnormalities prior to
  insertion; confirm catheter position with a CXR (if IJ or subclavian)
  prior to use
- Anticoagulation will be required in most patients requiring RRT
  - Avoid anticoagulation in patients with coagulopathy
- CVVH fluid balance should be prescribed: there are three possibilities:
  - Net balance to the patient is negative: useful in fluid overload, an
    hourly negative balance of 50–100 ml is usually sufficient (higher
    rates may be used, but the patient should be monitored for
    cardiovascular decompensation
  - Net balance to the patient is even: the CVVH machine will
    have to be adjusted regularly to ensure that any fluid boluses
    (e.g. from drugs) are removed
  - Balance to the *machine* is even: net balance to the *patient* will be
    positive as any fluid boluses will accumulate

**Further management**
- The underlying cause of the ARF should be actively sought and treated
- Many drug doses will require adjustment where ARF or CRF is present, discuss with pharmacy and/or nephrology specialists
- Monitor U&Es, including magnesium and phosphate
- Monitor the patient's temperature
- RRT may be discontinued intermittently in stable patients to look for evidence of renal recovery
  - Return of UOP
  - Maintenance of acid–base and electrolyte balance
  - 'Plateau' development of elevated creatinine and urea, and their eventual decrease

**Pitfalls/difficult situations**
- Consultation with the renal physicians may be required in situations where chronic renal supportive therapy is likely to be required, particularly if longer-term dialysis is unlikely to be appropriate
- Complications of CVVH (see p. 277)
- ARF with deranged urea and creatinine commonly persists for 2–3 weeks, and in some cases renal function never recovers
- In patients not receiving RRT furosemide infusions may be used to improve urine output; this will not alter outcome, but may improve fluid-balance management
- Polyuria is common in the recovery phase of ATN; care must be taken to avoid hypovolaemia
- IV contrast is known to cause contrast-induced nephropathy (CIN); where its use is essential in patients at risk of ARF ensure adequate hydration, consider giving acetylcysteine 150 mg/kg prior to contrast and use iso-osmolar radio contrast; prophylactic CVVH may also be used post contrast exposure
- Hypothermia can occur in patients undergoing CVVH and aggressive rewarming may be required
  - Pyrexia may be masked by CVVH-induced hypothermia

**Further reading**

Hilton R (2006). Acute renal failure. *BMJ* **333**, 786-90.
Forni LG, Hilton PJ (1997). Continuous hemofiltration in the treatment of acute renal failure. *N Engl J Med* **337**, 712–14.
Concise UK CKD guidelines. Available online at: www.renal.org
&#x2338; OHCC pp. 62, 330, 332. OHEA p. 316.

# ① **Haemofiltration complications**

### Cardiac arrest

In the event of a cardiac arrest clamp off the vascular access catheter lumens and stop CVVH, *unless* it is caused by hypovolaemia (wash the filter blood back into the patient) or hyperkalaemia (keep the filter running).

### Cardiovascular collapse/hypotension

Hypotension commonly occurs on commencement of CVVH (especially where extra-corporeal circuits are sterilized chemically, rather than with steam). Hypotension normally resolves rapidly, but may require colloid boluses (250 ml IV) and/or low-dose inotrope boluses (metaraminol IV 0.5–1mg). Where patients are shocked or cardiovascularly unstable consider commencing inotrope infusions prior to starting CVVH. Exclude bleeding (from the circuit, or as a result of anti-coagulation).

### Metabolic derangement

CVVH will usually correct hyperkalaemia within a few hours and control metabolic acidosis within a day. If this does not occur, consider whether potassium-releasing, or acidosis-causing, processes are still at work.

Potassium supplements are commonly added to the replacement fluid after the first day to prevent the development of hypokalaemia. Persistent lactataemia may be improved by using lactate-free replacement fluid.

### Pressure alarms

CVVH machines vary in design, but pressure alarms may include

- Transmembrane pressure (TMP) or filter pressure (FP): increasing pressures indicate filter clotting; check ACT and consider a further heparin bolus, or predilution if it is available, or change filter
- Arterial and venous pressures: high blood flow is desirable (≥200 ml/min) as this will deliver high ultrafiltration rates; this relies upon having good vascular access. High arterial pressures often indicate problems with hypovolaemia, hypotension, or line malposition or kinking; consider rotating, flushing, or changing the line. High venous pressures are often associated with line clotting
- Blood-leak or air-in-the-circuit alarms may also be present; the circuit should be fully inspected and problems corrected

### Filter clotting

Unless there is a contraindication to anticoagulation (coagulopathy, thrombocytopenia, imminent or recent surgery), an IV heparin infusion (~500–1000 units/hour) should be used to minimize filter clotting. INR and APTT should be checked first. A loading dose of 500–2000 units may be given. The lowest dose possible to maintain filter patency should be given. Target APTTR is 1.5–2.5 normal; target ACT is 150–180 s.

### Over anticoagulation

If over anticoagulation occurs heparin should be stopped until APTT returns to normal. If it is associated with major haemorrhage consider giving protamine IV (5 mg slowly, then review).

Epoprostenol (Flolan®) IV 5.2 ng/kg/min is an alternative if bleeding is a problem, but can cause hypotension.

### Indications for renal replacement therapy

- Significant fluid volume overload (e.g. causing, or likely to cause, pulmonary oedema)
- Hyperkalaemia (≥7.0 mmol/L, or rapidly increasing)
- Significant metabolic acidosis (pH ≤7.15)
- Symptomatic uraemia (usually >40 mmol/L)
- Haemodialysis may be indicated in some forms of poisoning (ethanol, methanol, ethylene glycol, salicylates, theophylline, lithium)

Patients who are known to be dialysis dependent prior to ICU/HDU admission should be treated with RRT before the above develop

High-volume haemofiltration has also been used as a treatment for severe sepsis/septic shock; its efficacy in this role remains unproven

### Modes of renal replacement therapy

- Continuous ambulatory peritoneal dialysis (CAPD)[*]
- Haemodialysis (HD)[†‡]
- Haemofiltration (HF)
  - Continuous arterio-venous haemofiltration (CAVH, CAVHF)[§]
  - Continuous veno-venous haemofiltration (CVVH, CVVHF)
  - Continuous veno-venous haemo-diafiltration (CVVHD, CVVHDF)

[*] CAPD is less effective in critically ill patients, is rarely possible where abdominal conditions exist, and may complicate other therapies (e.g. by splinting the diaphragm). It is only occasionally used in ICU/HDU.
[†] HD may precipitate haemodynamic instability in critically ill patients compared with CVVH.
[‡] Electrolyte imbalance, acidosis, and volume overload may be corrected more rapidly with HD.
[§] CAVH is only rarely used. Unlike CVVH, it does not require an extracorporeal pump and relies on systolic BP to drive blood, and is less efficient where shock is present (the risks associated with arterial cannulation are also present).

### Classification of chronic kidney disease

- Stage 1: kidney damage with normal or increased GFR[*] (≥90)
- Stage 2: kidney damage and mildly decreased GFR[*] (60–89)
- Stage 3: moderately decreased GFR[*] (30–59)
- Stage 4: severely reduced GFR[*] (15–29)
- Stage 5: kidney failure (established renal failure), GFR[*] <15

[*] GFR is measured in ml/min/1.73 m$^2$
Adapted from Concise UK CKD guidelines (www.renal.org)

# ☢ **Rhabdomyolysis/crush syndrome**

Rhabdomyolysis occurs when widespread muscle breakdown leads to the release of intracellular products (e.g. potassium, phosphate, myoglobin).

## Causes
- Trauma: crush injury (typically >1 hour), compartment syndrome (typically lower body), burns, electrocution
- Vascular occlusion (occasionally following vascular surgery)
- Muscle over-activity: seizures, dystonia, hyperpyrexia
- Immobility (especially associated with falls or overdoses)
- Toxins/drugs: ecstasy, envenomation
- Paraneoplastic syndromes

Patients at greater risk of developing ARF include those with:
  - More severe muscle injury, or hypotension/dehdration
  - CRF, diabetes, hypertension, cardiac failure, or vasculitis

## Presentation and assessment
Features of rhabdomyolyisis include:
- General: lethargy and malaise, low-grade pyrexia may be present
  - Other trauma, or skin erythema/blistering may indicate crush injury
- Neuromuscular: pain, tenderness, and stiffness
  - Tense swollen compartments may be present
  - Paralysis or paraesthesia of affected limb
- Cardiovascular: pale and pulseless peripheries may be present
  - Tachycardia and hypertension; hypotension occurs with reperfusion
  - ECG changes associated with hyperkalaemia: tall tented T waves, slurring of ST segments into T waves, small P waves, prolonged PR interval, widened QRS, complete heart block, asystole or VF
- Respiratory: tachypnoea/dyspnoea due to pain or metabolic acidosis
  - $PaCO_2$ is often <3.5 kPa because of compensatory hyperventilation
- Renal: characteristic dark-brown urine
  - Oliguria (<0.5 ml/kg/hour) or anuria; metabolic acidosis
- GI: nausea and vomiting may be present
- Neurological: altered mental state, decreased consciousness
- Other: hyperkalaemia, hypercalcaemia and hyperphosphataemia

## Investigations
- ABGs (metabolic acidosis with/without respiratory compensation)
- FBC, coagulation studies (DIC may be present)
- Serum CK (usually >200 IU/L in rhabdomyolysis; values >20 000 IU/L are not uncommon; CKMB should remain low)
- U&Es: high creatinine to urea ratio suggests rhabdomyolysis (>10 μmol/L to 1 mmol/L); serial measurements to monitor potassium levels
- LFTs (likely to be deranged)
- Serum magnesium, calcium, and phosphate
- 12-lead ECG (if hyperkalaemia suspected)
- Urine dipstick (myoglobin will show as positive for blood)
- Send urine for myoglobin
- Renal tract imaging may be required to differentiate between direct injury and rhabdomyolysis

**Differential diagnoses**
- Dermatomyositis/polymyositis
- Other causes of ARF

**Immediate management**

- Give $O_2$ as required; support airway, breathing, and circulation
- In the case of trauma, a crush injury, or unconsciousness
  - Use spinal precautions including hard collar, sandbags, and strapping (and in-line manual stabilization for intubation)
  - Complete a basic ABC primary survey
  - Obtain an 'AMPLE' history (see p. 2)
  - Assess neurological state and treat accordingly (see p. 158)
- Involve orthopaedic specialists in trauma or compartment syndrome
  - Manometry of the affected compartment may be required
  - Fasciotomy is indictated if diastolic blood pressure minus compartment pressure is <30 mmHg
- Hyperkalaemia may be temporarily controlled by insulin IV 15–20 units soluble insulin in 50 ml 50% dextrose over 30–60 minutes (may not work if muscle damage is profound)
  - Boluses of sodium bicarbonate 8.4% IV 25–50 ml may help to control hyperkalaemia and acidosis as a temporary measure
  - RRT may be required to treat hyperkalaemia, acidosis, or fluid overload (myoglobin is not removed by CVVH/HD)

*Methods aimed at avoiding ARF*
- Aggressive fluid loading is required, aiming for UOP >2 ml/kg/hour
  - Invasive monitoring will be required
- Urinary alkalinization with sodium bicarbonate 1.24% (IV 500 ml) aiming for a urine pH >6 may improve myoglobin excretion

**Further management**
- In severe cases of crush injury causing severe hyperkalemia and acidosis limb amputation may be required
- Regularly monitor U&Es, including magnesium and phosphate
- Perform secondary and tertiary surveys as soon as appropriate

**Pitfalls/difficult situations**
- Aggressive fluid resuscitation combined with ARF may lead to pulmonary oedema, typically >6 hours after injury
- Recognition of compartment syndromes in burn victims is difficult because of overlying soft tissue injury
- Open fractures may still cause a compartment syndrome
- Consider the possibility of rhabdomyolysis in all obtunded patients

**Further reading**

Hunter JD, Gregg K, Damani Z (2006). Rhabdomyolysis. *Br J Anaesth CEPD Rev* **6**, 141–3.
Gonzalez, D (2005). Crush syndrome. *Crit Care Med* **33**(Suppl), S34–41.
Tiwari A, *et al.* (2002). Acute compartment syndromes. *Br J Surg.* **89**(4):397–412, 2002.
📖 OHCC p. 528.

# Gastrointestinal and hepatic

# ☠ Gastrointestinal haemorrhage

Haemorrhage may occur in the upper or lower GI tract. Severity can vary greatly from trivial to immediately life-threatening.

## Causes
Upper GI
- Peptic ulcer disease may be pre-existing, or may develop as 'stress' ulceration which is associated with:
  - Critical illness and shock
  - Renal failure
  - Burns
  - NSAID, steroid, or SSRI use
- Oesophageal (or gastric) varices
- Malignancy
- Mallory–Weiss tear

Lower GI
- Infection or inflammation (e.g. diverticulitis)
- Malignancy
- Trauma
- Angiodysplasia

Minor gastric erosions may result in major GI bleeds where patients are anticoagulated, or suffering from coagulopathy or thrombocytopaenia.

## Presentation and assessment
Small GI bleeds may cause unexplained anaemia, whilst major bleeds may cause features associated with haemorrhage (see p. 114), including:
- General: pallor and anaemia
- Gastrointestinal: haematemesis or NG aspirate (classically 'coffee-ground')
  - Abdominal (commonly epigastric) pain
  - Nausea, vomiting, or diarrhoea
  - Melaena may occur with upper or lower GI bleeding, typically 24–48 hours after the commencement of the bleeding
  - Fresh PR blood (if source is below the ligament of Treitz)
- Cardiovascular: tachycardia, hypotension, increased capillary refill time
- Respiratory: tachypnoea/dyspnoea
- Renal: oliguria (<0.5 ml/kg/hour), metabolic acidosis
- Neurological: syncope, decreased consciousness

## Investigations
- Cross-match blood
- ABGs
- FBC, coagulation screen (including fibrinogen)
- U&Es, LFTs (urea is likely to be high)
- ECG
- CXR (subdiaphragmatic air will occur with perforation)
- GI endoscopy
- Angiography or radio-labelled bleeding scan

**Differential diagnoses**
- Haemoptysis
- Epistaxis/pharyngeal bleeding (swallowed blood may be regurgitated)
- Occult haemorrhage, or any cause of shock

**Immediate management**

- Give $O_2$ as required; support airway, breathing, and circulation
- Endotracheal intubation may be required to protect the airway where there is torrential bleeding and/or oesophageal manipulation (e.g. insertion of Sengstaken tube)
  - Induction of anaesthesia may provoke cardiovascular instability
- Obtain large-bore venous access (ideally 2 x 14 g cannula)
- Ensure blood is cross-matched, aggressively correct coagulopathies
- Circulatory resuscitation will be required
  - Start fluid resuscitation as clinically appropriate, initially with colloid followed by blood if required
  - Urinary catheterization and fluid balance monitoring is required
  - Invasive monitoring of CVP may be required
  - Inotropic/vasopressor support for circulation as necessary
- IV ranitidine or omeprazole are commonly started (there is no evidence that either improves acute outcome)
- For lower GI bleeding colonoscopy (or sigmoidoscopy for distal sources) is the investigation of choice
- For upper GI bleeding upper GI endoscopy is the investigation of choice, with endoscopic cautery, or sclerotherapy where possible
  - Oesophageal varices may respond to banding
  - NGTs should be inserted after endoscopy and left to drain
- Bleeding oesophageal varices may respond to the somatostatin analogue octreotide SC 100–200 µg 6-hourly, or IV 20–50 µg/hour
- Variceal bleeding may also be controlled by inserting a Sengstaken Blakemore (SSB) tube (or equivalent: Minnesota, Linton–Nachlas tubes)
  - Sedation may be required in order to tolerate Sengstaken tubes
- Massive bleeding, or re-bleeding after endoscopic intervention, may indicate the need for surgery or interventional radiology

**Further management**
- Careful cardiovascular monitoring and serial full blood count measurement should be undertaken
- Insert an NGT
- Prophylaxis against stress ulceration should include enteral feeding and avoidance of steroids, SSRIs, and NSAIDs where possible
  - Consider giving ranitidine IV (50 mg 8-hourly) or PO/NG (150 mg 12-hourly), or omeprazole IV 40 mg daily, or sucralfate NG (2 g 8-hourly)
- Transjugular intrahepatic porto-systemic shunting (TIPSS) may be considered for patients with oesophageal varices
- Consider CT/angiography in lower GI bleeding if patient stable
- Consider IV ciprofloxacin 800 mg daily for 7 days in variceal bleeding

## Pitfalls/difficult situations

- Patients should be stabilized before endoscopy but this is not always possible with ongoing bleeding
- Rise in urea and drop in haemoglobin may be the only initial sign that a bleed is present in the intubated patient
- In some cases the source of bleeding may not be found; angiography or labelled scans should be considered
- Lower GI bleeding may be treatable with angiographic embolization
- Aortoenteric fistulas may present with relatively small GI bleeds prior to a catastrophic haemorrhage

## Further reading

Barkun A, Bardou A, Marshall JK, et al. (2003). Consensus recommendations for managing patients with nonvariceal upper gastrointestinal bleeding. *Ann Intern Med* **139**, 843–57.

Jalan R, Hayes P (2000). UK Guidelines on the management of variceal haemorrhage in cirrhotic patients. British Society of Gastroenterology. *Gut* **46**(Suppl. III), III1–15.

📖 OHCC pp. 344, 346, 350.

# ⚠ **Acute severe pancreatitis**

Acute inflammation of the pancreas may cause local tissue destruction and a generalized inflammatory response causing distal organ failure.

## Causes

- Gallstones (up to 35% of cases)
- Alcohol (up to 40% of cases)
- Viral/bacterial infection (especially mumps, rubella, EBV, HIV)
- Medications, toxins: azathioprine, didanosine, pentamidine
- Trauma: blunt abdominal or iatrogenic (e.g. following ERCP)
- Vasculitis or ischaemia
- Hypercalcaemia, hypertriglyceridaemia
- Envenomation

## Presentation and assessment

Features of pancreatitis include:

- General: pyrexia, marked third-space loss
- Abdominal/gastrointestinal: abdominal pain (radiating to back)
  - Nausea and vomiting, diarrhoea may also occur
  - Cullen's sign (umbilical bruising), Grey–Turner's sign (flank bruising)
- Cardiovascular: tachycardia, hypotension
- Respiratory: tachypnoea/dyspnoea due to pain or metabolic acidosis
  - Respiratory distress may occur due to abdominal splinting or pleural effusion
- Renal: oliguria (<0.5 ml/kg/hour), metabolic acidosis
- Other: sepsis, multiple organ failure, hypocalcaemia, hyperglycaemia

## Investigations

- ABGs (metabolic acidosis is common)
- FBC, coagulation screen (DIC may develop)
- U&Es, LFTs
- Serum amylase and lipase (raised in pancreatitis, but moderate rises may be non-specific)
- Serum glucose, calcium, magnesium, phosphate
- Serum CRP
- Full septic screen (blood, urine, and sputum culture)
- CXR, AXR: raised hemidiaphragm, pleural effusions, basal atelectasis, or pulmonary infiltrates may be present
- US abdomen to evaluate the biliary tract
- CT abdomen (contrast-enhanced) to confirm diagnosis and assess severity; indications for CT include
  - Hyperamylasaemia, clinically severe pancreatitis, temperature >39°C
  - Ranson score >3, APACHE II >8
  - Failure to improve after 72 hours of conservative treatment
  - Acute deterioration

## Differential diagnoses

- Bowel obstruction/perforation
- Mesenteric ischaemia

- Cholecystitis
- Renal colic
- MI
- Pneumonia
- DKA

Immediate management

- Give $O_2$ as required; support airway, breathing, and circulation
- In severe cases respiratory support may be required using NIV or mechanical ventilation
  - Drainage of massive pleural effusions may improve lung function
- Aggressive fluid resuscitation is likely to be required
  - Urinary catheterization and fluid balance monitoring is required
  - Invasive monitoring of CVP may be required
  - CO monitoring will be required if CVS instability is present
  - Inotropic/vasopressor support for circulation as necessary
- Analgesia (morphine PCA or infusion) and anti-emetics should be prescribed
- Correct coagulopathy/electrolyte disturbance
  - Hypocalcaemia may be corrected with calcium chloride 10% IV (10 ml)
  - Hyperglycaemia is likely to require an IV insulin sliding scale
- The severity of the pancreatitis should be assessed using a scoring system (see p. 288)

Further management

- Regular reassessment of oxygenation/fluid balance is required
- Maintain strict glucose control
- Renal replacement therapy may become necessary
- NG tube enteral feeding is possible in most patients (80%) but a naso-jejunal tube may be needed; TPN may be used in patients in whom a 5 day trial of enteral feeding has failed
- Be vigilant for complications, including pancreatic necrosis, abscess or pseudocyst formation, diabetes mellitus, pancreatic encephalopathy, hypocalcaemia, and sepsis
- If gallstone obstruction is suspected, ERCP should be performed (ideally within 24–72 hours of onset)
  - Early cholecystectomy may be indicated
- Patients with >30% necrosis on CT may benefit from broad-spectrum antibiotics (e.g. imipenem)
- Surgical referral: indications for surgery include infected pancreatic necrosis or pancreatic abscess, persistent biliary peritonitis
- Consider repeating any CT scans at 48–72 hours from onset to delineate necrosis

## Pancreatitis severity scoring

### APACHE II score
Score >8 indicates a severe attack

### Ranson criteria (score 1 for each of the following)
- At presentation
  - Age >55
  - Blood glucose >11 mmol/L
  - White cell count >16 x 10$^9$/L
  - Lactate dehydrogenase (LDH) >400 IU/L
  - AST >250 IU/L
- Within 48 hours after presentation:
  - Haematocrit fall by >10%
  - Serum calcium <2 mmol/L
  - Base deficit >4 mmol/L
  - Blood urea rise >1 mmol/L
  - Fluid sequestration >6 L
  - PaO$_2$ <8 kPa

| | |
|---|---|
| Score 0–2 | <1% mortality |
| Score 3–4 | 15% mortality |
| Score 5–6 | 40% mortality |
| Score >6 | ~100% mortality |

### Modified Glasgow scale
- Age >55 years
- PaO$_2$ <8 kPa
- White cell count >15 x 10$^9$/L
- Serum calcium <2 mmol/L
- ALT >100 IU/L
- Lactate dehydrogenase (LDH) >600 IU/L
- Blood glucose >10 mmol/L
- Serum albumin <32 g/L
- Blood urea >16 mmol/L

A score of ≥3 within 48 hours predicts severe pancreatitis

### Computed tomography grading
A: Normal
B: Focal/diffuse enlargement
C: Gland abnormalities associated with peri-pancreatic inflammation
D: Two or more fluid collections and/or gas in or adjacent to pancreas

CT depiction of necrosis (especially in the head of pancreas) is associated with development of complications and death

### Other factors associated with severity/worse outcome
- Pleural effusion present on admission
- CRP >150 mg/L within first 48 hours of symptoms
- Obesity (BMI >30)
- Proven necrosis >30%
- Persistent organ failure

## Pitfalls/difficult situations

- Identifying severe cases early and patients who are likely to deteriorate rapidly enables rapid aggressive treatment and has better outcome
- CT scanning within 48 hours may underestimate necrosis but initial scan may help with differential diagnosis
- Timing of surgical intervention can be difficult: early intervention is associated with higher mortality, but infected pancreatitis and patients with worsening condition will need surgery
- There is little evidence at present that drug therapy such as octreotide is of any benefit

## Further reading

Whitcomb D (2006). Acute pancreatitis. *N Engl J Med* **354**, 2142–50.

Working Party of the British Society of Gastroenterology *et al.* (2005). UK guidelines for the management of acute pancreatitis. *Gut* **54**(Suppl III), III1–9

Balthazar EJ (2002). Acute pancreatitis: assessment of severity with clinical and CT evaluation. *Radiology* **223**, 603–13

Kingsnorth A, O'Reilly D (2006). Acute pancreatitis. *BMJ* **332**,1072–6.

OHCC p. 354.

# ① The acute abdomen

An acute abdomen (critical illness associated with marked abdominal signs, chiefly tenderness and rigidity) may be the cause of admission to ICU, or may occur whilst in critical care.

## Causes
- Generalized peritonitis due to perforated viscus: large bowel, small bowel, gastroduodenal ulcer
  - Anastamotic breakdown should be suspected in patients following surgery, especially where there was prior contamination and a primary anastamosis
  - Traumatic perforation should be suspected where there is penetrating injury, or where there is blunt trauma causing major bruising, or spine, rib, or pelvic fractures
- Generalized peritonitis due to other source of infection e.g. spontaneous bacterial peritonitis or in patients receiving CAPD
- Generalized peritonitis due to peritoneal irritation
  - Traumatic splenic rupture, ectopic pregnancy, or a ruptured AAA
- Localized peritonitis: diverticulitis, cholecystitis, appendicitis, abscess formation

## Presentation and assessment
Features associated with an acute abdomen
- General: pyrexia, marked third-space losses, shoulder-tip pain
- Abdominal/gastrointestinal
  - Abdominal pain causing rigidity and prostration, with rebound and guarding (bowel obstruction may cause colic)
  - Abdominal distension
  - Absent or altered bowel sounds
  - Anorexia or lack of NG absorbtion, or large NG aspirates
  - Nausea and vomiting, diarrhoea or bowel obstruction
  - Abdominal mass may be present
- Cardiovascular: tachycardia, hypotension
- Respiratory: tachypnoea/dyspnoea due to pain or metabolic acidosis
  - Respiratory distress may occur due to abdominal splinting
- Renal: oliguria (<0.5 ml/kg/hour), gradually worsening metabolic acidosis or lactataemia
- Other: sepsis, multiple organ failure, raised WCC

## Investigations
- Cross-match blood
- ABGs
- FBC, coagulation studies
- U&Es, LFTs
- Serum glucose
- Serum amylase, lipase
- Serum magnesium, phosphate, calcium
- Consider β-HCG
- ECG and cardiac enzymes

- Full septic screen (blood, sputum, urine)
- Send surgical samples for culture
- CXR (check for air under the diaphragm, basal atelectasis may be present)
- AXR (check for enlarged bowel or sentinel loops)
- US (may rapidly reveal presence of blood) or abdomen CT scan

**Differential diagnoses**

- MI
- Pneumonia
- Gastroenteritis
- Sickle cell crises
- Drug withdrawal

**Immediate management**

- Give $O_2$ as required; support airway, breathing, and circulation
- In severe cases endotracheal intubation and ventilation may be required to stabilize the patient prior to surgery
- Give analgesia
- Keep patient NBM and insert NGT
- Commence aggressive fluid resuscitation
  - Urinary catheterization and fluid-balance monitoring is required
  - Inotropic/vasopressor support for circulation as necessary
  - Invasive monitoring may be required
- Obtain surgical advice
  - Where the patient is cardiovascularly unstable and probably actively bleeding, treat as for haemorrhage (see p. 114) and consider rapid surgical intervention
  - Where infection is suspected the patient may proceed to laparotomy/laparoscopy once they have been optimized
- Commence antibiotics for suspected bowel perforation: piptazobactam IV 4.5 g 8-hourly and gentamicin IV 5 mg/kg daily

**Further management**

- If infection is present treat as for sepsis (see pp. 118, 322 and 346)
- Measure IAP and monitor for IAH (see p. 294)
- Enteral feeding may be possible after large bowel surgery; consider TPN after small bowel surgery

**Pitfalls/difficult situations**

- AXRs and erect CXRs are often difficult to obtain on ventilated patients; despite the associated risks of transfer abdomen CT scan may more appropriate
- Patients are often less stable immediately after surgery
- Heavily sedated (or paralysed) patients may not exhibit classical abdominal signs

**Further reading**
OHCC p. 348.

## ☼ Bowel ischaemia

Bowel ischaemia may present with subtle symptoms and is associated with a high mortality.

### Causes
- Mechanical: bowel volvulus, adhesions, and incarcerated hernias can all result in ischaemia
- Embolic: thrombus (especially associated with new onset AF), endocarditis, vegetation
- Venous thrombosis: procoagulant disorders, malignancy
- Prolonged hypotension/shock (particularly in patients known to have vascular disease)

### Presentation and assessment
Suspect further ischaemic bowel in any patient who has had a recent small bowel resection for ischaemia

Features associated with an acute abdomen
- General: mildly raised WCC, pyrexia (occurs late)
- Abdominal/gastrointestinal
  - Abdominal pain, initially without significant tenderness
  - Sudden diarrhoea or vomiting may occur with pain
  - Diarrhoea may be bloody
  - Nausea and abdominal distension may develop
  - Absent or altered bowel sounds
  - Anorexia or lack of NG absorbtion, or large NG aspirates
  - Ischaemic bowel may perforate
  - Incarcerated femoral or inguinal hernias may be present
- Cardiovascular: tachycardia (hypotension is a late finding)
  - AF may be present
- Respiratory: tachypnoea/dyspnoea due to pain or metabolic acidosis
- Renal: oliguria (<0.5 ml/kg/hour) and rapidly developing ARF are common
  - Metabolic acidosis and lactataemia develop rapidly
- Other: sepsis, multiple organ failure

Most abdominal signs (i.e. rigidity and distension) occur late, by which time hypotension and severe acidosis are commonly present

### Investigations
- Cross-match blood
- ABGs
- FBC, coagulation studies
- U&Es (potassium may be raised)
- LFTs (LDH and ALP commonly raised)
- Serum glucose
- Serum CK (often raised)
- Serum amylase (often mildly raised)
- Serum phosphate (commonly raised)
- Serum magnesium, calcium

- Full septic screen (blood, sputum, urine)
  - Send stool for culture (consider checking for FOB)
- ECG and cardiac enzymes
- CXR, AXR ('thumbprinting')
- US or CT abdomen (thickened bowel wall, pneumatosis intestinalis, mesenteric oedema)

**Differential diagnoses**

- Pancreatitis
- AAA
- Renal colic
- Bowel obstruction or perforation
- Infective colitis

**Immediate management**

- Give $O_2$ as required; support airway, breathing, and circulation
- Commence aggressive fluid resuscitation
  - Urinary catheterization and fluid-balance monitoring is required
  - Inotropic/vasopressor support for circulation as necessary
  - Invasive monitoring may be required
- Give analgesia
- Keep patient NBM and insert NGT
- Obtain surgical advice
  - Early identification of ischaemic bowel may allow angiography and embolectomy
  - Laparotomy and bowel resection is often required

**Further management**

- Avoid hypotension
- ARF and metabolic acidosis often develops rapidly postoperatively, requiring RRT
- Sepsis is common; antibiotics are likely to be required
- Measure IAP and monitor for IAH (see p. 294)
- Enteral feeding is occasionally possible after large bowel surgery, consider TPN after small bowel resection

**Pitfalls/difficult situations**

- Patients often become cardiovascularly unstable as the bowel is handled
- Incarcerated hernias are easy to miss
- Gut tonometry/microdialysis may offer a method of detecting ischaemic bowel early
- Vasopressors may exacerbate ischaemia
- Mortality is high (50–100%)

# ① Intra-abdominal hypertension

Rises in intra-abdominal pressure (IAP) can lead to abdominal compartment syndrome (ACS) where blood flow to retro-peritoneal and intra-peritoneal contents becomes compromised.

---

**Grades of intra-abdominal hypertension (IAH)**

- IAH grades       Intra-abdominal pressure
- Normal (non-ventilated)   0 (5–7 mmHg in ICU patients)
- Grade I (mild)       12–15 mmHg (16–20 cmH$_2$O)*
- Grade II (moderate)    16–20 mmHg (21–28 cmH$_2$O)
- Grade III (severe)     21–25 mmHg (29–35 cmH$_2$O)
- Grade IV (extreme)    >25 mmHg (>35 cmH$_2$O)

\* May be seen during mechanical ventilation, post surgery, and in the obese

---

## Causes

The risk factors for IAH include
- Blunt abdominal trauma (ACS can develop in up to 15% of patients)
- Abdominal surgery with primary closure
- Severe burns with eschar formation
- Prone positioning
- Bowel obstruction
- Haemoperitoneum, pneumoperitoneum
- Ascites or visceral oedema, infection, liver failure, pancreatitis, massive fluid resuscitation
- Peritonitis, intra-abdominal abscesses
- Tumour, haematoma, surgical packs
- Pelvic fracture

ACS exists if IAP remains >20 mmHg and new organ dysfunction occurs.

## Presentation and assessment

IAH can only be diagnosed by measuring IAP (see page 508). A high index of suspicion is required to initiate measurement. Features of IAH may include
- General: sepsis may develop (related to bacterial translocation)
- Abdominal/gastrointestinal: tense abdomen
  - Abdominal wounds may dehisce; fasciitis may occur
  - Hepatic function may become deranged
  - Anastamotic breakdown or bowel ischaemia may occur
- Cardiovascular: tachycardia, hypotension, decreased CO (due to IVC obstruction and increased afterload, all worse in hypovolaemia)
  - CVP and PAOP may remain high because of transmitted IAP
- Respiratory: respiratory distress may occur due to abdominal splinting
  - Reduced lung/chest wall compliance leads to increased airway pressures in ventilated patients
  - Hypercarbia (due to increased dead-space) and hypoxia
- Renal: oliguria and metabolic acidosis, despite adequate BP
  - ARF with raised urea and creatinine may develop
- Other: lactataemia may develop

**Investigations**
- ABGs
- FBC, coagulation studies
- U&Es, LFTs
- Serum amylase, serum glucose
- CXR (basal atelectasis)
- CT abdomen, slit-like IVC compression, tense retroperitoneal infiltration and increased AP to transverse diameter ratio may be present

**Immediate management**

- Give $O_2$ as required; support airway, breathing, and circulation
- Consider respiratory support with NIV or mechanical ventilation
- IAP should be measured (see p. 508)
  - Grade I        maintain normovolaemia
  - Grade II       hypervolaemic resuscitation
  - Grade III      surgical decompression
  - Grade IV       decompression and re-exploration
- Aggressive fluid resuscitation is likely to be required
  - Urinary catheterization and fluid-balance monitoring is required
  - Inotropic/vasopressor support for circulation as necessary
- Abdominal perfusion pressure (APP) should be calculated (MAP – IAP); APP should be maintained at ≥60 mmHg
- Sedation, supine body position, and neuromuscular blockade should be considered (to improve abdominal wall compliance)
- An NGT should be inserted to decompress intraluminal contents
- Consider dividing any eschars present on burns victims
- Consider paracentesis of abdominal fluid, or percutaneous drainage of haematomas or abscesses
- Surgical decompression is the treatment of choice for ongoing ACS; the abdomen may need to be left open

**Further management**
- Venous stasis is common; thromboprophylaxis should be used
- Regular repeated measurement of IAP should continue

**Pitfalls/difficult situations**
- Open abdomens following decompression may lead to fluid loss (up to 20 L/day) and hypothermia; enteral feeding is often still possible
- If left untreated ACS leads to MOF with ~100% mortality

**Further reading**

Malbrain M, Cheatham M, Kirkpatrick A, et al. (2006). Results from the International Conference of Experts on Intra-abdominal Hypertension and Abdominal Compartment Syndrome. I: Definitions. Int Care Med **32**, 1722–32.
Bailey J, Shapiro MJ (2000). Abdominal compartment syndrome. Crit Care **4**, 23–9.
http://www.wsacs.org/

# :O: **Fulminant hepatic failure**

Fulminant hepatic failure is defined as potentially reversible liver failure due to severe liver injury in the absence of pre-existing liver disease, and with encephalopathy occurring within 8 weeks of the first symptom. Hyper-acute liver failure exists if the encephalopathy appears within 7 days of jaundice, and acute liver failure exists if it appears within 8–28 days of jaundice.

## Causes

- Drugs: paracetamol (the most common cause); other drugs include sulphonamides, NSAIDs, phenytoin, isoniazid, MAOIs, ecstasy
- Infection: HAV, HBV, HCV, CMV, EBV, and HSV
- Toxins: *Amanita phalloides* (mushroom), carbon tetrachloride,
- Alcohol
- Autoimmune hepatitis
- Malignancy : lymphoma, metastases
- PET/HELLP syndrome
- Vascular: Budd–Chiari syndrome, veno-occlusive disease, hypotensive ischaemia
- Other: Wilson's disease, Reye's syndrome, neuroleptic hyperthermia

## Presentation and assessment

Hepatic failure may be associated with a history of viral illness, or drug (paracetamol) or alcohol intake.

Signs of chronic liver failure are not commonly present unless the present illness is 'acute-on-chronic'; the usual presentation of hepatic failure is due to one of the complications of liver failure

- General: jaundice
- Cardiovascular: vasodilatation, hyperdynamic circulation, lowered blood pressure (predominantly diastolic), and tachycardia
  - Increased cardiac output and decreased SVR
  - Spikes of hypertension may indicate cerebral oedema
- Respiratory: hypoxia due to increased shunt fraction
  - Pulmonary aspiration or atelectasis (unconscious patient) and/or chest infection
  - ARDS (up to 10% patients)
- Abdominal/GI: abdominal pain and retching (particularly with paracetamol poisoning)
  - Splenomegaly is typically absent in most cases; its presence may indicate Wilson's disease or lymphoma
- Renal: hepatorenal syndrome may develop (see p. 302)
- Neurological: encephalopathy (by definition, see p. 300)

Features associated with a worse prognosis include

- Bleeding complications: GI bleeding is common; subconjuctival haemorrhage (in paracetamol poisoning); prolonged PT and low-grade DIC
- Metabolic complications: hypoglycaemia, hyponatraemia, hypokalaemia, hypophosphataemia, lactic acidosis
- Infections: pneumonia, UTI, or sepsis

**Investigations**

- Group and save
- ABGs
- FBC, coagulation screen
- U&Es, LFTs (albumin may be normal initially)
- Serum glucose (monitor hourly)
- Drug screen (paracetamol)
- Viral serology (HAV–IgM, HbsAg; HBcore–IgM; EBV, CMV, HSV)
- Full septic screen (blood, urine, sputum)
- ECG, CXR
- Liver ultrasound (secondaries, lymphoma, venous patency)
- Liver biopsy (rarely required)

**Differential diagnoses**

- Sepsis
- Poisoning
- Causes of encephalopathy (see p. 192)

**Immediate management**

- Give $O_2$ as required; support airway, breathing, and circulation
- Endotracheal intubation and mechanical ventilation are likely
  to be required in grade 3 or 4 encephalopathy
- Insert large peripheral venous cannulae for volume expansion
  - Start volume expansion with colloids
  - Urinary catheterization and fluid-balance monitoring is required
  - Inotropic/vasopressor support for circulation as necessary
  - Invasive monitoring will be required; FFP cover may be required
    for central line insertion
- Check blood sugar and correct hypoglycaemia (aim for >3.5 mmol/L)
  - Glucose 25%, 25 ml IV
  - A continuous infusion of high-dose glucose (i.e. 50% glucose at
    10–50 ml/hour, ideally given via a central line) may be required

**Further management**

- Discuss all cases with a liver transplant unit: transfer to a regional
  unit may be indicated; liver transplant may be indicated
- MARS may be used as a bridge to transplant
- Give N-acetylcysteine IV (see p. 440) in paracetamol poisoning
- Penicillamine and vitamin E may be required in Wilson's disease
- Aggressively treat any infection; antibiotics and antifungals may be
  recommended as prophylaxis if there is no evidence of infection
- Monitor for glucose, DIC, metabolic acidosis, and electrolyte
  imbalance, and correct abnormalities
- Correct coagulopathies with vitamin K IV (10 mg once only);
  FFP and platelets if required
- Enteral feeding should be commenced; TPN should be used
  in the presence of ileus
- Manage encephalopathy (p. 158) and renal failure (p. 272)

## Pitfalls/difficult situations

- The presence of ARDS, renal failure, and grade 4 encephalopathy are associated with worse prognosis
- The cause of the hepatic failure may not be clear, or hepatic failure may be due to 'acute-on-chronic' condition
- Distribution and metabolism of the drugs will be altered; consult hepatologists and pharmacists on dose adjustments

## Further reading

Riaz Q, Gill MD, Sterling MD (2001). Acute liver failure. *Gastroenterology* **33**, 191–8.
Lai WK, Murphy N (2004). Management of acute liver failure. *Br J Anaesth CEPD Rev* **4**, 40–3.
&#x1F4D5; OHCC pp. 358, 360, 364.

**Transplant criteria for patients with acute liver failure**

- Paracetamol overdose
  - pH <7.30 (irrespective of grade of encephalopathy)
  
  **or**
  - PT >100 s (INR >6.5) and serum creatinine >300 μmol/L (3.4 mg/dl) with grade III or IV encephalopathy
- Non-paracetamol
  - PT >100 s (INR >6.5), irrespective of encephalopathy grade
  
  **or three of**
  - PT >50 s (INR >3.5)
  - Unfavourable aetiology (non-paracetamol, not Hep A or B)
  - Jaundice to encephalopathy >7 days
  - Age <10 years or >40 years
  - Bilirubin >300 μmol/L (>17.6 mg/dl)

Adapted from Chang AJ, Dixit V, Saab S (2003). Fulminant hepatic failure. *Curr Treat Options Gastroenterol* **6**, 473–9.

# :✪: Hepatic encephalopathy

Hepatic encephalopathy covers a spectrum of altered cerebral function secondary to hepatic failure.

## Causes

Acute fulminant hepatic failure can cause hepatic encephalopathy, as can chronic liver failure decompensation due to infection, GI bleed, or trauma.

## Presentation and assessment

- History of jaundice
- Grade 1: mild drowsiness, impaired cognition
- Grade 2: increasing drowsiness, confusion but conversant
- Grade 3: obeys simple commands but marked confusion
- Grade 4: responds only to painful stimuli or not responsive

Cerebral oedema is more common with grade 3/4 hepatic encephalopathy. Systemic hypertension, pupillary abnormalities, decerebrate posturing, hyperventilation, seizures, and loss of brainstem reflexes may occur.

## Investigations (see p. 297)
Also include

- Serum glucose
- Culture: blood, urine, sputum, and ascitic fluid
- CT head scan
- Consider EEG (slow voltage waveforms)

## Differential diagnoses

- Meningitis/encephalitis, stroke, intracranial haematoma
- Hypoxia or hypercapnia
- Endocrine abnormality: hypopituitarism, myxoedema, Addison's disease
- Hypo- and hyperthermia
- Electrolyte disturbance: hyponatraemia, hypoglycaemia, hyper- and hypo-osmolar states

## Immediate management

- Give $O_2$ as required; support airway, breathing, and circulation
- Endotracheal intubation and mechanical ventilation will be required if GCS <9 or if the patient is not protecting their airway
- Insert an NG tube and drain any blood in stomach
- Give lactulose to achieve two to three bowel motions per day
- Correct electrolyte imbalance and hypoglycaemia
- Correct coagulopathy before invasive procedures
- Consider metronidazole 500 mg PO 8-hourly
- Consider early ICP monitoring in grade 3/4 encephalopathy; maintain CPP >50 mmHg
  - Nurse with 30° head-up tilt
  - Aggressively treat any seizures according to protocol (p. 166)

**Further management**
- Maintain adequate nutrition (protein restriction is not recommended)
- Treat raised ICP with mannitol (100 ml 20%) unless renal failure present in which case use haemofiltration
- Avoid sedation if possible (it may be required for ICP control)
- Thiopental infusion may be required to reduce cerebral metabolic rate if there is persistent seizure activity
- Consider L-ornithine, L-aspartate administration (seek expert help)

**Pitfalls**
- Cerebral oedema requires a high index of suspicion to detect (irreversible brain injury is associated with ICP >30 mmHg, or CPP <40 mmHg)
- Early referral to a specialist centre is important

**Further reading**
Kunze K (2003). Metabolic encephalopathies. *J Neurol* **245**, 1150–9.
OHCC p. 362.

# ☼ Hepatorenal syndrome

Hepatorenal syndrome is the development of renal failure in patients with severe liver disease in the absence of any other identifiable cause of renal pathology.

## Causes

Hepatorenal syndrome may
- Occur spontaneously in the setting of progressive liver failure
- Be associated with spontaneous bacterial peritonitis (SBP), sepsis, and large paracentesis without albumin replacement
- Arise from compensatory renal vasoconstriction secondary to systemic vasodilatation

Two types of hepatorenal syndrome exist
- Type 1: acute form—rapidly progressive renal failure occurs spontaneously in patients with severe liver disease (may be associated with SBP)
- Type 2: chronic form—deterioration occurs over months, typically in patients with diuretic-resistant ascites

## Presentation and assessment

The diagnosis of hepatorenal syndrome requires the exclusion of other causes of renal failure in patients with liver disease. General signs and symptoms may include fatigue/malaise, systemic vasodilatation, hypotension, high cardiac output, and evidence of liver failure/ascites.

The diagnostic criteria for HRS include
- Chronic or acute liver disease with advanced hepatic failure and portal hypertension
- Low GFR, as indicated by serum creatinine >225 μmol/L or creatinine clearance <40 ml/min
- Absence of shock, ongoing bacterial infection, or recent treatment with nephrotoxic drugs. Absence of excessive fluid losses (including GI bleeding)
- No sustained improvement in renal function following expansion with 1.5 L of isotonic saline
- Proteinuria <0.5 g/day, and no ultrasonagraphic evidence of renal tract disease

Additional critera NOT required for diagnosis but commonly present
- urine volume <500 ml/day
- urine sodium <10 mmol/L
- urine osmolality >plasma osmolality
- urine RBC <50 per high field
- serum sodium <130 mmol/L

## Investigations (see p. 297)

Also include
- ABGs
- FBC, coagulation studies
- U&Es, LFTs
- Urinary osmolality and electrolytes

- Culture: blood, urine, sputum, ascitic fluid
- ECG
- Echocardiography
- Abdominal ultrasound

**Differential diagnoses**
- Hypovolaemia
- GI bleed
- Sepsis
- Paracetamol overdose
- Acute tubular necrosis
- Glomerulonephritis

**Immediate management**

- Give $O_2$ as required; support airway, breathing, and circulation
- Aggressive fluid resuscitation is likely to be required
  - Consider volume expansion 1.5 L salt-poor albumin
  - Urinary catheterization and fluid-balance monitoring is required
  - Invasive CVP and BP monitoring will be required
  - Consider cardiac output monitoring
  - Inotropic/vasopressor support for circulation as necessary
- Consider giving terlipressin IV 2 mg 12-hourly
- Exclude reversible causes/precipitating factors
- Insert nasogastric tube
- Monitor and correct any electrolyte imbalance
- Commence a non-nephrotoxic broad-spectrum antibiotic

**Further management**
- Refer to a nephrology specialist
- Avoid/stop any nephrotoxic drugs
- Consider paracentesis (giving 10 g albumin replacement for every litre of ascites drained)
- Diuretics, octreotide, and *N*-acetylcysteine have all been used, but there is little evidence that they improve outcome
- Renal replacement therapy can be used to support the patient until the liver recovers. Patients often need dialysis until liver transplantation
- Liver transplantation is the treatment of choice
- TIPSS may be of benefit

**Pitfalls/difficult situations**
- Volume status is difficult to assess; seek expert help

**Further reading**
Dagher L, Moore K (2001). The hepatorenal syndrome. *Gut* **49**, 729–37.
Arroyo V, Gines P, Gerbes AL, et al. (1996). Definition and diagnostic criteria of refractory ascites and hepatorenal syndrome in cirrhosis. International Ascites Club. *Hepatology* **23**, 164–76.
Ortega R, Gines P, Uriz J, et al. (2002). Terlipressin therapy with and without albumin for patients with hepatorenal syndrome: results of a prospective, nonrandomized study. *Hepatology* **36**, 941–8.

# Haematology

# ☼ Clotting derangement

Abnormally delayed blood clotting may occur because of deficiencies in the amount and/or function of blood constituents, including coagulation factors and platelets. Clinically, this may lead to problems with bleeding.

## Causes

In the critically ill, deranged haemostasis is often multifactorial.

*Coagulation factor deficiency*
- Acquired
  - Dilution secondary to massive transfusion
  - Liver failure
  - Consumption, e.g. DIC, extracorporeal circulation
  - Drugs, e.g. heparin, warfarin
  - Nutritional deficiency, particularly vitamin K
  - Autoantibodies, e.g. lupus anticoagulant, anti-factor VIII antibody
  - Primary fibrinolysis, e.g. burns, neurosurgery, prostatectomy, malignancy
  - Amyloid (factor X deficiency)
- Inherited
  - Haemophilia A (factor VIII deficiency) and B (factor IX deficiency, *Christmas disease*)
  - von Willebrand's disease (factor VIII deficiency and platelet dysfunction)

*Thrombocytopenia*
- Reduced platelet production
  - Marrow infiltration by malignancy
  - Marrow failure, e.g. critical illness, sepsis, viruses
  - Nutritional deficiency, e.g. vitamin $B_{12}$, folate
  - Drugs, including cytotoxics and alcohol
- Increased platelet consumption
  - DIC (see p. 312)
  - Immune destruction, e.g. heparin-induced thrombocytopenia (HIT) (see p. 310), idiopathic thrombocytopenic purpura (ITP), HIV
  - Drugs, e.g. penicillins, thiazides, anticonvulsants, antituberculous drugs
  - Hypersplenism
  - Extracorporeal circuits
- Dilution: massive transfusion

*Platelet dysfunction*
- Drugs, e.g. aspirin, NSAIDs, clopidogrel, abciximab
- Uraemia
- Liver failure
- Leukaemias
- Inherited platelet disorders (rare), e.g. Glanzmann's disease, Bernard–Soulier syndrome

**Presentation and assessment**
- Haemorrhage, including intra-operative failure to achieve haemostasis
- Oozing from wounds and drain sites
- Spontaneous bleeding, bruising, or purpura (atypical sites such as muscles and joints may be involved)
- Incidental finding on haematological investigation

**Investigations**
Consideration of the patient's history and clinical state, along with the results of the initial haematological investigations, should help to guide diagnosis of any clotting derangement. Basic investigations should include
- G&S
- FBC
- Coagulation screen (including fibrinogen)
- FDPs, D-dimers
- U&Es
- LFTs

Involvement of a haematologist is required in many cases as more specialized haematological tests may be indicated.

---

**Clotting function tests**

Prothrombin time (PT) (normal 12–14 s)
- Assesses factor VII activity: extrinsic coagulation pathway
- Prolonged in liver disease

Activated partial thromboplastin time (APTT) (normal, 25–35 s)
- Assesses factors VIII, IX, XI, XII: intrinsic coagulation pathway
- Normal PT and prolonged APTT suggests an inherited defect

Thrombin time (TT) (normal, 10–12 s)
- Assesses thrombin and fibrinogen: common clotting pathway

Platelet count
- Thrombocytopenia: platelet count $<150 \times 10^9$/L
- No assessment of platelet function

Fibrinogen (normal, 2–4 g/L)
- Reduced in DIC

Fibrin degradation products (normal <10 mg/L)
- Increased in DIC

D-dimer
- Formed by converting fibrinogen to cross-linked fibrin
- Raised in DIC

---

**Differential diagnoses**
- Meningococcal and streptococcal septicaemia, infective embolic rashes
- Ongoing bleeding
- Excessive anti-coagulation
- Laboratory error, or sample contamination (i.e. from IV drip arm)

## Immediate management

Give $O_2$ as required; support airway, breathing, and circulation
- If the patient is clinically shocked, begin immediate fluid resuscitation (see p. 114)
- Maintain a high index of suspicion for 'surgical bleeding', or for large-vessel bleeding
  - In post-operative patients
  - Following trauma
  - Following invasive procedures and line insertion
- Send urgent blood for cross-match, FBC, platelet count, 'coagulation screen' (PT, APTT, and TT), and fibrinogen assay
- Maintain normothermia (hypothermia impairs coagulation)

### Management of haemorrhage with coagulopathy

Coagulopathy (prolonged TT, APTT, PT/elevated INR)
- Stop any anticoagulant drugs
- Rapid reversal of clotting factor deficiency may be achieved by giving fresh frozen plasma (FFP) 10–15 ml/kg, aim for INR <1.5 in the bleeding patient
- If fibrinogen is low (<1.0 g/L), often associated with massive transfusion and DIC, give cryoprecipitate 10–15 units
- Warfarin overdose
  - Consider FFP or prothrombin complex concentrate (concentrated factors II, VII, IX, and X)
  - Give vitamin K IV 10 mg (takes ~12 hours to be effective)
- Heparin overdose (is rapidly excreted with normal renal function)
  - Consider protamine IV slowly (over 10 minutes): 1 mg for every 80–100 units heparin

Thrombocytopenia
  - A platelet count <50 × $10^9$/L in a bleeding patient should be urgently treated with transfusion of platelets
  - One adult dose (5 units) will raise the count by ~10 × $10^9$/L
  - 'Anti-platelet' drugs should be stopped; irreversible drugs such as clopidogrel or aspirin mean that transfusion may be necessary despite apparently normal platelet numbers
  - Desmopressin has been used after cardiac surgery to increase platelet function

Massive transfusion consumptive coagulopathy
- Liaise with haematologists
- Repeat coagulation studies every 2 hours or after every 4–6 units of packed red cells and give
  - FFP (12 ml/kg or 2 bags[*]) if PT or APTT >1.5 times normal, or if more than 4–6 units of stored blood is transfused
  - Platelet concentrates (0.5–1 unit/10 kg body weight) or one to two adult doses[†]) if the count is <50 × $10^9$/L
  - Cryoprecipitate (1 pack/10 kg body weight) if fibrinogen <0.8 g/L
  - Consider using recombinant factor VIIa

[*] One bag of FFP contains ~300 ml
[†] One adult dose of platelets = 5 units

**Further management**
- Ongoing transfusion necessitates regular coagulation studies and platelet counts, as does critical illness
- Ongoing bleeding in the face of normal coagulation studies and platelet numbers should prompt a thorough search for a *surgical* cause
- Discussion with a haematologist is recommended
- Hypocalcaemia should be corrected; calcium is an important cofactor in the coagulation cascade
- Thrombocytopenia/platelet dysfunction
  - Associated critical illness and infection should be treated, nutritional deficiencies addressed, and other potential causes of thrombocytopenia considered
  - Involvement of a haematologist is indicated if no cause is apparent as bone marrow biopsy may be required to secure a diagnosis
  - Immune thrombocytopenia is treated with IV immunoglobulin and steroids
  - Specialist haematology input and testing is often required to diagnose and quantify abnormal platelet function
  - Dialysis and desmopressin are used in the setting of platelet dysfunction secondary to uraemia
  - All patients with a platelet count <20 × 10⁹/L are at risk of spontaneous haemorrhage, and transfusion should be considered (some centres use a trigger of <10 × 10⁹/L in the absence of fever or bleeding)
  - Platelets should be transfused where the count is <50 × 10⁹/L and procedures (i.e. lumbar puncture) are planned, or is <100 × 10⁹/L and high-risk surgery (i.e. neurosurgery or spinal surgery) is planned

**Pitfalls/difficult situations**
- Irreversible 'anti-platelet' drugs, particularly aspirin and clopidogrel, should be stopped 5–7 days before surgery and invasive procedures (to allow a new cohort of platelets to be produced); other NSAIDs may be stopped 1–2 days before
- FFP and cryoprecipitate take up to 30 minutes to thaw
- Platelets are held centrally and may take up to 2 hours to reach peripheral hospitals
- If possible avoid procedures such as NGT or urinary catheter insertion in patients with coagulopathy
- Minor trauma may be associated with catastrophic bleeds in coagulopathic patients

**Further reading**
DeLoughery TG (2002). Thrombocytopenia in critical care patients. *J Intensive Care Med* **17**, 267–82.
📖 OHCC pp. 396, 398, 406.

# ⑦ **Haemoglobin transfusion triggers**

A conservative blood transfusion policy should be used within critical care. Suggested transfusion triggers are as follows:

| | |
|---|---|
| Active ischaemic heart disease | 10 g/dl |
| Ongoing bleeding | 8–10 g/dl |
| All other cases | 7 g/dl |

It is also suggested that patients with burns, cerebrovascular disease, or head injury should share a transfusion trigger of 8–10 g/dl.

Where major haemorrhage is predicted in a critically ill patient(e.g. a patient with critical illness who has to undergo a major surgical procedure such as cardiac bypass operation or liver surgery) consider

- Administering antifibrinolytics before activation of the coagulation cascade by surgery: aprotinin IV 2 million units loading dose followed by 0.5 million units/hour (hypersensitivity occurs in 0.5% of patients; do not repeat within 6 months)
- Alternatively, give tranexamic acid IV (loading dose 50–125 mg/kg)
- Perioperative cell salvage

# ⑦ **Heparin-induced thrombocytopaenia**

Critically ill patients are commonly exposed to heparin, e.g. DVT prophylaxis, invasive line flushes. In up to 30% of patients heparin induced thrombocytopaenia (HIT) may ensue. The incidence is less with low molecular weight heparins (LMWHs).

HIT occurs 4–14 days after the introduction of heparin, most commonly after a surgical insult (especially cardiac surgery), but can be hyperacute and occur within 24 hours of exposure in patients previously exposed to HIT within the past 100 days.

HIT causes a fall in platelet count of >30% (though rarely reaches absolute values <10×10$^9$/L) but causes a hypercoagulable state. Patients are at high risk of thrombotic events or skin necrosis.

Heparin should be stopped and an alternative anticoagulant commenced, such as danaparoid or a hirudin. Warfarin should be *avoided* as it can lead to further skin necrosis.

Where HIT is suspected blood should be sent for HIT antibody tests

## Further reading

Napolitano LM, Warkentin TE, AlMahameed A, Naswary SA (2006). Heparin-induced thrombocytopaenia in the critical care setting: diagnosis and management. *Crit Care Med* **34**, 2898–911.
📖 OHCC pp. 182, 400, OHEA p. 328.

**Table 9.1 Coagulants/antifibrinolytics**

| | Administration | Compatability | Indication | Dosing |
|---|---|---|---|---|
| Fresh frozen plasma (FFP) | Use a 170 μm filter Use within 2 hours | Use ABO-compatible plasma | Deficiencies of factors II, V, VII, IX, X, and XI; reversal of warfarin; massive transfusion; antithrombin III deficiency; | If INR or APTTR >1.5 infuse 15 ml/kg |
| Cryoprecipitate (CPT) | Use a 170 μm filter | | Haemophilia A; von Willebrand disease; factor XIII deficiency; following massive transfusion | Infuse 10–15 units if fibrinogen <0.8 g/L |
| Platelet concentrate (PC) | Use a 170 μm filter Shelf life 5 days | ABO-*incompatible* platelets are safe | Thrombocytopenia or platelet abnormality and bleeding; bleeding prophylaxis in severe thrombocytopenia; following massive transfusion | If platelets <50 × 10⁹/L infuse 1unit/10 kg body weight |
| Vitamin K | | | Antagonism of warfarin; hepatic coagulopathies | 1–10 mg IM or slow IV bolus |
| Factor VIIa | | | Licensed: haemophilia A or B with inhibitors to factors VIII or IX; congenital factor VII deficiency Unlicensed: massive blood transfusion, trauma | 100 μg/kg repeated at 1–2-hourly intervals if required |
| Protamine | | | Reversal of unfractionated heparin | 1 mg neutralizes 80–100 units of heparin slow IV |
| Tranexamic acid | | | Menorrhagia; haemophilia (prior to surgery); cardiac surgery, to minimize blood loss; minimize surgical blood loss; reversal of thrombolytic therapy | 10–20 mg/kg slow IV injection two to four times daily |

# ☼ Disseminated intravascular coagulation

Disseminated intravascular coagulation (DIC) is a 'consumptive' coagulo-pathy characterized by abnormal widespread intravascular coagulation and fibrinolysis leading to loss of coagulation factors and platelets. Both bleeding and microvascular thrombosis causing organ damage can occur.

## Causes
There are many causes of DIC, including
- Sepsis (60% of cases)
- Trauma (especially crush injury and tissue necrosis) and burns
- Obstetric emergencies: severe pre-eclampsia, abruption, amniotic fluid embolism, IUFD
- Anaphylaxis
- Transfusion reactions and haemolysis
- Malignancy: e.g. mucinous adenocarcinomas, promyelocytic leukaemia
- Liver failure
- Heat stroke
- DKA
- Autoimmune disease

## Presentation and assessment
A diagnosis of DIC is often suggested by widespread bleeding and deranged coagulation, low fibrinogen, and platelet count. Assay of fibrin degradation products (FDPs) may also be helpful.

*Acute DIC*
- Bleeding may predominate
  - Petechiae and ecchymoses (purpura fulminans)
  - Oozing puncture sites and mucous membranes
  - Haemorrhage, typically GU, GI, pulmonary, or intracranial
- Microvascular thrombi may predominate affecting any organ, typically
  - Skin (ischaemia)
  - Kidneys (ARF, oliguria)
  - Lungs (hypoxia, dyspnoea, cyanosis)
  - Brain (delirium, coma)
  - Other affected organs may include GIT, liver, heart, and pancreas

*Chronic DIC*
- Bleeding may be milder; embolic events may still occur
- Chronic DIC may be clinically silent, disturbing laboratory values only

## Investigations

- FBC (decreased platelets)*
- Blood film/smear may show schistocytes (90% of chronic DIC and 50% of acute DIC), leucocytosis with a left shift, and thrombocytopenia
- Coagulation studies (prolonged PT, APTT, and TT)*
- Fibrinogen (decreased)*
- FDPs, D-dimers (both increase)

## Differential diagnoses

- ITP
- TTP
- HELLP
- HIT
- Bone marrow failure from any cause

### Immediate management

- Give $O_2$ as required; support airway, breathing, and circulation
- Maintain adequate oxygenation and intravascular volume (minimize the effects of any thromboses)
- The initial treatment is aimed at correcting the underlying cause
- Manage haemorrhage appropriately (see p. 114)
    - Replace platelets and fibrinogen (with cryoprecipitate) as required to treat haemorrhage, or before any invasive procedures

## Further management

- Involvement of a haematology specialist is essential
    - Plasma exchange may be considered
    - Activated protein C may be used in sepsis, but may exacerbate any bleeding tendency
- Continue monitoring the clinical and laboratory parameters
- Once the trigger for DIC is removed FDP levels should fall, and fibrinogen levels should rise in 3–6 hours if liver function is adequate

## Pitfalls/difficult situations

- Heparin has been used as a treatment for DIC, but its use remains controversial

## Further reading

Senno SL, Pechet L, Bick RL (2000). Disseminated intravascular coagulopathy (DIC): pathophysiology, laboratory diagnosis, and management. *J Intensive Care Med* **15**, 144–58.

---

* A chronic compensated form can exist with 'supranormal' values of PT and APTT; normal or mildly elevated fibrinogen; normal or slightly low platelets.

# ⓘ Neutropenia

Neutropenia is defined as a neutrophil count $<2 \times 10^9$/L, although there may be some racial variation. Counts $<1 \times 10^9$/L are associated with incr-eased risk of infection.

## Causes

A low index of suspicion for neutropenia should be maintained in any patient with severe infection or trauma, having radio- or chemotherapy, having anti-thyroid drugs, or with autoimmune disease.

*Acquired*
- Cytotoxic drug therapy
- Marrow infiltration by malignancy
- Idiopathic aplasia and myelodysplasia
- Severe infection, especially viral and tropical infections, brucellosis, TB
- Radiotherapy
- Drugs: antithyroid drugs (e.g. carbimazole), sulphonamide antibiotics
- Hypersplenism
- Autoimmune destruction, e.g. SLE, rheumatoid arthritis
- Felty's syndrome (rheumatoid arthritis, splenomegaly, and neutropenia)
- Severe trauma
- Nutritional deficiency, particularly vitamin $B_{12}$ and folate

*Inherited*
- Congenital agranulocytosis (*Kostmann's syndrome*): presents in infancy
- Cyclic neutropenia (cyclic variations in cell counts over a period of several weeks)

## Presentation and assessment

Neutropenia is asymptomatic, unless symptoms and signs of infection are present (see p. 322). It may be an incidental finding during unrelated investigations.

## Investigations

Unexplained neutropenia requires urgent investigation. Haematological guidance is necessary as further testing may include blood films and bone marrow biopsy.

## Differential diagnoses
- Sampling error/laboratory error

## Immediate management

- Give $O_2$ as required; support airway, breathing, and circulation
- Drugs which may be implicated should be stopped
- Investigate and treat infection/sepsis urgently
  - Parenteral antimicrobial therapy is crucial and microbiological advice must be sought in the context of the neutropenic patient
  - See Chapter 10 for suggestions regarding empirical antibiotic therapy

## Further management

- Measures should be instigated to protect the neutropenic patient from infective complications
  - Isolation of the patient, particularly if the neutrophil count $<1 \times 10^9$/L
  - Strict infection control procedures should be enforced ('reverse-barrier' nursing)
  - Minimize invasive procedures
  - Fastidious patient hygiene
  - Regular mouthwashes, e.g. hydrogen peroxide 2-hourly
  - Candida prophylaxis
  - High-calorie diet avoiding foods at risk of microbial contamination, e.g. salads
  - Closely monitor for signs of infection, with regular bacteriological screening
- Recombinant human granulocyte-colony stimulating factor (rhG-CSF) may be used to improve bone marrow neutrophil production

## Pitfalls/difficult situations

- Neutropenia *secondary* to severe infection places the patient in a poorer prognostic group
- Neutropenia secondary to radio- or chemotherapy often has to be tolerated as a side effect of necessary therapy, and measures to avoid infective complications (see above) should be instituted
- Atypical infections are more common in this population; blind broad-spectrum antibiotics may be required initially

## Further reading

Penack O, Beinert T, Buchheidt D. et al. (2006). Management of sepsis in neutropenia: Guidelines of the Infectious Diseases Working Party (AGIHO) of the German Society of Hematology and Oncology (DGHO). *Ann Hematol*; **85**, 424–33.
📖 OHCC p. 408.

## ☼ Severe haemolysis

Severe haemolysis causes premature destruction of RBCs resulting in compromised organ function

### Causes
If RBC survival falls below 120 days, bone marrow production can compensate in chronic conditions. Severe haemolysis is usually related to an acute haemolytic condition or decompensation.

*Acquired*
- Immune
  - Autoimmune: warm or cold antibody mediated; may be idiopathic or secondary, e.g. lymphoma, SLE
  - Isoimmune, e.g. transfusion reaction
  - Drug induced, e.g. high-dose penicillin, methyldopa
- Non-immune
  - Traumatic, e.g. prosthetic valves
  - Microangiopathic/haemolytic uraemic syndrome (HUS)
  - HELLP syndrome (see p. 420)
  - Infection related, e.g. sepsis, malaria

*Inherited*
- Haemoglobinopathies, e.g. sickle cell disease (see below), thalassaemia
- Membrane disorders, e.g. hereditary spherocytosis
- Enzyme defects (rare), e.g. G6PD (decompensation with haemolysis; anaemia and jaundice may occur after sulfonamide administration)

### Presentation and assessment
Common presentations of haemolysis resulting in ICU admission are
- Transfusion-related haemolysis
  - Presentation may range from chest pain, SOB, headache, and rigors to cardiovascular collapse and multi-organ failure
- Sickle cell crises
  - Crises are characterized by pain (ischaemia), classically in long bones and soft tissues but any site may be involved
  - Chest symptoms, neurological involvement, renal impairment, GI sequelae, thrombocytopenia, and liver failure may supervene
- Other causes of haemolysis may present with cardiovascular collapse; severe anaemia; coagulopathy or DIC; jaundice; acute renal failure
- Splenomegaly suggests reticuloendothelial (extravascular) haemolysis

Critically ill patients frequently have secondary bone marrow suppression. Therefore compensation for ongoing haemolysis may be compromised and resulting anaemia severe.

### Investigations
- Cross-match
- ABGs
- FBC (blood film may reveal fragmented cells, RBC trauma, or sickle cells; immature RBC forms, e.g. reticulocytes, suggest a compensatory increase in marrow production)

- Haptoglobins (reduced)
- U&Es, LFTs (elevated unconjugated bilirubin)
- Urine dipstick, urinalysis (urinary urobilinogen)
- Plasma and urine assays of free Hb (raised in intravascular haemolysis)
- Direct Coombs testing identifies antibody/complement-coated RBCs, indicating an immune aetiology
- Consider Hb electrophoresis (to diagnose haemoglobinopathies) and bone marrow biopsy

### Differential diagnoses
- Liver failure
- Sepsis
- Haemorrhage

### Immediate management
- Give $O_2$ as required; support airway, breathing, and circulation
- Aggressive fluid resuscitation may be required
- Obtain a full history and examination, e.g. sickle cell disease, recent transfusion (of ABO incompatible blood), or drugs
- Stop any potentially implicated drugs or transfusions
- Transfuse blood in the severely anaemic, aiming for Hb >7 g/dl

*Transfusion-related haemolysis.*
- Transfusion should be *stopped immediately* and the collapsed patient resuscitated.
- Patient identity, blood product, and documentation should be carefully re-checked.
- Liaison with haematology is imperative and return of the blood product, patient blood sampling, and official reporting is mandatory

*Sickle cell disease*
- Management centres around oxygenation, maintaining circulating volume, peripheral perfusion, and normothermia.
- Adequate analgesia is essential and opioids are commonly required
- Transfusion is indicated if Hb <6 g/dl

### Further management
- After initial stabilization, further management will be dictated by identification of the haemolytic process
- Supportive measures may be required, e.g. blood component transfusion, haemofiltration

### Further reading
OHCC pp. 402, 404, OHEA pp. 266, 330.

# ① **Vasculitic crises**

Vasculitis may be primary or secondary and causes destructive inflammatory changes to the blood vessel walls, characteristically affecting different calibre vessels depending on aetiology.

## Causes
Causes of vasculitic crises (i.e. involving organ impairment), include
- Primary
  - Wegener's granulomatosis
  - Microscopic polyarteritis
  - Goodpasture's syndrome/anti-GBM disease
- Secondary
  - SLE
  - Weil's disease
  - Infective endocarditis
  - Malignancy
  - Rheumatoid arthritis
  - Drug reactions
  - Type 2 cryoglobulinaemia (commonly associated with HCV)

## Presentation and assessment
Infection may precipitate a vasculitic crisis in predisposed individuals. Secondary vasculitis may present alongside the symptoms and signs of the primary illness. Presenting features may include
- General: pyrexia, weight loss and malaise
  - Rashes and nodules
  - Myalgia, arthralgia/arthritis
  - Epistaxis and nasal discharge
- Respiratory: cough, dyspnoea, haemoptysis
- Renal: ARF, haematuria, proteinuria
- Neurological: confusion, fits, focal neurological impairment
  - Peripheral polyneuropathy

Vasculitis should be suspected in any patient with unexplained deterioration in the presence of coexisting chronic rheumatological disease, HCV, malignancy, or new drug therapy.

## Investigations
- ABGs
- FBC, coagulation screen (DIC may supervene)
- U&Es, LFTs
- Serum CK (elevated with muscle involvement)
- Serum ESR and CRP
- Septic screen (blood, urine, sputum) if infection/sepsis suspected
- ANCA (classically positive in Wegener's and microscopic polyarteritis)
- ANA/dsDNA. (positive in SLE)
- Anti-GBM
- Urine dipstick
- ECG
- CXR

- Echocardiogram if infective endocarditis is suspected
- Consider renal biopsy

Expert guidance from rheumatology, renal, or respiratory physicians will be suggested by the pattern of involvement, and will direct investigation.

**Differential diagnoses**
- Sepsis

**Immediate management**
- Give $O_2$ as required; support airway, breathing, and circulation
- Stop any potentially implicated drugs
- Airway or pulmonary haemorrhage (see pp. 36 and 82) may require ventilatory support
- Pulmonary oedema may occur requiring treatment (see p. 86)
- Cardiac monitoring will allow early identification of arrhythmias
- Invasive haemodynamic monitoring should be considered and careful fluid-balance measurement undertaken
- Seizures should be treated appropriately (see p. 166)
- Infection and sepsis should be sought and treated aggressively according to local microbiological guidelines

**Further management**
- Primary vasculitis treatment centres around immunosuppression and steroid therapy.
- Plasma exchange may be of benefit in renal disease; expert involvement is obligatory
- Management of secondary vasculitis will involve treatment of the underlying pathology
- RRT may be required for acute renal failure (see p. 277)
- Correct any electrolyte abnormalities

**Pitfalls/difficult situations**
- In certain conditions blindness and/or deafness may occur
- Tracheal involvement may lead to development of subglottic stenosis and airway compromise

**Further reading**
📖 OHCC pp. 492, 494.

# Infections

## ☼ Sepsis (see also septic shock, p. 118)

Inflammation resulting in the systemic inflammatory response syndrome (SIRS) may be caused by many diseases that result in admission to critical care. When the cause is infection sepsis may develop (see below).

> **Definitions of SIRS and sepsis**
> - Systemic inflammatory response syndrome (SIRS): response to a variety of clinical insults manifesting by two or more of the following:
>   - Temperature >38°C or <36°C
>   - Heart rate >90 beats/min
>   - Respiratory rate >20 breaths/min or $PaCO_2$ <4.3 kPa
>   - White cell count >12000 cells/mm$^3$, <4000 cells/mm$^3$, or >10% immature (band) forms
> - Sepsis: SIRS criteria in presence of infection

The incidence of bacteraemia in hospital admissions is approximately 7 per 1000 admissions. Of these, 20% develop septic shock which has a mortality of 40–60%.

### Causes

*Causes of SIRS include:*
- Infection
- Trauma or burns
- Pancreatitis
- Infarction: myocardial, intracerebral, bowel, pulmonary embolism
- Drug and alcohol withdrawal
- Massive blood transfusion

*Sepsis*

Infections causing sepsis may be either community or hospital acquired (or, as a subset, ICU acquired). Infecting organisms may be either endogenous (i.e. derived from gut or throat) or exogenous (e.g. *Acinetobacter*, *Pseudomonas*, and MRSA). Common sites of infection include:
- Respiratory (~38%)
- Device-related (~5%)
- Wound/soft tissue (~9%)
- Genito-urinary (~9%)
- Abdominal (~9%)
- Endocarditis (~1.5%)
- CNS (~1.5%)

Common conditions and interventions may lead to the disruption of natural defences against infection
- Trauma or burns
- Major surgery (especially GI, genito-urinary surgery, or surgery of infected areas)
- Intestinal obstruction/distension
- Gut ischaemia or perforation

- Tracheal intubation or tracheostomy
- Indwelling urinary catheters and wound drains
- Intravascular catheters
- IV infusions of fluids, drugs and nutrition

In immunocompromised patients atypical, multiple, and fungal infections may be seen. Common causes of a compromised immune system include:
- Malnutrition
- Alcohol/drug abuse
- Multiple trauma
- AIDS
- Drug treatment: chemotherapy, steroids
- Prolonged systemic disorders: including renal failure, hepatic failure, malignancy, multiple infections
- Radiation injury
- Major surgery
- Multiple blood transfusions

Presentation and assessment

Presentation of infections, SIRS, and sepsis varies according to site and type of infection, host defence and comorbidity. Non-localizing signs and symptoms of infections may include:
- General: pyrexia (or hypothermia, particularly in the elderly or immunocompromised), sweats, rigors
- Respiratory: tachypnoea and hypoxia
- Cardiovascular: tachycardia (bradycardia may be a pre-terminal sign)
  - Peripheral vasodilatation (warm peripheries), or peripheral shutdown (cold peripheries), usually as late manifestation
  - Hypertension or hypotension
  - Decreased JVP, CVP, or PAOP
  - Cardiac output monitoring may reveal increased cardiac output (although it may decrease in severe sepsis) and decreased systemic vascular resistance
  - Arrhythmias, particularly AF, atrial flutter, or VT
  - Occasionally cardiac: angina or ischaemia
  - Peripheral/dependent oedema
- Neurological: agitation, confusion, diminished consciousness, syncope
- Renal: oliguria, raised urea and creatinine
  - Metabolic acidosis
- Gastrointestinal: anorexia, nausea and vomiting
- Haematology: raised or lowered WCC; DIC
- Other: raised inflammatory markers (CRP, ESR, PCT)

Patients with sepsis may develop:
- Severe sepsis: sepsis with evidence of organ dysfunction, hypoperfusion, or hypotension, including oliguria, alteration in consciousness, or metabolic acidosis
- Septic shock: sepsis associated with hypotension (systolic blood pressure <90 mmHg, or >30 mmHg below normal resting pressure, or MAP <60 mmHg) which does not respond to volume resuscitation in the presence of perfusion-related complications
- Multi-organ dysfunction syndrome or failure (MODS or MOF)

**Factors associated with poor prognosis in sepsis**

- Age >70 years
- Multi-organ (>2) failure
- ARDS
- Leucopenia
- Hypothermia
- DIC

**Investigations**

Most investigations are indicated to monitor complications

- ABGs
- FBC, coagulation screen (including D-dimers and fibrinogen)
- U&Es, LFTs
- Serum calcium, magnesium, phosphate
- Serum glucose
- ECG

Some investigations may also confirm the likelihood of sepsis, locate the source, or identify the organisms involved

- CRP and/or ESR
- Serum procalcitonin is used in some centres to help differentiate inflammation from infection
- Serum (and urine) antigen tests may be available for some organisms
- Bacteriology: one or more of the following
  - Septic screen: blood*, urine, and sputum cultures
  - Wound swabs
  - Nose and throat swabs
  - Drain fluid
  - Stool
  - CSF (lumbar puncture may also reveal other findings (p. 208))
  - If any invasive lines are removed, line tips should be sent for culture
  - Some institutions take brush samples from CVCs
  - Bronchoalveolar lavage (BAL) samples
  - Speculum examination and vaginal swabs
- CXR
- Ultrasound and/or CT scan of chest, abdomen (including renal and hepatic), head, or pelvis for evidence of a collection
- Echocardiography (trans-thoracic (TTE), or trans-oesophageal (TOE)) for suspected endocarditis or to assess any LV dysfunction

**Differential diagnoses**

- Malignancy
- Connective tissue diseases
- Drug withdrawal
- Infarction: myocardial, intracerebral, bowel, pulmonary embolism
- Inflammation: hepatitis, pancreatitis, trauma or burns

* Blood cultures should be taken from every invasive line, as well as 1–2 percutaneous venous samples; percutaneous venous stabs should be taken from different sites to minimize the risk of skin contamination

Immediate management

- Give $O_2$, titrate $SaO_2$ to >96%
- Airway: endotracheal intubation may be required
  - Where infection threatens airway patency
  - Where there is decreased consciousness (GCS ≤8)
  - To facilitate mechanical ventilation
- Ensure breathing/ventilation is adequate
  - Fatigue may lead to respiratory failure; CPAP, and/or non-invasive BiPAP may be indicated
  - In severe shock mechanical ventilation may be needed to optimize oxygenation
  - Respiratory infections may also compromise breathing and require mechanical ventilation
- Circulatory support should be commenced in patients with hypotension or elevated serum lactate
  - Large peripheral venous cannulae are required
  - Arterial and/or central venous cannulation should be undertaken as soon as feasible, checking coagulation studies and platelets first
- Resuscitate with crystalloids/colloids, aiming for the following (ideally within 6 hours)
  - CVP 8–12 mmHg
  - MAP ≥65 mmHg
  - Urine output ≥0.5 ml/kg/hour
- Consider dobutamine up to 20 µg/kg/min if venous oxygen saturation <70%, or if cardiac output is low despite fluid resuscitation
- Vasopressor therapy with norepinephrine 0.05–3 µg/kg/min or dopamine 0.5–10 µg/kg/min (via a central catheter) is indicated when fluid challenge fails to restore adequate blood pressure/organ perfusion
  - Central venous or mixed venous oxygen saturations ≥70%
- Consider transfusing packed red blood cells if Hb <7g/dl (10 g/dl if there is cardiac ischaemia or ongoing haemorrhage), or to achieve a haematocrit ≥30% if venous oxygen saturation <70% despite a CVP of 8–12 mmHg
- Consider measurement of CO (e.g. oesophageal Doppler, LidCO) and SVR to optimize fluid resuscitation and inotropic support

*Infection identification and control*

- Treat any identifiable underlying cause, make a full survey for likely sources of infection, take a focused clinical history, and review notes and charts where possible
- Take all appropriate cultures: ensure one or two percutaneous blood culture samples; also sample blood from each intravascular catheter
- Commence appropriate antibiotics ideally within first hour of treatment: respiratory (see p. 332), abdominal (see p. 346), wound/soft tissue (see p. 348), genitourinary (see p. 344), endocarditis (see p. 336), CNS (see p. 340)
- Remove intravascular access devices that are a potential infection source after establishing other vascular access
- Arrange surgery, if required, to remove focus of infection

**Further management**
- Admit the patient to suitable critical care facility
- Continue invasive monitoring and assessment of respiratory and circulatory status
- Monitor and treat complications, including ARDS, DIC, metabolic acidosis, and electrolyte imbalance

*Infection*
- Use infection control procedure where resistant or highly infectious agents are suspected
- Report any notifiable diseases (see p. 378)
- Reassess antimicrobial regimen within 72 hours and adjust according to culture results; following advice from microbiology, aim to
  - De-escalate antimicrobial therapy from broad-spectrum to targeted therapies
  - Monitor for superadded or ICU-acquired infections (e.g. ventilator-associated pneumonia (VAP))
- Where there is no improvement repeat all cultures and consider adding therapy for unusual organisms, including antivirals and antifungals
  - Consider changing indwelling catheters and vascular lines for suspected secondary ICU infections
- Consider combination therapy for neutropenic patients and those with *Pseudomonas* infections

*Adjunctive therapies*
- Activated protein C (see p. 122–123 for indications/contraindications)
- Low-dose steroids: consider steroids (hydrocortisone 50–75mg IV 6-hourly for 7 days with or without fludrocortisone 50 µg PO daily); avoid high-dose steroids
  - Consider performing a short synacthen (250 µg ACTH) stimulation test; discontinue steroids in patients where cortisol increase is >9 µg/dl

*Treat or prevent complications*
- Vasopressor-resistant septic shock (VRSS) may occur where hypotension and tissue hypoperfusion cannot be corrected with standard vasopressor/inotropic therapy; consider
  - Vasopressin infusion 0.01–0.04 units/min IV infusion
  - Alternatively consider terlipressin 1 mg IV 8-hourly
  - Methylene blue IV has been reported to improve haemodynamics and tissue perfusion
- Respiratory
  - ARDS: use a lung-protective ventilation strategy (see p. 50)
  - Ventilator-associated pneumonia: raise the bed head 45° unless contraindicated
  - Use a weaning protocol
- Renal
  - Do not use 'renal dose' dopamine
  - Correct any metabolic acidosis; use continuous veno-venous haemofiltration (CVVH) or intermittent haemodialysis if necessary
  - Avoid bicarbonate therapy for lactic acidaemia if pH ≥ 7.15

- Haematology
  - Do not use erythropoietin to treat sepsis-related anaemia
  - Do not use fresh frozen plasma to correct laboratory clotting abnormalities unless there is bleeding or invasive procedures are planned
  - DIC: correct fibrinogen if bleeding, or risk of bleeding
  - ARDS: minimize the use of blood products by following a restrictive transfusion policy for blood (see p. 310; aim for ≥7.0 g/dl where there is no bleeding or coronary artery disease) and for platelets (see p. 309) (transfuse if <5 × $10^9$/L, OR if 5–30 × $10^9$/L and there is a bleeding risk, OR if <50 × $10^9$/L and surgery or invasive procedures are planned)
  - Do not use antithrombin therapy
- Other measures
  - Consider antipyretics and/or peripheral cooling for pyrexia
  - Consider giving pethidine 25 mg IV to treat rigors
  - Provide stress ulcer prophylaxis (e.g. ranitidine 50 mg IV 8-hourly)
  - Sedation use a protocol and sedation score and avoid neuromuscular blockers if possible
  - Consider DVT prophylaxis with low-dose unfractionated heparin or low molecular weight heparin; use compression stockings or an intermittent compression device where heparin is contraindicated
  - Maintain strict glycaemic control where possible
  - Enteral nutrition may help maintain integrity of the gut mucosal barrier
  - TPN may be required in the presence of ileus

## Pitfalls/difficult situations

- Cause/source of infection may not be clear; consider non-obvious locations (retro-peritoneal space, vertebrae)
- Fungal infections are often overlooked; suspect in cases of secondary infections and in immunocompromised patients
- DIC may be difficult to treat; seek expert haematology advice
- Patients with impaired renal function or on renal replacement therapy often require alterations to any specified regimens; discuss with pharmacy or microbiology
- Antimicrobial regimens may also have to be adapted for patients with confirmed penicillin allergy
- Mixed pictures of shock often occur with sepsis coexisiting with other causes such as cardiac failure
- New infections are common in patients already admitted to critical care and are often picked up via routine blood sampling (e.g. raised WCC on FBC) or on X-rays performed for other reasons (e.g. CXR to check CVC position); have a low threshold for suspecting vascular access catheters as a source for bacteraemia
- Organisms are often not found in culture (in up to 40% of cases)

## Further reading

Dellinger RP, Carlet JM, Masur H, et al. (2004). Surviving Sepsis Campaign guidelines for management of severe sepsis and septic shock. *Intensive Care Med* **30**, 536–55.
www.survivingsepsis.org
Ⓜ OHCC pp. 480–4, 486.

# ⓘ Pyrexia of unknown origin

Classical definition pyrexia of unknown origin (PUO) is that of a temperature >38°C for 2 weeks. Within intensive care, any temperature ≥38.5°C should trigger a review of the patient.

## Causes

In the ICU setting infection is the primary cause of pyrexia. Patients are at increased risk of infection where there is:
- Use of invasive lines or endotracheal intubation (or tracheostomy)
- Immunosuppression from any cause
- Prolonged ICU stay, ICU overcrowding, reduced staff numbers

*Infections*
- Catheter (CVC, PAOP, arterial line) related sepsis
- UTI, urinary catheter related sepsis
- Ventilator-associated pneumonia (VAP)
- Intra-abdominal collections
- Colitis (especially *Clostridium difficile*)
- Sinusitis (especially if using nasogastric or naso-endotracheal tubes)
- 'Occult', unusual, or difficult to culture infections such as
  - Infective endocarditis (IE)
  - Viruses (including CMV), Fungal (especially *Candida*), TB

*Other causes of pyrexia*
- Malignancy: lymphoma, leukaemia, solid cell tumours (especially renal)
- Connective tissue diseases: SLE, RA, PMR, sarcoid, vasculitis
- Drug-related (both administration and withdrawal, e.g. alcohol)
- Infarction: myocardial, intracerebral, bowel, pulmonary embolism
- Inflammation: SIRS, ARDS, hepatitis, pancreatitis, burns, post-surgery
- Blood transfusion

## Presentation and assessment

Pyrexia may be associated with other evidence of infection, including:
  - Tachypnoea, tachycardia, rigors, sweats
  - Complications of sepsis (see p. 323)
  - Raised WCC and inflammatory markers

## Investigations

- FBC and differential (check for eosinophils), U&Es, LFTs
- Blood culture from all lines and peripheral 'stab' samples
- Samples for culture with/without microscopy/Gram stain
  - Samples from all drains and any effusions that can be tapped
  - Sputum (ideally BAL or protected specimen if intubated)
  - Swabs from nose, throat, naso-pharynx, and perineum
  - Urine (also do a dipstick test)
  - If diarrhoea is present stool culture and *C.difficile* toxin testing
- CXR
- Consider trans-thoracic or trans-oesophageal echocardiography (TTE or TOE) if endocarditis is suspected

- Consider US of abdomen
- Consider CT of any suspect area (especially after major surgery)
- Consider sinus X-rays, autoantibody screens, GI endoscopy, BM biopsy

**Differential diagnoses**
- Exclude measurement errors (check core temperature if possible)

**Immediate management**

- Give $O_2$ as required; support airway, breathing, and circulation
- Review the patient's history including drug history, sexual history, travel, occupation, and exposure to animals
- Look for any obvious site of infection including
  - Eyes, ears, mouth
  - PR/PV (especially to exclude the presence of tampons)
  - Cannulae: epidural and catheter entry sites for redness/pus
  - Skin, especially the back of the patient and buttocks
- Check for enlarged lymph nodes
- Review all previous investigations, looking for changes in inflammatory markers, WCC, increased insulin requirements, alteration in oxygen requirements, increased lactate, reduced absorption of feed
- If the patient is unwell, start empirical treatment with different broad-spectrum antibiotics to those used previously, covering for HAIs (e.g. imipenem IV 500 mg 6-hourly and vancomycin IV 500 mg 6-hourly)

**Further management**
- Remove as many non-essential invasive devices as possible
- Consider inserting new CVCs (at new sites), especially if blood drawn from a line produces a positive blood culture; culture old line tips
- If blood cultures remain negative but the patient is still clinically unwell, continue broad-spectrum antibiotics for 48 hours and review
- Consider introducing antifungal medications if the patient condition is deteriorating and the fever remains high
- Treat with antipyrexial agents with/without surface cooling if there is limited cardiovascular reserve or brain injury, or pyrexia is >39.5°C

**Pitfalls/difficult situations**
- Pyrexia precedes other signs for ≥3 days in some infections, including viral hepatitis, EBV, measles, leptospirosis, typhoid
- TTE is often technically difficult on mechanically ventilated patients
- Hypothermia may also be associated with infection
- If temperature persists despite 5–7 days of adequate antibiotic cover, consider stopping all antibiotics for 12 hours, re-culturing from all sites, and starting different antibiotics
- CVVH often causes low temperatures and can mask signs of fever
- Patients may become colonized, but not infected, with organisms
- Consider the possibility of rare/tropical infections and biological agents

**Further reading**
Marik PE (2005). Fever in ICU. *Chest* **117**, 855–86.
📖 OHCC p. 518.

# ☠ **Airway infections** (see also p. 30)

## Causes

- Pharyngeal, retropharyngeal, or peri-tonsillar abscess
- Ludwig's angina or deep-neck infections
- Diphtheria
- Epiglottitis

## Presentation and assessment

General signs and symptoms of infection (p. 323) may be accompanied by

- Tachypnoea, dyspnoea, hypoxaemia, and cyanosis
- Stridor
- 'Hunched' posture: sitting forward, mouth open, tongue protruding
- 'Muffled' or hoarse voice, sore throat, painful swallowing, drooling
- Neck swelling
- Trismus

## Investigations (see p. 324)

Also consider

- Lateral soft tissue neck X-ray may demonstrate swelling and loss of airway cross-section ('thumb-print' and 'vallecula' signs)
- Laryngoscopy (indirect or fibreoptic) performed by a skilled operator
- CT or MRI of head and neck

## Immediate management

Follow guidelines on p. 31

- Give O₂ as required; support airway, breathing, and circulation
- Airway intubation may be required in severe cases, and is likely to be a high-risk procedure requiring senior supervision
- Consider IV hydrocortisone 200 mg IV 8-hourly

### Suggested empirical antimicrobials

- Cefuroxime 1.5 g IV 8-hourly with metronidazole 500 mg IV 8-hourly
- Alternatives include co-amoxiclav 1.2 g IV 8-hourly
- In severe infections consider adding chloramphenicol
- For diphtheria consider erythromycin 0.5–1 g IV 6-hourly

# ☼ Pneumonia (see also p. 58)

## Causes

- Community-acquired pneumonia (CAP)
- Aspiration pneumonia
- Atypical pathogens (e.g. *Mycoplasma*, *Chlamydia*, *Legionella*, viruses, fungi)
- Hospital-acquired pneumonia (HAP) or healthcare-associated pneumonia (HCAP)
- Ventilator-acquired pneumonia (VAP)

## Presentation and assessment

Signs and symptoms of infection (see p. 323) may be accompanied by:
- Increasing respiratory distress, tachypnoea, dyspnoea
- Cough, purulent sputum, haemoptysis, or pleuritic chest pain
- Features of coexisting disease (e.g. COPD or bronchiectasis)
- CXR changes of collapse, consolidation or parapneumonic effusion

CURB-65 score (see p. 59) may be used to assess pneumonia severity

Aspiration should be suspected in patients where there is:
- Neurological injury or decreased consciousness level
- Difficulty swallowing (e.g. stroke, Parkinson's disease)
- NG feeding

Atypical pathogens should be suspected where the following are present:
- Younger patients
- Dry cough
- Multisystem involvement (e.g. headache, abnormal LFTs, elevated serum creatine kinase)
- A history of travel, pets, high-risk occupations, comorbid disease
- Immunosuppressive disease or therapy

HAP should be suspected in patients where:
- Symptoms occur ≥48 hours after hospital admission
- The patient is readmitted ≤10 days after discharge from hospital
- Residence in a nursing home or extended care facility where there is recent or prolonged antibiotic use (e.g. leg ulcer treatment)

HCAP should be suspected where the patient is or has been:
- Resident in a nursing home or extended care facility
- Receiving care for a chronic condition

VAP may be present in mechanically ventilated patients where there is:
- Worsening oxygenation
- Increased sputum production
- Indices of infection (pyrexia, WCC, CRP, culture results)
- CXR changes on routine films
- Inability to maintain endotracheal cuff pressure >20 cmH$_2$O and/or raise the head of the patient to 30°–40°
- Clinical pulmonary infection scores (CPIS) scores >6 (see box opposite)

Multiple drug resistance (MDR) may be present if:
- There is a failure to respond to appropriate antibiotics (especially β-lactam-producing antibiotics)
- The patient has been on prolonged antibiotic therapy
- Immunosuppressive disease or therapy have been used
- HAP/VAP are suspected
- HCAP is suspected and there has been:
  - Treatment as an inpatient in the previous 6 months
  - Chronic dialysis
  - Prolonged antibiotic usage (especially wound care)
  - The patient, their relatives, or the place where they are treated are known to be associated with multidrug-resistant pathogens
  - Long-term urinary catheter or invasive lines are present

---

**Clinical pulmonary infection scores (CPIS)**

Temperature
- ≥36.5 C and ≤38.4 C — 0 points
- ≥38.5 C and ≤38.9 C — 1 point
- ≥39 C or ≤36.4 — 2 points

White cell count
- ≥4 × 10$^9$/L and ≤11 × 10$^9$/L — 0 points
- <4 × 10$^9$/L or >11 × 10$^9$/L — 1 point
- (Band form ≥50% — *add 1 point*)

Tracheal secretions
- No tracheal secretions — 0 points
- Non-purulent tracheal secretions — 1 point
- Purulent tracheal secretions — 2 points

Culture of tracheal aspirate
- Lght quantity/no growth — 0 points
- Moderate or heavy quantity — 1 point
- (Same bacteria on Gram stain — *add 1 point*)

Oxygenation: $PaO_2/FiO_2$
- >32 kPa (240 mmHg) — 0 points
- ARDS present[*] — 0 points
- ≤32 kPa (240 mmHg)/no ARDS present — 2 points

CXR findings
- No infiltrate — 0 points
- Diffuse (or patchy) infiltrate — 1 point
- Localized infiltrate — 2 points

Progression of pulmonary infiltrate on CXR
- No progression — 0 points
- Progression (CHF/ARDS excluded) — 2 points

[*] ARDS: $PaO_2/FiO_2$ ≤ 26.7 kPa (200 mmHg), PAOP ≤18 mmHg, and bilateral CXR infiltrates
Adapted from Pugin J, et al. (1991) Am Rev Resp Dis, **143**, 1121–9; Singh N et al. (2000). Am J Resp Crit Care Med, **162**, 505–11.

**Investigations** (see p. 59 and 324)
Also consider
- FBC, U&Es, LFTs, CRP, CK
- CXR
- Sputum for Gram stain and culture (if TB suspected request AFBs)
- Bronchoscopy samples (or protected endobronchial specimen or brush) for:
  - Culture, including *Legionella* culture
  - Immunofluorescence for *Chlamydia*, influenza A and B, parainfluenza, adenovirus, respiratory syncytial virus, *Pneumocystis carinii*
  - In VAP qualitative cultures of endotracheal secretions may differentiate colonization from infection (>10⁶ CFU/ml)
- Serology for viral/atypical testing (and samples 7–10 days after admission)
- Throat swabs for viral infections: influenza A and B, parainfluenza, adenovirus, respiratory syncytial virus
- Urine for *Legionella* and pneumococcal antigen
- Pleural fluid (if aspirated) for microscopy and culture

**Immediate management**

Follow guidelines on p. 59
- Give O₂ as required; support airway, breathing, and circulation
- Severe pneumonia is likely to require respiratory support: either non-invasive ventilation or mechanical ventilation with endotracheal intubation

**Suggested empirical antimicrobials**
- CAP: co-amoxiclav IV 1.2 g 8-hourly and clarithromycin IV 500 mg 12-hourly
  - If associated with influenza add flucloxacillin IV 2 g 6-hourly
- Aspiration pneumonia: co-amoxiclav IV 1.2 g 8-hourly and metronidazole IV 500 mg 8-hourly
  - For severe in-hospital aspiration add gentamicin IV 5 mg/kg daily
- Atypical pathogens suspected: co-amoxiclav IV 1.2 g 8-hourly and clarithromycin IV 500 mg 12-hourly (in *Legionella* consider adding rifampicin IV 600 mg 12-hourly); in immunocompromised patients, or where any of the following are suspected, treat accordingly
  - *Pneumocystis carinii*: co-trimoxazole IV 120 mg/kg/day
  - Fungal infections: amphotericin B IV 0.25–1 g 6-hourly
  - Viral infections: herpes, aciclovir IV 10 mg/kg 8-hourly; CMV, ganciclovir IV 5 mg/kg 12-hourly; RSV, nebulized ribavirin 20 mg/ml
- HAP/HCAP/VAP: avoid previously used antibiotics
  - Consider ceftazidime IV 2 g 8-hourly and gentamicin IV 5 mg/kg daily with/without flucloxacillin IV 2 g 6-hourly
- MDR organisms suspected: add
  - MRSA: vancomycin IV 500 mg 6-hourly or linezolid IV 600 mg 12-hourly
  - Resistant *Acinetobacter*: amikacin IV 7.5 mg/kg 12-hourly

**Further management**
- Report notifiable diseases such as *Legionella* (see p. 352)
- Complications such as empyema may require surgical treatment

**Further reading**
BTS (2001). BTS Guidelines for the management of community acquired pneumonia in adults *Thorax* **56**(Suppl 4), iv1–64.

Macfarlane JT, Boldy D, Boswell T, *et al.* (2004). Update of BTS pneumonia guidelines: what's new? *Thorax* **59**, 364–6.

ATS (2005). Guidelines for the management of adults with hospital-acquired, ventilator-associated, and healthcare-associated pneumonia: American Thoracic Society Documents. *Am J Resp Crit Care Med* **171**, 388–416.

OHCC p. 288.

# ① **Endocarditis**

### Causes
- Underlying aortic or mitral valve disease, or rheumatic disease
- Prosthetic heart valves
- IV drug use (right-sided endocarditis)

### Presentation and assessment
General signs and symptoms of infection (see p. 323) may be accompanied by:
- Dental infections
- Osler's nodes, Janeway lesions, splinter haemorrhages, purpuric lesions, Roth spots
- Splenomegaly
- Glomerulonephritis, microscopic haematuria
- Infarcts (lung, heart, brain)
- Metastatic abscesses
- Heart murmurs

### Investigations (see p. 324)

Also consider
- Serial blood cultures
- Serial CRP measurements
- Serology (especially for *Coxiella burnetti*, *Bartonella*, *Chlamydia*, *Candida*, *Aspergillus*)
- Urine dipstick
- ECG
- Trans-thoracic/trans-oesophageal echocardiography
- Tissue sample culture (following surgery)

### Immediate management

Follow guidelines on p. 325
- Give $O_2$ as required; support airway, breathing, and circulation
- Treat heart failure (see p. 124) and arrhythmias (see pp. 136 and 140)

**Suggested empirical antimicrobials**
- Gradual-onset: benzylpenicillin IV 2.4 g 6-hourly and gentamicin IV 5 mg/kg daily
- Associated with IV drug use: flucloxacillin IV 2 g 6-hourly and gentamicin IV 5mg/kg daily
- Prosthetic valves or severe infection/complications: vancomycin IV 500 mg 6-hourly, gentamicin IV 5 mg/kg daily, and rifampicin IV 600 mg 12-hourly
- If immunocompromised add amphotericin B IV 0.25–1 g 6-hourly

**Further management**
- Surgery may need to be considered where there is:
  - Gross valve regurgitation causing haemodynamic compromise
  - Prosthetic valve endocarditis
  - Perivalvular abscesses or very large vegetations
  - Resistant organisms (e.g. MRSA)

**Further reading**
Beynon RP, Bahl VK, Prendergast BD (2006). Infective endocarditis. *BMJ* **333**, 334–9.

# ⓘ Mediastinitis

## Causes
- Oesophageal perforation (traumatic, post-surgical anastamotic breakdown, spontaneous (Boerhaave syndrome))
- Tracheal perforation
- Mediastinal extension of dental or neck infection

## Presentation and assessment
General signs and symptoms of infection (see p. 323) may be accompanied by:
- History of coughing or choking (Boerhaave syndrome)
- Recent oesophageal surgery or endoscopy
- Increasing respiratory distress, tachypnoea, dyspnoea
- Signs associated with pneumothorax or hydrothorax (i.e. percussion note and auscultation changes), most commonly left-sided

## Investigations (see p. 324)

Also consider:
- CXR (may show pneumomediastinum, pneumothorax, or hydrothorax)
- CT scan of chest
- Water-soluble contrast swallow (or barium swallow)

## Immediate management

Follow guidelines on p. 325
- Give $O_2$ as required; support airway, breathing, and circulation
- Keep patient NBM
- Insert intercostal chest drain(s) as indicated by X-ray findings

### Suggested empirical antimicrobials
- Piptazobactam IV 4.5 g 8-hourly and gentamicin IV 5 mg/kg daily and fluconazole IV 400 mg daily

## Further management
- Thoracic surgical advice should be sought

# ☼ Meningitis and encephalitis

(see also p. 192)

## Causes

The most common causative agents are *Streptococcus pneumoniae* and *Neisseria meningitidis*, and viral infections. *Haemophilus influenzae* has become rare as a consequence of mass HiB innoculation. *Listeria* and fungal infections e.g. *Cryptococcus*) are common in immunocompromised patients. *Staphylococcus aureus* and *Staphylococcus epidermis* are common following surgery.

## Presentation and assessment (see also p. 192)

General signs and symptoms of infection (p. 323) may be accompanied by:
- Meningeal signs: headache, neck stiffness, vomiting, photophobia, and lethargy
- Raised ICP: focal neurological signs, seizures, altered mental state, decreased consciousness, papilloedema

## Investigations (see p. 324)

Also consider:
- Blood cultures
- Serum PCR
- Throat swab
- Rash scrapings or skin pustule aspirates for culture/PCR
- Head CT scan (and/or MRI)
- LP (opening pressure, CSF for urgent Gram stain and microscopy, PCR, protein, glucose (with paired plasma sample))
- If *Cryptococcus* or *Toxoplasmosis* are present consider HIV testing

## Immediate management

Follow guidelines on p. 194
- Give $O_2$ as required; support airway, breathing, and circulation
- Treat the systemic effects of meningococcal sepsis as appropriate (p. 350)
- Treat decreased consciousness (p. 158) and seizure activity (p. 166)
- Give dexamethasone 10 mg IV 6-hourly with first dose of antibiotic

**If you suspect bacterial meningitis do not delay treatment.** Antibiotic therapy should be commenced immediately. If meningococcal disease is suspected, benzylpenicillin may have already been given by the GP or the admitting physicians

### Suggested empirical antimicrobials
- Ceftriaxone 2 g IV 12-hourly
- If viral meningitis is suspected add aciclovir IV 10 mg/kg 8-hourly
- If following neurosurgery add flucloxacillin IV 2 g 6-hourly (vancomycin IV 500 mg 6-hourly if MRSA)
- In immunocompromised patients consider adding amoxicillin IV 1 g 6-hourly and gentamicin IV 5 mg/kg daily and amphotericin B IV 0.25–1 g 6-hourly and aciclovir IV 10 mg/kg 8-hourly

**Further management**
- Report notifiable diseases (p. 378)
- If bacterial meningitis present consider prophylaxis for staff

# ☼ Intracerebral abscess

## Causes
Intracerebral abscesses are most commonly caused by haematogenous spread of infections and are associated with endocarditis and dental sepsis. Intracerebral abscess may also complicate neurosurgery, penetrating injury, or meningitis.

## Presentation and assessment
General signs and symptoms of infection (see p. 323) may be accompanied by signs and symptoms associated with meningitis (see p. 192)

## Investigations (see p. 324)

Also consider:
- Blood cultures
- Surgical aspirates
- Drain fluid culture
- LP is contraindicated

## Immediate management

Follow guidelines on p. 325
- Give $O_2$ as required; support airway, breathing, and circulation
- Give dexamethasone 10 mg IV 6-hourly if mass effect is present

### Suggested empirical antimicrobials
- Ceftriaxone IV 2 g 12-hourly and metronidazole IV 500 mg 8-hourly
- If following neurosurgery add flucloxacillin IV 2 g 6-hourly (vancomycin IV 500 mg 6-hourly if MRSA)
- In immunocompromised patients consider adding amoxicillin IV 1 g 6-hourly and gentamicin IV 5 mg/kg daily; consider adding treatment for toxoplasma

## Further management
- Neurosurgical referral is required

## Further reading
Chadwick DR Viral meningitis British Medical Bulletin; 75&76: 1–14.
📖 OHCC p. 374.

# ⓘ **Urological infections**

### Causes
- Urinary tract infection (UTI) may be upper (pyelonephritis) or lower (cystitis)

### Presentation and assessment
General signs and symptoms of infection (p. 323) may be accompanied by:
- Back pain or renal colic; suprapubic pain
- Dysuria, urinary frequency
- Haematuria, cloudy urine
- In the elderly the only symptom may be altered mental state

Infection is more common in patients with stones (or following surgery for renal calculi), indwelling catheters, neurogenic bladder, diabetes or immunosuppression.

### Investigations (see p. 324)

Also consider:
- U&Es
- Urine for culture (mid-stream urine (MSU) or catheter-specimen urine (CSU)): catheterized patients will have evidence of colonization without infection (a positive culture typically has >$10^5$ organisms/ml)
- Urine dipstick (positive if nitrates or leucocyte esterases are present)
- Renal tract imaging to identify calculi or hydronephrosis
  - Pelvic X-ray (kidney ureter bladder (KUB))
  - Intravenous urogram (IVU)
  - US kidney or CT abdomen

### Immediate management
Follow guidelines on p. 325
- Give $O_2$ as required; support airway, breathing, and circulation
- Analgesia is likely to be required, especially if colic is present

#### Suggested empirical antimicrobials
- Community-acquired infection: co-amoxiclav IV 1.2 g 8-hourly
- Severe or hospital-acquired infection: piptazobactam IV 4.5 g 8-hourly and gentamicin IV 5 mg/kg daily
- Immunocompromised: consider adding fluconazole IV 200 mg daily

### Further management
- Urological referral is required if ureteric obstruction occurs

### Pitfalls/difficult situations
- Consider TB (send early morning urines for AFBs), schistosomiasis, or fungal infections
- Aggressively treat bacteriuria in the presence of pregnancy or a transplanted kidney
- If neurogenic bladder is possible perform a full neurological assessment

# ⚠ Abdominal infections

## Causes

Abdominal infections include peritonitis caused by gut perforation, cholangitis/cholecystitis, and colitis (commonly caused by *Clostridium difficile*).

## Presentation and assessment (see also pp. 290 and 323)
General signs and symptoms of infection may be accompanied by:
- Recent history of abdominal operation
- Abdominal pain, rebound, guarding; bowel obstruction, or diarrhoea
- Nausea and vomiting; anorexia (or failure to absorb NG feed)
- Jaundice

## Investigations (see p. 324)
Also consider
- ABGs (metabolic acidosis, lactate)
- Serum LFTs, CRP, amylase, or lipase
- Cultures of surgical/radiological aspirates, tissue samples, or drain fluid
- Stool for culture and *C.difficile* toxin
- CXR (sub-diaphragmatic air may be present)
- CT abdomen; US abdomen
- Lower GI endoscopy (if colitis suspected)

---

### Immediate management

Follow guidelines on p. 325
- Give $O_2$ as required; support airway, breathing, and circulation
- Analgesia may be required
- Abdominal catastrophe is likely to require aggressive fluid and/or inotrope resuscitation
- Surgical referral is required for a patient with an acute abdomen
  - Laparotomy may be required
  - US or CT-guided percutaneous abscess drainage may be possible

### Suggested empirical antimicrobials
- Perforation/peritonitis: piptazobactam IV 4.5 g 8-hourly and gentamicin IV 5 mg/kg daily
  - Consider adding fluconazole IV 400 mg daily
  - If previous CAPD consider adding vancomycin IV 500 mg 6-hourly
- Cholangitis: ceftriaxone IV 2 g 12-hourly
- Suspected *C.difficile*: metronidazole PO/NG 400 mg 8-hourly or vancomycin PO/NG 125 mg 6-hourly
  - If there is no NG access then use metronidazole IV 500 mg 8-hourly

---

## Further management
- ERCP may be indicated for obstructive jaundice

## Further reading
Starr J (2005). *Clostridium difficile* associated diarrhoea: diagnosis and treatment. *BMJ* **331**, 498–501.
📖 OHCC pp. 340, 352.

# ① Skin and orthopaedic infections

## Causes
- Septic arthritis
- Abscess formation or wound infection
- Cellulitis
- Necrotizing fasciitis

## Presentation and assessment
General signs and symptoms of infection (see p. 323) may be accompanied by:
- A medical history of immunocompromise, chronic disease (e.g. diabetes or renal failure), or IV drug use
- Recent skin trauma (often very mild); recent joint replacement
- Obvious abscesses; frank pus in wounds, wound drains, or urine
- Skin or joint erythema and swelling
- Crepitus
- Vesicles or blistering
- Lymph node enlargement
- Pain

Necrotizing fasciitis occurs when infection spreads along the superficial and deep fascial planes, most commonly on the legs, abdomen, perineum, or groin (Fournier's gangrene affects men involving scrotum, perineum, or penis) causing:
- Rapidly progressive cellulitis (over hours)
- Skin may become grey and necrotic in appearance
- Severe pain, although affected skin is often anaesthetized
- Systemic disturbance, often severe, including septic shock, DIC, ARF, metabolic acidosis

## Investigations (see p. 324)
Also consider:
- Serum CK
- Serum CRP and ESR
- Synovial fluid microscopy, Gram stain, and culture (for septic arthritis)
- Blood cultures
- Pus or debrided skin samples for cultures
- Skin biopsy is suspected necrotising fasciitis
- Joint X-rays
- Soft tissue X-ray or CT scan (may reveal tissue necrosis or emphysema)
- US imaging of hips may be required in hip septic arthritis
- MRI may be useful in detecting osteomyelitis

## Immediate management

Follow guidelines on p. 325
- Give $O_2$ as required; support airway, breathing, and circulation
- Analgesia may be required
- Surgery may be required
  - Surgical debridement will be required for necrotizing fasciitis
  - CT imaging for suspected necrotizing fasciitis should not delay surgical exploration
  - Arthroscopy/joint washout may be required for septic arthritis

### Suggested empirical antimicrobials
- Septic arthritis: vancomycin IV 500 mg 6-hourly and ceftriaxone IV 2 g 12-hourly
- Severe surgical wound infection: vancomycin IV 500 mg 6-hourly and gentamicin IV 5 mg/kg daily and metronidazole IV 500 mg 8-hourly
- Cellulitis: benzylpenicillin IV 1.2 g 6-hourly and flucloxacillin IV 2 g 6-hourly (change flucloxacillin to vancomycin IV 500 mg 6-hourly for MRSA)
- Necrotizing fasciitis: benzylpenicillin IV 1.2 g 6-hourly and gentamicin IV 5 mg/kg daily and metronidazole IV 500 mg 8-hourly

## Further management

- Repeated surgery/surgical debridement may be required
- Tetanus immunoglubulin with/without tetanus vaccine may be required
- Hyperbaric oxygen may promote wound healing in severe wound/soft tissue infections

## Pitfalls/difficult situations

- A high mortality is associated with necrotizing fasciitis and surgical debridement is often severe/radical
- Osteomyelitis may complicate trauma or joint/infection
- Compartment syndrome may complicate necrotizing fasciitis
- STDs are associated with septic arthritis
- A high index of suspicion for contaminated wounds is required (e.g. rabies, botulism, tetanus)

## Further reading

Coakley G, Mathews C, Field M, *et al.* (2006). BSR & BHPR, BOA, RCGP and BSAC guidelines for management of the hot swollen joint in adults. *Rheumatology* **45**, 1039–41.

# ☻ Meningococcal sepsis

*Neisseria meningitidis* can cause a variety of clinical syndromes; the most deadly is meningococcal sepsis.

## Causes

Risk factors for meningococcal sepsis include:
- Communal living (e.g. university halls of residence and army barracks)
- Overcrowding and social deprivation
- Smoking or recent URTI (increased risk of nasopharyngeal carriage)
  - Passive smoking is a risk factor for invasive disease
- Complement deficiencies (increased risk of re-infection)

## Presentation and assessment

Meningitis and meningoencephalitis may occur without septicaemia (see pp. 192 and 340) or can be associated with systemic sepsis (the signs and symptoms of meningitis are often the more pronounced of the two).

Systemic sepsis without meningitis may occur
- General: rapidly deteriorating influenza-like presentation with
  - Pyrexia, myalgia,
  - Rash: purpuric (or sometimes petechial) lesions on abdomen and/or lower limbs, coalescing into ecchymoses
- Respiratory: tachypnoea and hypoxia; pulmonary oedema may develop, especially associated with aggressive fluid resuscitation
  - ARDS may develop
- Cardiovascular: tachycardia
  - Cardiovascular compromise may develop rapidly
  - Pericarditis may develop
- Neurological: agitation, confusion, diminished consciousness
- Renal: oliguria, raised urea and creatinine (ARF may develop)
  - Metabolic acidosis
- Gastrointestinal: anorexia, diarrhoea, nausea and vomiting
- Haematology: DIC
- Musculoskeletal: septic arthritis may occur

## Investigations (see also p. 324)
- ABGs: compensated metabolic acidosis with elevated lactate levels
- FBC: WCC may be high or low; Hb and platelets may be low
- Coagulation studies, including fibrinogen (DIC may be present)
- Serum glucose (often low)
- U&Es, LFTs
- Blood culture (two sets as *N.meningitidis* may be difficult to culture)
- Blood EDTA bottle for antigen detection and PCR
- CT brain (if reduced consciousness and focal neurological signs)

*Lumbar puncture is not indicated for patients with meningococcal sepsis.*

## Differential diagnoses
- Bacterial sepsis from *Streptococcus pneumoniae* or *Haemophilus influenzae*
- Toxic shock syndrome
- Viral haemorrhagic fevers (especially if there is a history of travel)

## Immediate management

- Give $O_2$ as required; support airway, breathing, and circulation
- Airway: endotracheal intubation may be required
  - Where there is decreased consciousness (GCS ≤8)
  - To facilitate mechanical ventilation
- Ensure breathing/ventilation is adequate
  - Mechanical ventilation may be needed to optimize oxygenation in severe shock or pulmonary oedema
- Circulatory support should be commenced
  - Large peripheral venous cannulae are required
  - Fluid boluses will be required to treat hypotension (pulmonary oedema is common, particularly once ≥30 ml/kg of IV fluid boluses have been given)
  - Inotropic/vasopressor support is likely to be required
  - Use early goal-directed treatment (CVP 8–12 mmHg; MAP ≥65 mmHg; UOP ≥0.5 ml/kg/hour; $ScvO_2$ or $S\bar{v}O_2$ ≥70%)
  - Arterial and/or central venous cannulation should be undertaken as soon as feasible, checking coagulation studies and platelets first

**If you suspect meningococcal septicaemia do not delay treatment**
Antibiotic therapy should be commenced immediately. If meningococcal disease is suspected, benzylpenicillin may have already been given by the GP or the admitting physicians.
- Antimicrobial treatment: ceftriaxone 2 g IV 12-hourly

## Further management

- Transfer to HDU/ICU
- Cardiac output monitoring is likely to be required as there is often a larger degree of myocardial depression with meningococcal sepsis than with other types of sepsis
  - Calcium replacement may improve myocardial function
- Consider treatment with activated protein C (see p. 122–123)
- Renal replacement therapy is likely to be required
- Modify antimicrobial treatment according to blood culture results and microbiological advice
- Sepsis care bundles should be implemented, including tight glucose control, low-dose steroids, DVT prophylaxis, and GI prophylaxis
- Check limbs regularly as DIC and purpura fulminans can cause occlusion of vessels and amputation may be required

## Pitfalls/difficult situations

- The speed of onset from innocuous symptoms to death can be <2 hours and delay in antibiotic administration may be fatal
- The rash may present as a maculopapular rash

## Further reading

Baines PB, Hart CA (2003). Severe meningococcal disease in childhood. *Br J Anaesth* **90**, 72–83.

# ⓘ **Legionnaire's disease**

(see also Pneumonia, pp. 58 and 322)

This rare, but life-threatening, pneumonia is caused by *Legionella pneu-mophilia* (90%), or *Legionella mcdadei* (5–10%) and accounts for 2–5% of community-acquired pneumonias.

## Causes

*Legionella* is spread by exposure to aerosolized infected water
- Contaminated water-storage tanks
- Air conditioning units

Legionnaire's disease is more common in:
- The middle-aged or elderly
- Smokers
- Chronic alcoholics
- Patients with chronic illness (e.g. diabetes, COPD, or renal failure)
- Males are twice as likely to be affected as females

## Presentation and assessment

*Legionella* is often contracted abroad and there is increased prevalence in the summer and autumn (patients often return from their holidays unwell). The incubation period is 2–10 days.

Systemic complications are more common than in other pneumonias, and may be out of proportion to the degree of respiratory involvement. Signs and symptoms may include:
- General: influenza-like presentation with fevers, sweats, and rigors
- Respiratory: tachypnoea and hypoxia
  - Dry cough
  - Pleuritic chest pain is common
- Cardiovascular: tachycardia
  - Cardiovascular compromise may develop (more common than in other pneumonias)
- Renal: oliguria, raised urea and creatinine (ARF may develop)
- Gastrointestinal: abdominal pain, vomiting, and diarrhoea are common
- Neurological: confusion, diminished consciousness, focal cerebellar signs

## Investigations (see also p. 324)
- ABGs
- FBC (a moderate increase in WCC with a lymphopenia may occur)
- U&Es (hyponatraemia and raised urea and creatinine are common)
- LFTs (often deranged and with low albumin)
- Serum CK (occasionally raised)
- Serum CRP
- Blood cultures × 2 (organism is difficult to grow and must be specifically requested; can take 10 days to culture)
- Sputum, endotracheal aspirate, or BAL for immunofluorescence testing
- Urinary antigen testing: highly specific
- Serum for *Legionella* antigen
- CXR (rapidly progressive patchy shadowing)

Differential diagnoses
- Other organisms which cause CAP
- Always consider TB as a cause of pneumonia in patients with multisystem involvement who fail to respond to conventional treatment

Immediate management
- Give $O_2$ as required; support airway, breathing, and circulation
  - Assess degree of pneumonia according to CURB-65 score (see p. 59)
  - Respiratory support/mechanical ventilation is commonly required
- Send appropriate blood tests (see Investigations)
- Treat as community-acquired pneumonia
  - Commence co-amoxiclav IV 1.2 g 8-hourly and clarithromycin IV 500 mg 12-hourly
  - When diagnosis is confirmed add rifampicin IV 600 mg 12-hourly

Further management
- Transfer to HDU/ICU
- Fluoroquinolones may be used in immunosuppressed patients
- Antibiotics should be continued for 14–21 days
- *Legionella* is not a notifiable disease, but public health should be informed
- Sepsis care bundles should be implemented, including tight glucose control, low-dose steroids, DVT prophylaxis, and GI prophylaxis

Pitfalls/difficult situations
- Patients are often disproportionately sicker than those with CAP
- Hypoxia and confusion may make patients non-compliant with therapy
- 20% of patients develop ARDS
- Pericardial and myocardial involvement may occur
- Systemic involvement, especially liver and neurological changes, makes the diagnosis more likely

Further reading

Hoare Z, Lim WS (2006). Pneumonia: update on diagnosis and management. *BMJ* **332**, 1077–9.

# ☼ Tetanus

Tetanus is caused by a neurotoxin, tetanospasmin, released by *Clostridium tetani*, a Gram-positive anaerobic bacillus. The toxin is irreversible and prevents neurotransmitter release, causing muscle rigidity, muscle spasm, and autonomic instability. Recovery occurs with nerve terminal regrowth.

## Causes

Four forms of tetanus are described: local, cephalic, neonatal, and generalized (the most common form). Risk factors include:
- Inadequate or no previous vaccination history
- Penetrating trauma (often trivial)
- Drug abusers, especially if SC or IM injectors

## Presentation and assessment

Symptom onset occurs 2–60 days after inoculation. Often the injury is trivial. Signs and symptoms may include:
- General: sore throat, hypersecretion (saliva, bronchial), hyperpyrexia
- Neuromuscular
  - Early symptoms include neck stiffness, dysphagia, and trismus
  - Muscle spasms develop in facial muscles, 'risus sardonicus' (facial muscles are often affected first because of shorter axonal pathways)
  - Later spasms become more widespread with neck and back rigidity with/without hyperextension
  - Spasms are often triggered by innocuous stimuli; they are extremely painful and can damage muscles, tendons, joints, and bones
- Respiratory: spasms can cause laryngospasm and/or ventilation may be impaired, causing respiratory arrest
- Cardiovascular: autonomic instability develops a few days after spasms have commenced and can cause tachycardia and hypertension, bradycardia, asystole, and profound hypotension
- Gastrointestinal: ileus
- Neurological: seizures may occur

## Investigations

Tetanus is a clinical diagnosis
- ABGs (may show high lactate and metabolic acidosis)
- FBC
- U&Es, LFTs, serum CK
- Blood cultures/wound swabs (30% of wound cultures grow organism)
- X-rays of any suspected fracture sites

## Differential diagnoses

- Acute dystonic reactions
- Epilepsy
- Chorea
- Meningitis/encephalitis or SAH
- Strychnine poisoning
- Rabies
- Drug withdrawal states

Immediate management

- Give $O_2$ as required; support airway, breathing, and circulation
- Consider elective endotracheal intubation and mechanical ventilation: the most common cause of death is from laryngospasm and respiratory muscle paralysis
- Nurse in a dark room with minimal stimulation
- Control muscle spasm and autonomic instability
  - Heavy sedation with diazepam (or midazolam) and morphine is required (doses may be very high)
  - Refractory spasms may require neuromuscular blockade

**Prevent further toxin damage and release**
- Give human tetanus antitoxin IM 5000–10 000 IU
  - One dose is required as the half-life is 23 days; it neutralizes circulatory toxin, but not that bound intra-neuronally
  - Side effects include fevers, shivers, and hypotension; the rate of infusion should be slowed if this occurs
- Reduce toxin load by debriding any infected tissue
- Give metronidazole IV 500 mg 8-hourly for 7–10 days to eradicate any remaining bacterium

Further management

- Secondary agents which may be used for muscle spasms include baclofen, dantrolene, and chlorpromazine
- Refractory autonomic instability may respond to:
  - Clonidine (centrally acting $\alpha_2$-adrenergic agonist)
  - Magnesium sulphate infusion: 20 mmol/hour adjusted to achieve plasma concentrations of 2.5–4.0 mmol/L
- Prolonged mechanical ventilation may require a trachoestomy
- Treatments aimed at reducing complications of neuromuscular weakness or paralysis include:
  - Respiratory infections: regular physiotherapy and tracheal toilet
  - NG or PEG feeding, gastric ulcer prophylaxis
  - DVT/PE: compression stockings or LMWH
  - Skin damage, joint contractures: pressure area care, physiotherapy
  - Bowel care may be needed
- Watch for nosocomial infections, fractures, or rhabdomyolysis
- Immunization is required in the convalescent period
- Public health need to be informed as tetanus is a notifiable disease

Pitfalls/difficult situations

- Clinical suspicion is important to institute early effective management
- Sudden cardiac arrest is common and may be due to high catecholamine levels or a direct effect of the toxin on the myocardium
- Recovery of function may take months

Further reading

Cook TM, Protheroe RT, Handel JM (2001). Tetanus a review of the literature. *Br J Anaesth* **87**, 477–87.
📖 OHCC p. 390.

# :⚙: Botulism

Botulism is caused by the toxin of *Clostridium botulinum*. The main effects of the toxin are on the nervous tissue where it blocks the presynaptic release of acetylcholine at neuromuscular junctions, parasympathetic terminals, and autonomic ganglia. The toxin has six subtypes (A–F), but A, B, and E cause the illness.

## Causes

*Clostridium botulinum* may be:
- Food borne (symptoms start within 18 hours of ingestion of contaminated food)
- Associated with IV or SC/IM ('popping') drug abuse with black tar containing heroin (this leads to subcutaneous wounds that promote growth of the organism)

## Presentation and assessment

Signs and symptoms include:
- General: fatigue, dry mouth, dilated pupils
- Neurological: dizziness
- Neuromuscular: progressive muscular weakness leading to symmetrically descending paralysis
    - Extra-ocular muscles (blurred vision), followed by pharyngeal and then upper and lower limb muscles in severe cases
    - Paraesthesiae may occur
- Respiratory: respiratory failure due to muscle weakness may occur in severe cases
- Gastrointestinal: nausea, vomiting, constipation, ileus

Poor prognosis is indicated by limb and respiratory weakness, age >20 years, and illness caused by type A toxin

## Investigations

- ABGs
- FBC
- U&Es, LFTs
- Blood cultures
- Serum and stool assay for *Clostridium* toxin
- Pulmonary function tests
- ECG
- CXR
- Tensilon test to exclude myasthenia gravis
- Nerve conduction studies to exclude Guillain–Barré syndrome
- EMG studies will show abnormal patterns

## Differential diagnoses

- Guillain–Barré syndrome
- Spinal cord injury (especially epidural abscess or haematoma)
- Periodic paralysis
- Tick paralysis

Immediate management

- Give $O_2$ as required; support airway, breathing, and circulation
- Airway may become compromised if the protective reflexes of the upper airway are compromised; early intubation must be considered
- Assess adequacy of ventilation using FVC and $FEV_1$
  - If FVC <15 ml/kg, or FVC < predicted TV, or failure to expectorate secretions occurs, supportive ventilation is indicated
  - Repeat PFTs 4-hourly
  - Other indications for ventilation may include hypercapnia and/or CXR (pneumonia, atelectasis)

**Prevent further toxin damage and release**
- Give 10 000 units of trivalent anti-toxin immediately (and then every 4 hours); contact DOH duty officer for out-of-hours supply
  - Anticipate minor allergic reactions and keep antihistamines and steroids ready for administration
- Consider gastric lavage or enemas to remove toxins (patients with bulbar weakness require endotracheal intubation before lavage)

Further management

- Transfer to HDU/ICU
- Continuing assessment and management of airway and breathing problems
  - Treatment of pneumonia if present
  - Continue administration of anti-toxin
  - Guanidine hydrochloride, an acetylcholine agonist, can be given orally at 30 mg/kg/day in divided doses

Pitfalls/difficult situations

- Dilated and non-reactive pupils in an alert patient is a distinguishing feature of botulism; however, the pupils may remain dilated but reactive

Further reading

📖 OHCC p. 390.

# ☼ Toxic shock syndrome

Toxic shock syndrome is caused by toxin-producing Gram-positive organisms (staphylococci or streptococci). The site of infection is often localized, and the systemic manifestations are the result of the toxins.

## Causes
- Associated with menstruation and/or use of vaginal tampons
- Drug-induced
- Any wound infection (post-operative)

## Presentation and assessment
Presenting signs and symptoms are those of acute onset sepsis (see p. 323), and may be accompanied by:
- General: fever, diffuse macular rash (may be similar to drug reaction)
- Cardiovascular: rapidly progressive tachycardia and hypotension
- Gastrointestinal: diarrhoea
- Haematological: DIC
- Multi-organ dysfunction

## Investigations
- ABGs
- FBC (leucocytosis is common), coagulation screen (for DIC)
- U&Es, LFTs (LFT dysfunction is present in up to 40% of cases)
- Serum CK (often elevated) and CRP
- Cultures: blood cultures (rarely positive), vaginal swabs, throat swabs, urine culture, wound swabs
- ECG and CXR

## Differential diagnoses
- Any cause of sepsis, including meningococcal septicaemia

**Immediate management** (as for sepsis p. 325)
- Give $O_2$ as required; support airway, breathing, and circulation
- Ensure breathing/ventilation is adequate
  - Mechanical ventilation may be needed to optimize oxygenation
- Circulatory support should be commenced
  - Large peripheral venous cannulae are required
  - Fluid boluses will be required to treat hypotension
  - Inotropic/vasopressor support is likely to be required
  - Use early goal-directed treatment (CVP 8–12 mmHg, MAP ≥65 mmHg, UOP ≥0.5 ml/kg/hour, $ScvO_2$ or $S\bar{v}O_2$ ≥70%)
  - Arterial and/or central venous cannulation should be undertaken as soon as feasible, checking coagulation studies and platelets first

**Treatment of infection**
- Remove the source of infection: wound drainage (or removal of foreign body, including tampons) may have to be undertaken while the patient is still being resuscitated
- Give flucloxacillin IV 2 g 6-hourly

**Further management**

As for sepsis and septic shock (see pp. 326 and 120)

**Pitfalls/difficult situations**

- Immediate removal of source of infection is crucial
- Rapid onset of syndrome requires rapid response for resuscitation
- Multidisciplinary involvement will be required
- Rash may be similar to acute drug reactions

# ① Panton–Valentine leucocidin (PVL) infections

PVL toxin, which is capable of destroying white blood cells, is carried by ≤ 2% of *Staphylococcus aureus* strains (both MRSA and MSSA). Skin and soft tissue infection are common, although septic arthritis and community-acquired necrotizing pneumonia can occur.

## Presentation and assessment

General signs and symptoms of infection (see p. 323) may be accompanied by:
- Abscesses, cellulitis, and tissue necrosis affecting children/young adults
- Diarrhoea and vomiting
- Marked leucopenia
- Pneumonia with CXR changes (infiltrates with effusions, and later cavitation) with/without haemoptysis

## Investigations (see p. 324)

Also consider
- FBC
- Serum CK and CRP (likely to be extremely high)

### Immediate management

Follow guidelines on p. 325
- Give O₂ as required; support airway, breathing, and circulation
- Where multi-organ failure is present consider:
  - Activated protein C
  - Intravenous immunoglobulin (IVIG)

**Suggested empirical antimicrobials**
- PVL-associated SA infection: flucloxacillin IV 2 g 6-hourly and linezolid IV 600 mg 12-hourly and rifampicin IV 600 mg 12-hourly

## Further management

- Apply infection control measures where pneumonia is present (surgical masks for endotracheal intubation and closed tracheal suctioning)

## Enteric fever (typhoid)

# ⚠ Enteric fever (typhoid)

Enteric fever is caused by infection with *Salmonella enterica typhi* or *Salmonella enterica paratyphi*. It is endemic in Africa, South America, and the Indian subcontinent.

## Causes

- Spread is mostly faeco-oral and can be food or water-borne
- Chronic carrier state can be present in 1–3% of infected patients a year after treatment of acute illness

## Presentation and assessment

The incubation period is 7–21 days; occurrence a month after return from an endemic area is rare. General signs and symptoms of infection (see p. 323) may be accompanied by:

- General: malaise, headache (a very common symptom), chills, sweats, myalgia, sore throat, and cough
  - Gradual rise of temperature in the first week
  - Erythematous lesions which blanch on pressure (rose spots) appear on upper abdomen in up to 30% of patients
  - Cervical lymphadenopathy
- Cardiovascular: tachycardia is relatively uncommon
- Respiratory: pneumonia may occur
- Gastrointestinal: anorexia, pain, nausea, vomiting, constipation, diarrhoea can all be seen (constipation occurs early, diarrhoea late)
  - Jaundice
  - Acute abdomen due to bowel perforation may occur, typically in the second or third week of infection
  - Splenomegaly or hepatomegaly may be seen
- Neurological: coma, seizures, encephalopathy, and meningism occur in up to 5% of patients
- Renal: UTIs may occur

5–10% of patients present with toxic shock or multi-system dysfunction

## Investigations (see also p. 324)

Also consider

- FBC
  - <7 days: raised WCC may be seen
  - >7 days: marrow suppression may occur with decreased Hb, WCC, and platelets
- U&Es
- LFTs (commonly deranged in the first 7 days)
- CXR/AXR (sub-diaphragmatic gas may be seen in bowel perforation)
- CT head scan will be required if neurological complications are present
- Cultures
  - <7 days: blood cultures positive in up to 90% of patients
  - >7 days: blood cultures are generally negative, but urine and stool cultures are likely to be positive
  - Bone marrow cultures may be appropriate, but are more invasive
- Serology

## Differential diagnoses

- Malaria
- Meningitis/encephalitis
- Diarrhoea-causing illnesses: e.g. *C.difficile* colitis, cholera, *Shigella*

### Immediate management

- Give $O_2$ as required; support airway, breathing, and circulation
- Aggressive fluid resuscitation is likely to be required
- Inotropic support may be required ion some cases
- Invasive monitoring may be required in unstable patients
- In severe toxaemia consider steroids (dexamethasone IV 3 mg/kg followed by 1 mg/kg 6-hourly for eight doses)

### Suggested empirical antimicrobials

- Give ceftriaxone IV 2 g 12-hourly
- Alternatively ciprofloxacin IV 400 mg 12-hourly

## Further management

- Supportive measures will be required, as in sepsis (see p. 326)
- Careful management of electrolyte balance is required
- Antipyretic therapy may be required
- Typhoid is a notifiable disease; public health must be informed
- Continuing assessment and management of complications is required
  - Pneumonia
  - UTIs
  - Cholecystitis
  - Haemolytic anaemia
  - Meningitis
  - Peripheral neuropathy
  - Osteomyelitis
  - Intestinal perforation and/or intestinal haemorrhage; may require surgery

## Pitfalls/difficult situations

- Chloramphenicol has been standard antibiotic therapy, but outbreaks of drug resistance have occurred

## Further reading

Bhutta ZA (2006). Current concepts in the diagnosis and treatment of typhoid fever. *BMJ* **333**, 78–82.

# ① Malaria

Malaria is caused by a bite from the infected female *Anopheles* mosquito. After a variable time in the liver, injected sporozoites invade RBCs, destroying them and releasing merozoites. The destruction of RBCs and the immune response to foreign proteins causes a profound physiological disturbance and the clinical features of malaria.

## Causes

Malaria is caused by *Plasmodium vivax*, *Plasmodium ovale*, *Plasmodium malariae*, or *Plasmodium falciparum* (potentially the most dangerous of the malaria-causing organisms).

Risk factors for malaria include:
- Travel to endemic areas
- Inadequate prophylactic measures (or the co-administration of enzyme-inducing medications)

Severity is increased in:
- People in non-endemic areas (i.e. travellers)
- Children
- Pregnant women

## Presentation and assessment

History will include travel to, or through, endemic areas (although 'airport malaria' can occur, typically among baggage handlers and ground-crew). Incubation period is typically 7–10 days, but can be longer.

Signs and symptoms may include:
- General: fever (not always the classical tertian or quartan fever)
  - Rigors, chills, and sweats
  - Muscular aches and pains
  - Jaundice or anaemia may be clinically apparent
- Respiratory: tachypnoea (hypoxia or pulmonary oedema may develop)
- Cardiovascular: tachycardia (cardiovascular compromise may develop)
- Renal: oliguria, raised urea and creatinine (ARF may develop)
  - Metabolic acidosis
- Gastrointestinal: abdominal pain, anorexia, nausea and vomiting
  - Hepatosplenomegly may be found
- Neurological: confusion, behavioural changes, diminished consciousness, headache (cerebral malaria)
  - Upper motor neurone signs may occur

Severe malaria is defined as parasitaemia with one or more of:
- Impaired consciousness *or* multiple convulsions
- Respiratory distress *or* pulmonary oedema
- Circulatory collapse
- Severe anaemia *or* abnormal bleeding
- Haemoglobinuria
- Jaundice
- Hypoglycaemia
- Metabolic acidosis

Investigations
- ABGs (metabolic acidosis is common)
- FBC (thrombocytopenia and/or anaemia may be seen)
- Blood film (thick and thin films) for parasite recognition and count
  - Often two or three films are needed over a period of several hours to confirm diagnosis
  - Regular films are needed throughout treatment to assess effectiveness of therapy
  - Parasite count: <2% mild; 2–5% moderate; >5% severe
- Coagulation screen, including D-dimers and fibrinogen (DIC may occur)
- U&Es (renal failure may occur)
- LFTs (elevations in AST and bilirubin reflect haemolysis)
- Serum glucose (needs rechecking hourly)
- Blood culture (other infections may be present)
- Urinalysis
- CT head scan may be required to exclude other diagnoses

Differential diagnoses
- Influenza
- Meningitis
- Viral haemorrhagic fevers
- Hepatitis
- Leptospirosis
- Typhoid

Immediate management
- Give $O_2$ as required; support airway, breathing, and circulation
- Obtain IV access and rehydrate as necessary
- Check serum glucose; if hypoglycaemic give 20–50 ml of 50% dextrose

Treatment of parasitaemia
- Quinine IV 20 mg/kg over 4 hours (maximum dose 1400 mg); then 10 mg/kg over 4 hours every 12 hours for 5 days (monitor ECG)
  - Quinine can be given orally when the patient is able to absorb effectively
- Alternatively artesunate IV 2.4 mg/kg at 0, 12, and 24 hours, and then daily (use if heart disease or very high parasitaemia are present, or if quinine resistance is suspected, i.e. travel in Southeast Asia)
- Both regimens are followed by either one dose of Fansidar® (pyrimethamine and sulfadoxine ) or a 7 day course of doxycycline 100 mg daily

Further management
- Transfer to HDU/ICU
- Monitor the effectiveness of therapy with 4-hourly blood films to show a reduction in parasite count
- Invasive monitoring is required in severe malaria

- Exchange transfusion may be considered for patients with severe disease and very high parasite counts
- Consider using antipyretics with/without surface cooling
- Complications include ARF, ARDS, DIC, hypoglycaemia, metabolic acidosis, and seizures
  - Seizures should be treated aggressively (see p. 166): check glucose and U&Es; once other causes have been excluded cerebral malaria is the most probable cause (which is a poor prognostic marker)
- Infections occur alongside malaria (Gram-negative sepsis is particularly common and often precipitates circulatory collapse)
  - If clinical suspicion exists consider commencing broad-spectrum antibiotics after blood cultures

## Pitfalls/difficult situations

- Deterioration can occur rapidly (within hours)
- Presentation with hypoglycaemia, convulsions, or acidosis is associated with a poorer outcome
- Do not reduce the dose of drugs if renal failure is present
- Complications can occur with even low levels of parasitaemia
- Sometimes the parasite is difficult to find; treat on clinical suspicion and treat for the most severe form (*P.falciparum*)

## Further reading

Whitty CJM, Lalloo D, Ustianowski A (2006). Malaria: an update on the treatment of adults in non-endemic countries. *BMJ* **333**, 241–5.

Pasvol G (2006). The treatment of complicated and severe malaria. *Br Med Bull* **75–76**, 29–47.

OHCC p. 490.

## :⚙: Viral haemorrhagic fevers

Viral haemorrhagic fevers (VHFs) are a group of illnesses endemic in Africa, South America, and various regions of Asia. The main complicating feature is haemorrhage. Suspected cases occur within 21 days of leaving the endemic area. All cases should be discussed with an infectious diseases specialist regarding isolation and handling of blood and specimens.

### Causes

There many different types of VHF, including:
- Argentine, Bolivian, Brazilian, and Venezuelan haemorrhagic fevers
- Crimean–Congo haemorrhagic fever (CCHF)[*]
- Chikungunya
- Dengue fever
- Ebola[*]
- Hantaan
- Kyasanur Forest disease
- Lassa fever[*]
- Marburg fever[*]
- Olmsk haemorrhagic fever
- Rift Valley fever
- Yellow fever

These are high-risk infections as person-person spread can occur.

[*] These are high-risk infection as person-to person spread can occur

**Table 10.1** Viral haemorrhagic fevers

| | Spread | Incubation period | Common area of origin |
|---|---|---|---|
| Crimean-Congo haemorrhagic fever | Contact with infected livestock or ticks<br>Human to human transmission | 1–12 days | East and West Africa, but also Dubai, Iraq, Pakistan, India, Turkey, Greece, Albania, Afghanistan |
| Dengue fever | Mosquito to human transmission<br>It can also spread as an epidemic | 3–15 days | Asia and Africa |
| Ebola virus fever | It can also spread as an epidemic<br>Human to human transmission | 2–21 days | Zaire, Sudan, Côte D'Ivoire, Gabon |
| Lassa fever | Rodent to human<br>Human to human transmission | 3–21 days | West Africa |
| Marburg fever | Human to human transmission | 3–16 days | Uganda |
| Yellow fever | Mosquito to human transmission | 3–15 days | Equatorial regions of Africa and South America |

**Table 10.2** Presentation and assessment

| Infection | Signs and symptoms |
|---|---|
| Crimean–Congo haemorrhagic fever | High-grade pyrexia; malaise; headache; pain in limbs and loins; anorexia, nausea, vomiting and abdominal pain; haemorrhagic complications; CNS involvement occurs in 15–20% of cases |
| Dengue fever | The first exposure leads to systemic illness resembling viral fever; the second exposure to a different serotype leads to haemorrhagic complications. |
| | High-grade pyrexia; headache; joint pains; maculopapular rash |
| | Second exposure: haemorrhagic shock (presentation will depend on the site of bleeding and amount of blood loss) |
| Ebola virus fever | High-grade pyrexia; sore throat; headache; joint pains; abdominal pain; vomiting; maculopapular rash; haemorrhagic complications |
| Lassa fever | High-grade pyrexia; sore throat (pharyngitis); retrosternal pain; proteinuria; haemorrhagic complications (presentation will depend on the site of bleeding and amount of blood loss) |
| Marburg fever | Similar to Ebola |
| Yellow fever | In first 3 days of onset: high-grade pyrexia; headache; muscle pains; vomiting |
| | In the following days: haemorrhagic complications; jaundice; relative bradycardia; renal failure; DIC; multi-system dysfunction |

**Investigations** (see also p. 324)

Also consider
- ABGs
- FBC (leucopenia may be present)
- Coagulation screen
- U&Es (renal failure may occur)
- LFTs
- Thick and thin blood films (thick films are not recommended) to identify malaria
- Diagnostic PCR and serological tests (paired testing of acute and convalescent sera is recommended)
- CXR

Wherever possible closed sampling systems should be used
- No fingerprick tests should be undertaken where VHF is suspected
- The point of testing of samples (including ABGs) should be discussed with an infectious diseases expert
- Any samples taken must be classed as high risk and treated according to local protocols

**Differential diagnoses**
- Malaria (the most common alternative diagnosis)
- Typhoid
- Leptospirosis
- Viral hepatitis
- Rheumatic fever

**Immediate management**
- Give $O_2$ as required; support airway, breathing, and circulation
- A full and detailed history should be taken, documenting any travel, contact with animals, outdoor activities, or medical work (including post-mortem work)
- Isolation and protection should be implemented as an initial precaution
    - VHF agents with person-to-person spread (CCHF, Ebola, Lassa, Marburg) all require high-security isolation
    - Protective measure should include a protective gown and a waterproof protective apron, latex gloves, a particulate filter facemask, and eye protection; the exception to this would be individuals in a deliberate aerosol release exposure zone
    - Scrupulous handwashing is required as normal
    - Decontamination
- In severe toxaemia, treat as septic shock (see p. 118)
    - Severe shock is common and will require aggressive fluid resuscitation with/without inotropes
- Ribavirin has been used for the treatment of Lassa fever and CCHF

**Further management**
- Supportive measures as in sepsis are required
- Continuing assessment and management of complications; obtain haematological advice on blood and blood product replacement
- The involvement of an infectious diseases specialist is essential
- VHF infection is considered a notifiable disease; public health must be informed

**Pitfalls/difficult situations**
- Malaria must be excluded, but concurrent viral infection may occur
- Toxaemia and haemorrhagic complications carry high mortality
- Late transmission of Marburg and Lassa fever may occur
- The disposal of dead bodies should be treated as a biohazard risk

**Further reading**
http://www.cdc.gov/ncidod/dvrd/spb/index.htm
Advisory Committee on Dangerous Pathogens (1996). *Management and Control of Viral Haemorrhagic Fevers.* HMSO, London.
http://www.hpa.org.uk/infections

# ☼ Severe acute respiratory syndrome (SARS) and avian influenza (H5N1)

SARS is caused by the SARS-associated coronavirus (SARS-CoV). Avian influenza is spread by the H5N1 strain of influenza A

## Presentation and assessment

SARS should be considered where there is a history of recent (<10 days) travel to an area where SARS may re-emerge (e.g. Hong Kong, mainland China, Vietnam) combined with fever, cough or respiratory distress, and CXR infiltrates. Contact with a patient known to have SARS should also prompt consideration of the diagnosis.

Avian influenza should be considered in any patient with fever and respiratory compromise who has had close contact (<1 m) with potentially infected birds or close contact with an infected patient.

Symptoms may include fever, cough, sore throat, rhinorrhoea, myalgia, conjunctivitis, diarrhoea, and respiratory distress.

## Investigations

Should include:
- FBC (lymphopenia is common)
- Coagulation studies (APTT commonly increased in SARS)
- U&Es, LFTs (commonly deranged)
- Serum CK and CRP (both may be raised)
- Blood and sputum cultures
- Test for atypical pneumonia pathogens
- CXR
- Other samples
  - SARS: serum for antibody testing, or sputum/nasopharyngeal aspirates for PCR
  - H5N1: nasopharyngeal aspirate, throat swab, endotracheal aspirate, or BAL should be taken for PCR, immunofluorescence, or viral culture

## Immediate management

- Give $O_2$ as required; support airway, breathing, and circulation
- Treatment is supportive
- Isolate patient and use strict infection precautions: gown, gloves, eye protection, and high filtration mask
- Treat as for pneumonia (see p. 58)
- Consider starting treatment with oseltamivir for H5N1

## Further reading

Health Protection Agency website: http://www.hpa.org.uk
Centers for Disease Control and Prevention website: http://www.cdc.gov/
Kamming D, Gardam M, Chung F (2003). Anaesthesia and SARS. Br J Anaesth 90, 715–18.

# ⚠ HIV and critical illness

Human immunodeficiency virus (HIV) causes a chronic incurable destruction of the immune system with consequential opportunistic infections causing acquired immune deficiency syndrome (AIDS).

The outcome of HIV-positive patients admitted to ITU with non-HIV-related illnesses is the same as those who are HIV-negative.

## Causes

HIV infection is caused by the viruses HIV1 and HIV2, both of which can be transmitted by sexual contact, blood-to-blood or mucous membrane contact, or vertical transmission. Individuals at high risk of HIV infection include:
- Men who have sex with men
- IV drug abusers
- People who have had sex with individuals from areas of high prevalence (e.g. sub-Saharan Africa)
- Sex workers
- Healthworkers who suffer needlestick injuries
- People who received transfusions of infected blood products (no longer a significant risk factor in Western countries)

## Presentation and assessment

HIV infection can be subdivided into three separate categories
- Category A: asymptomatic persistent generalized lymphadenopathy, or acute HIV infection
- Category B: clinical conditions associated with a defect in cell-mediated immunity (e.g. oropharyngeal candidasis, oral hairy leukoplakia, ITP, multiple episodes of shingles)
- Category C (AIDS): confirmed HIV test and a CD4+ T-lymphocyte count of <200 cells/μl or a CD4+ percentage <14, or a CD4+ T-lymphocyte count of <200 cells/μl and an AIDS-related illness

Patients with HIV infection are likely to require critical care involvement because of:
- Diseases affecting immunocompetent individuals (HIV infection is incidental)
- Severe pneumonia (especially *Pneumocystis carinii*[*] pneumonia (PCP))
- Neurological disease (toxoplasmosis, *Cryptococcus*, primary CNS lymphoma, and progressive multifocal leucoencephalopathy)
- Drug reactions
  - NRTI drugs have been associated with hepatitis, lactic acidosis, bone marrow suppression and pancreatitis
  - nNRTI drugs are associated with TEN (see p. 464)
  - PI drugs are associated with GIT upset and pancreatitis
- Liver failure (hepatitis B or C co-infection can accelerate morbidity associated with HIV and increase the likelihood of liver failure)

---

[*] Also known as *Pneumocystis jirovercii*

### Investigations

Investigations will vary according to presenting disease, but consider:
- ABGs
- FBC, coagulation studies
- U&Es, LFTs
- Serum CRP
- HIV testing (see Pitfalls), CD4+ count, and HIV viral load
- BAL immunofluoresence (for PCP)
- Consider serology for CMV, *Toxoplasma*, and *Cryptococcus*
- CXR
- CT or MRI head scan if there is a neurological presentation
- LP (if ICP is not raised): send sample for protein, glucose, culture, Gram staining, Indian ink for *Cryptococcus*, TB, viral panel (e.g. HSV, EBV, VZV, J-C virus) cytology

---

#### AIDS-related illness

- Candidiasis of bronchi, trachea, or lungs, or of the oesophagus
- Cervical cancer, invasive
- Coccidioidomycosis, disseminated or extrapulmonary
- Cryptococcosis, extrapulmonary
- Cryptosporidiosis, chronic intestinal (duration >1 month)
- Cytomegalovirus disease (other than liver, spleen, or nodes)
- Cytomegalovirus retinitis (with loss of vision)
- Encephalopathy, HIV-related
- Herpes simplex: chronic ulcer(s) (duration >1 month); or bronchitis, pneumonitis, or oesophagitis
- Histoplasmosis, disseminated or extrapulmonary
- Isosporiasis, chronic intestinal (duration >1 month)
- Kaposi's sarcoma
- Lymphoma, Burkitt's (or equivalent term)
- Lymphoma, immunoblastic (or equivalent term)
- Lymphoma, primary, of brain
- *Mycobacterium avium* complex or *Mycobacterium kansasii*, disseminated or extrapulmonary
- *Mycobacterium tuberculosis*, any site (pulmonary or extrapulmonary)
- *Mycobacterium*, other species or unidentified species, disseminated or extrapulmonary
- *Pneumocystis carinii* pneumonia
- Pneumonia, recurrent
- Progressive multifocal leucoencephalopathy
- *Salmonella* septicemia, recurrent
- Toxoplasmosis of brain
- Wasting syndrome due to HIV

Adapted from 1993 Revised Classification System for HIV Infection and Expanded Surveillance Case Definition for AIDS Among Adolescents and Adults, National Center for Infectious Diseases, Division of HIV/AIDS

## Immediate management

- Give $O_2$ as required; support airway, breathing, and circulation
- The treatment for all HIV-related conditions is supportive

*PCP*

- Suggested by dry cough, gradual onset of breathlessness, desaturation on exercise, and diffuse shadowing on CXR
- NIV may be required; mechanical ventilation should also should be considered depending on stage of disease
- Pneumothoraces are common
- Antibiotic therapy should provide cover for common pneumonia-causing organisms as well as PCP
  - Co-amoxiclav IV 1.2 g 8-hourly and clarithromycin IV 500 mg 12-hourly and co-trimoxazole IV 120 mg/kg/day for 21 days
- If hypoxia is present give steroids (prednisolone PO 40 mg daily, or methylprednisolone IV 1 g daily)

*Neurological disease*

- Treatment and management is as for meningitis/encephalitis (pp. 192 and 340)
- Suggested antimicrobials include ceftriaxone 2 g IV 12-hourly and amoxicillin IV 1 g 6-hourly and amphotericin B IV 0.25–1 g 6-hourly and aciclovir IV 10 mg/kg 8-hourly

## Further management

- Involve the HIV team early to help with differential diagnoses and management
- Highly active anti-retroviral therapy (HAART) is rarely given in the acute setting, but may considered by the HIV team (who will supervise its prescription)
  - Immune reconstitution syndrome may occur in severely ill patients
  - Many medications are difficult to give (usually administered PO)
  - HAART drugs have multiple drug interactions

## Pitfalls/difficult situations

- Unusual or multiple infections may be seen
- Common infections can present in atypical ways
- HIV testing
  - Consent is required; where patients are unable to consent but knowing the patient's HIV status is in the patient's immediate clinical interests (i.e. it is likely to affect differential diagnosis and treatment decisions), then testing may be undertaken
  - Disclosure of the result to close contacts at risk of the infection is allowed but should ideally wait until the patient is able to give consent; where the patient is unlikely to survive disclosure is also allowed; follow the advice of the local HIV team
  - Disclosure to relatives who are not at risk is not allowed, even after death of the patient

- Needlestick injuries: post exposure prophylaxis should not be delayed while awaiting consent for HIV testing
- TB is common in HIV patients and is more infectious

### Further reading

General Medical Council (1997). *Serious Communicable Diseases.* GMC, London.

Rosen MJ (2006). Critical care of the immunocompromised patient: human immunodeficiency virus. Crit Care Med **34**(Suppl), S245–50.

Huang L (2006). Intensive care of patients with HIV. *N Engl J Med* **355**, 173–81.

www.hopkins-hivguide.org

📖 OHCC p. 488.

---

### Potential HIV exposure

Potential HIV exposure can occur as a result of percutaneous injury (e.g. needlestick injury) or exposure of broken skin or mucous membranes to another body fluid

Non-bloodstained saliva, urine, vomit, and faeces are *all considered safe*

#### Immediate management
- Stop the procedure

*For skin injuries*
- Encourage bleeding (do not suck wounds)
- Wash wound with soap and water
- Cover with a waterproof dressing

*For eye and mouth splash incidents*
- Irrigate with plenty of water

#### Further management
- Complete an incident form
- Check the patient: are they considered to be at high risk of carrying HIV? For example, someone who is known to have
  - HIV (or is ill with suspected HIV infection
  - Had sexual contact with someone who is HIV-positive
  - Refused an HIV test
  - Used drugs
  - Had male homosexual sex
  - Worked in the sex industry
  - Lived in, or travelled to, Africa
- Contact occupational health or infectious diseases department, according to local guidelines and follow their instructions which may include
  - Consenting patient for blood tests
  - Attend for blood testing yourself
  - Taking prophylactic retroviral therapy

# ⑦ **Notifiable diseases**

The attending medical practitioner, either in the patient's home or at a surgery or hospital, has the responsibility of reporting the disease to the Health Protection Agency (HPA) Centre for Infections (CFI). Typically this is done via the hospital departments of microbiology or infectious diseases.

The notifications system is intended to speed up the detection of possible outbreaks and epidemics – clinical *suspicion* of a notifiable infection is all that is required.

## Management

- If one of the notifiable diseases listed opposite is suspected the following details must be submitted
  - Name, age, and sex of the patient
  - The premises where the patient is
  - The patient's suspected disease or poisoning
  - The approximate date of onset
  - The day on which the patient was admitted
  - The address of the premises from which the patient came
  - Whether or not the patient's suspected disease, or poisoning, may have been contracted in hospital

**List of notifiable diseases**

- Acute encephalitis
- Acute poliomyelitis
- Anthrax
- Cholera
- Diphtheria
- Dysentery
- Food poisoning
- Leptospirosis
- Malaria
- Measles
- Meningitis
  - Meningococcal
  - Pneumococcal
  - Haemophilus influenzae
  - Viral
  - Other
- Meningococcal septicaemia (without meningitis)
- Mumps
- Ophthalmia neonatorum
- Paratyphoid fever
- Plague
- Rabies
- Relapsing fever
- Rubella
- Scarlet fever
- Smallpox
- Tetanus
- Tuberculosis
- Typhoid fever
- Typhus fever
- Viral haemorrhagic fever
- Viral hepatitis
  - Hepatitis A
  - Hepatitis B
  - Hepatitis C
  - Other
- Whooping cough
- Yellow fever

Leprosy is also notifiable, but directly to the HPA, CfI, IM&T Department

# Surgical patients

# ! Post-operative sepsis

Patients often develop SIRS in the post-operative period because of increased cytokine levels caused by surgical tissue trauma. This usually subsides within 48 hours. A persistent inflammatory response, or the development of end-organ dysfunction, may indicate the development of sepsis.

## Causes

A number of factors predispose patients to developing post-operative sepsis, including:

- Pre-operative infections unrelated to surgical operation (e.g. chest infections)
- Pre-operative infections related to, or requiring, surgical treatment (e.g. perforated abdominal viscus)
- Intra-operative peritoneal contamination with gut flora
- Gut ischaemia (e.g. thromboembolic events or volvulus)
- Reperfusion injuries(e.g. aortic cross-clamping or other major vascular surgeries)
- Immunocompromised patients
- Genitourinary surgery (especially where an indwelling catheter has been present, or where mucosa is damaged, e.g. by a calculus)
- Surgery on infected area (e.g. patients with burns or abscesses)

Pneumonia is more common
- Following chest surgery
- With prolonged immobility
- Where pain prevents coughing or deep breathing

**Presentation and assessment** (see also p. 322)
- Pyrexia may be associated with other evidence of infection, including:
  - Tachypnoea, tachycardia, rigors, sweats
  - Complications of sepsis (see p. 322)
  - Raised WCC and inflammatory markers
- Features of sepsis and end-organ dysfunction may be present
- After contaminated gut surgery, sepsis should be monitored for, particularly in the first 72 hours

## Investigations
- ABGs
- FBC, coagulation screen
- U&Es, LFTs, serum amylase
- Serum glucose, phosphate, magnesium, calcium
- CRP
- Consider samples for culture with/without microscopy/Gram stain
  - Blood from all lines and a peripheral 'stab'
  - Samples from all drains and any effusions that can be tapped
  - Sputum (ideally BAL or protected specimen if intubated)
  - Urine (also do a dipstick test)
  - If diarrhoea is present stool culture and *Clostridium difficile* toxin testing

- ECG
- CXR (and plain films of joints if appropriate)
- Consider US of abdomen
- Consider CT of any suspect area (especially after major surgery)

**Differential diagnoses**

- SIRS
- MI
- PE
- Haemorrhage
- Ongoing ischaemia (e.g. bowel ischaemia)

**Immediate management** (see also sepsis, p. 325)

- Give $O_2$ as required; support airway, breathing, and circulation
- Invasive monitoring will be required to guide fluid management
- Keep the patient NBM initially (in case surgery required)
- Inform surgical team as urgent removal of infective source
  may be required
- Assess blood loss and cross-match blood for transfusion if necessary

**Further management**

- Institute sepsis care management
- Consider:
  - Open wound drainage
  - Continuous wound irrigation
  - Multiple laparotomies for repeated washouts
- In some conditions (e.g. necrotizing fasciitis) repeated surgical
  debridement may be required
- Monitor and treat any complications of sepsis

**Pitfalls/difficult situations**

- Multi-organ failure may occur if the source of infection is not
  aggressively treated

**Further reading**

Monkhouse D (2006). Postoperative sepsis. *Curr Anaesth Crit Care* **17**, 65–70.

# ⚠ Wound dehiscence

This is partial or complete opening of the surgical wound. Manifestations and management will depend on the site.

## Causes

Predisposing factors include:
- Wound infection
- Tension in the surgical incision site
- Tissue oedema
- Bleeding and haematoma formation
- Tension due to collection of fluid, i.e. ascites
- Tension due to swollen organ, i.e. intestinal obstruction, ileus
- Persistent coughing
- Inadequate pain relief
- Poor tissue strength: malnutrition, malignancy
- Poor surgical technique

## Presentation and assessment

Wound dehiscence may present as:
- Opened wound noticed during dressing change
- Excessive soiling of the dressings noticed
- Inappropriate pain
- Signs of fluid/blood loss: tachycardia/hypotension

Later signs may include:
- Wound infection
- DIC
- Generalised sepsis

## Investigations

- ABGs
- FBC (low haematocrit and raised WCC)
- Coagulation screen
- U&Es (electrolyte abnormalities due to excessive fluid loss)
- LFT (protein/albumin likely to be low)
- ECG
- Consider CXR, AXR
- Consider US scan of wound, to detect any fluid collection

## Immediate management

- Give $O_2$ as required; support airway, breathing, and circulation
- Invasive monitoring will be required to guide fluid management
- Keep the patient NBM initially (in case surgery required)
- Inform surgical team as urgent surgical closure may be indicated
- Assess blood loss and cross-match blood for transfusion if necessary
- Cover wound with sterile dressing
- In mechanically ventilated patients consider deepening sedation or commencing neuromuscular blockade to decrease likelihood of expulsion of abdominal contents

**Further management**

- Continuing invasive monitoring and assessment of fluid status
- Continuing monitoring and correction of electrolyte imbalance
- Watch for DIC; correct abnormalities
- Watch for sepsis
- Surgical closure of wound, or insertion of packs, or drainage of collection may be required
  - After re-closure of abdominal wound, pain relief will be extremely important: consider epidural infusion of local anaesthetics and opioids; involve pain management team early
  - Re-closure of abdominal wound may also cause splinting of diaphragm; respiratory support is likely to be required
- Avoid and treat predisposing factors (see above)

**Pitfalls/difficult situations**

- Sepsis and multi-organ failure may occur because the open wound is prone to infections: strict sterile precautions are required
- Insensible fluid losses may be difficult to assess
- Patients are at high risk of developing MRSA infections

# :⊙: Major post-operative haemorrhage

The loss of blood from the site of surgery may be obvious (drains) or concealed. Hypotension and underperfusion of organs secondary to intravascular loss of blood may occur.

## Causes
- Massive transfusion coagulopathy
- Clip/suture migration
- Unnoticed haemostasis failure

## Presentation and assessment (see also haemorrhage, p. 114)
- Look for blood loss in the drains from surgical site
- Dressings may be soaked in blood
- Signs and symptoms of compression may appear (bleeding into neck leading to airway compression)
- Abdominal distension after intra-abdominal surgery
- Decreased GCS, signs of raised ICP (p. 190), after neurosurgery

Other signs and symptoms associated with haemorrhage (p. 114) may include tachycardia*, peripheral vasoconstriction, hypotension, oliguria, and thirst. Later signs of haemorrhage include signs and symptoms associated with organ failure i.e. dyspnoea, myocardial failure, drowsiness.

Wound drains
- Wound drains which continue to put out >100 ml/hour over 3 hours should be reviewed. However
  - Drains do not always drain
  - A large amount of blood may be concealed in the abdomen or thorax
  - Abdominal signs may be unreliable in post-operative patients
- Base any decision to investigate for haemorrhage on the clinical condition of the patient as well as wound drainage

## Investigations
- Serial physical examinations
- Cross-match blood
- ABGs
- FBC (and repeated bedside Hb testing if possible)
- Coagulation studies, including fibrinogen
- U&Es, LFTs
- ECG
- CXR
- Consider CT scan

## Differential diagnoses
- SIRS/sepsis
- MI
- PE
- Ongoing ischaemia (e.g. bowel ischaemia)

* Tachycardia fails to develop in up to 10% of individuals

**Immediate management** (see also haemorrhage, p. 116)

- Give $O_2$ as required; support airway, breathing, and circulation
- Where peri-airway bleeding/swelling occurs remove any clips and haematoma; consider early endotracheal intubation (see p. 36)
- Intra-thoracic bleeding may necessitate mechanical ventilation
- Keep the patient NBM initially (in case surgery required)
- Call surgeons as the patient may require immediate re-exploration
- Consider if patient is stable for transfer to the theatre
- Assess blood loss and cross-match blood for transfusion if necessary
- Control external haemorrhage: compression/elevation of the bleeding site
- Start restoring intravascular volume using colloids (gelofusine) initially
- Aggressively correct any coagulopathy
  - FFP (12 ml/kg) if PT or PTT >1.5 times normal, or if more than 4 units of stored blood is transfused
  - Platelet concentrates (1 pack/10 kg body weight) if the count is <50 x $10^9$/L
  - Cryoprecipitate (1 pack/10 kg body weight) if fibrinogen <0.8 g/L
- Inotropic support may be required initially
- Invasive monitoring will be required to guide fluid management, but should not delay urgent surgery

**Further management**

- Continue with respiratory support until cardiovascular stability is established
- Look for/manage complications of massive blood transfusion: hypothermia, hypocalcaemia, hyperkalaemia, coagulation factor depletion, thrombocytopenia, metabolic acidosis

**Pitfalls/difficult situations**

- Lack of clinical improvement despite adequate resuscitation should alert to
  - Other sites of bleeding/continuing bleeding
  - Pneumothorax or cardiac temponade
- Use of inotropes may mask the extent of hypovolaemia
- Massive blood loss: involve haematologists for guidance on appropriate blood and component therapy
- Adhere strictly to the cross-checking procedures for blood replacement to prevent inadvertent mismatched transfusion
- Large volumes may be suddenly 'dumped' into wound drains on turning patients and do not necessarily indicate new/sudden haemorrhage

**Further reading**

📖 OHEA pp. 424, 434, 438.

# ☠ Haemorrhage after cardiac surgery

Haemorrhage after cardiac surgery may be obvious (drains) or concealed (haemothorax). It may result in tamponade requiring surgical repair on the ICU.

## Causes
- Inadequate intra-operative haemostatis
- Rebound heparinization
- DIC (post cardiopulmonary bypass)
- Platelet dysfunction due to cardiopulmonary bypass and/or heparinization

## Presentation and assessment
- May present as sudden haemodynamic instability, arrhythmias, or shock
- Look for blood loss in the drains from surgical site (>400 ml in the first hour)
- Signs and symptoms of cardiac tamponade may rapidly appear (raised CVP/JVP, decreased cardiac output with hypotension and acidosis)

Other signs and symptoms associated with haemorrhage (p. 114) may include tachycardia[*], peripheral vasoconstriction, hypotension, oliguria, and thirst. Later signs of haemorrhage include signs and symptoms associated with organ failure, i.e. dyspnoea, myocardial failure, drowsiness.

## Investigations
- Cross-match blood
- ABGs
- FBC (and repeated bedside Hb testing if possible)
- Coagulation studies, including fibrinogen
- Activated coagulation time
- Plain radiographs
- Echocardiograph to exclude cardiac temponade
- US to establish haemothorax (drains may be blocked by a clot)

## Differential diagnoses
- MI
- Haemorrhage from elsewhere (GI bleed nay occur)
- Pneumothorax

---

[*] Tachycardia fails to develop in upto 10% of individuals

Immediate management

- Give $O_2$ as required; support airway, breathing, and circulation
- Consider early endotracheal intubation
- Control of haemorrhage
  - Insert two large-bore (16 gauge) IV cannulae
  - Start restoring intravascular volume using colloids initially
  - Transfuse blood as soon as feasible
- Sudden collapse and no response to rapid fluid infusion is an indication for re-exploration—call surgeons
- Consider protamine 1 mg/kg IV if rebound heparinization is suspected

Further management

- Desmoprssin, aprotonin, or aminocaproic acid may be of value; consult cardiac surgeons and haematologists
- Continue with respiratory support until cardiovascular stability is established
- Assess intravascular fluid status (CVP line) and cardiac contractility (CO monitoring)
- Inotropic support may be required initially
- Correct haematocrit, electrolyte abnormality
- Lack of clinical improvement despite adequate resuscitation should alert to
  - Other sites of bleeding/continuing bleeding
  - Pneumothorax or cardiac temponade
- Look for/manage complications of massive blood transfusion: hypothermia, hypocalcaemia, hyperkalaemia, coagulation factor depletion, thrombocytopenia, metabolic acidosis

Pitfalls/difficult situations

- Platelet dysfunction may take a long time to correct
- Massive blood loss: involve haematologists for guidance on appropriate blood and component therapy
- Adhere strictly to the cross-checking procedures for blood replacement to prevent inadvertent mismatched transfusion

# TUR syndrome

TUR syndrome occurs in patients undergoing prostatic surgery, and is due to excessive absorption of the non-electrolyte solution into the blood. It causes hyponatraemia and fluid overload which can manifest any time intra- or post-operatively.

## Causes

Factors predisposing the patient to TUR syndrome include:
- Prolonged surgery
- Irrigation under pressure >70 cmH$_2$O
- Opening of venous channels: inadequate haemostasis
- Extensive surgical field

## Presentation and assessment

In an awake patient signs and symptoms may include:
- Headache
- Dizziness, confusion
- Shortness of breath
- Nausea
- Visual disturbance

Later signs include:
- Decreased level of consciousness, seizures,
- Cardiovascular collapse and ECG changes
  - Bradycardia, wide QRS complex, elevated ST segments, ventricular tachycardia

## Investigations

- ABGs (Na$^+$ may be measured on ABGS, acidosis may be present)
- FBC
- U&Es (to confirm evidence of hyponatraemia, and to monitor progress)
- LFTs
- ECG
- CXR
- Consider head CT scan if Na$^+$ normal

## Differential diagnoses

- Urosepsis
- MI/LVF
- PE
- Haemorrhage

**Immediate management**

- Give $O_2$ as required; support airway, breathing, and circulation
- Endotracheal intubation and mechanical ventilation may be required if GCS <8, hypoxia is not corrected by face mask or CPAP, or frank pulmonary oedema is present
- Consider CPAP in cases with breathlessness due to pulmonary oedema (see also p. 86)
- Establish invasive monitoring as soon as possible to guide further fluid management
- Give furosemide 1 mg/kg IV: repeat doses may be required
- Consider giving mannitol 50—100 ml IV if the patient is symptomatic but does not have pulmonary oedema
- Correct hyponatraemia
  - Use saline 0.9% for gradual correction of hyponatraemia if $Na^+$ >120 mmol/L
  - Use hypertonic saline if $Na^+$ <120 mmol/L
- Correct hypokalaemia
- Treat arrhythmias if they cause haemodynamic compromise (see pp. 136 and 140)
- Adrenaline or dobutamine infusions may be required for inotropic support in ventricular failure

**Further management**

- Continuing invasive monitoring and assessment of fluid status
- Continuing monitoring and correction of electrolyte imbalance
- CVVH may be required if oliguria occurs secondary to prolonged hypotension
- Obtain haematological advice if DIC develops

**Pitfalls/difficult situations**

- Neurological complications may lead to long-term sequelae
- Multi-organ failure may occur if the condition is not treated rapidly

**Further reading**

📖 OHEA p. 270.

# ☼ Bronchopleural fistula

A communication between bronchus and pleural cavity, i.e. a bronchopleural fistula, may develop after lung surgery.

## Causes

Predisposing factors to the development of post-operative bronchopleural fistulae include:

- Excessive and prolonged positive pressure ventilation after lobectomy or pneumonectomy
- Infection of bronchial stump
- Following empyema drainage
- Disruption of suture line on bronchus
- Immunocompromised patients
- Steroids: poor tissue healing

## Presentation and assessment

- Appearance of, or sudden increase in, air coming out of the chest drain on the side of operation
- Collapse of the remaining lung
- Pneumothorax with or without tension (see p. 78)
- Hypoxia
- Breathlessness (if awake)
- Inability to deliver adequate tidal volume on the ventilator because of leak of air through fistula (in a ventilated patient)
- Respiratory failure
- Cardiovascular instability

## Investigations

- ABGs
- FBC
- U&Es, LFTs
- ECG
- CXR

## Differential diagnoses

- MI/LVF
- PE

**Immediate management**

- Give $O_2$ as required; support airway, breathing, and circulation
- Exclude a tension pneumothorax (p. 78); treat the pneumothorax
- Ensure working chest drain
- Positive pressure ventilation will be difficult to achieve: use large tidal volumes in the short-term, or convert volume-controlled ventilation to pressure-controlled ventilation
- Involve the anaesthetist and the surgeon
  - Bronchoscopy and insertion of a double-lumen tube may be required for independent lung ventilation (a range should be requested to be available: 37, 39, 41 Fr right- or left-sided)

**Further management**

- Repeated bronchoscopy may be required
- Surgical exploration and repair of fistula is the definitive treatment
- Early weaning from positive pressure ventilation will aid natural healing

**Pitfalls/difficult situations**

- Maintenance of adequate tidal volumes may be extremely difficult using conventional ventilators

**Further reading**

📖 OHEA p. 200.

# ① Post-operative pain

The extent of surgery, site of surgical incision, and type of organ involved, as well as any response to different management strategies, determine the type and severity of pain.

## Causes

In general
- Upper abdominal surgery and thoracic surgery cause severe pain
- Major joint surgeries also cause severe pain, particularly on movement
- Unstabilized fractures can be very painful

A number of factors may predispose to inappropriate intensity of post-operative pain, inluding:
- Pain threshold of an individual patient
- Known opiate tolerance
- Wound infection
- Wound tension

Pain should gradually diminish over the first 72 hours following surgery.

## Presentation and assessment

The patient will complain of pain, particularly during movement and coughing. Associated signs and symptoms may include:
- Tachycardia
- Hypertension
- Sweating
- Vasoconstriction (due to sympathetic stimulation)
- Anxiety, non-cooperation
- Increased rate of breathing
- Inadequate tidal volumes and respiratory insufficiency (abdominal and thoracic surgery)
- Inability to cough

Persistent lack of pain relief can lead to:
- Anxiety, depression
- Respiratory failure
- Impaired immunity: increased risk of infection and sepsis
- Poor mobility: prolonged recovery
- Poor tissue healing

## Differential diagnoses/investigations

Pain (especially when new) may occasionally be non-surgical in origin. Consider investigating the following
- Chest or abdominal pain: MI/angina, PE
- Shoulder-tip pain: diaphragmatic irritation (consider perforation or pneumothorax)
- Increasing abdominal pain: consider anastomotic breakdown, bowel ischaemia, obstruction
- Leg pain: compartment syndrome, ischaemia, DVT

### Immediate management

- Follow local guidelines and Involve the acute pain management team
- Analgesia is started intra-operatively and should be planned to continue into the post-operative period
- Assess pain using a 10-point scale (where 0 is 'no pain' and 10 is 'the worst pain imaginable'); aim for scores <3
  - As a minimum patients should be able to cough and deep breath
- Ensure regular adjunctive analgesics are prescribed alongside opioids or regional techniques: paracetamol and NSAIDs (if appropriate)
- Troubleshoot opioids or epidurals as below; consider intermittent regional anaesthetic blocks where pain is difficult to control

**Parenteral opioids**
- Patient-controlled analgesia (PCA) is the most common mode of opioid delivery after major surgery
- Check that the patient is able to use the handset
- Consider a bolus of opioid; discuss with the anaesthetist/pain team
- Give prophylactic anti-emetics if required
- Monitor for sedation and respiratory depression
- Remove the handset from any over-sedated patient

**Epidurals** (or other regional anaesthesia infusions)
- A low concentration of local anaesthetic (e.g. bupivacaine 0.125%) combined with fentanyl is infused into the epidural space
- Avoid concomitant administration of IV opioids if opioid-containing infusions are used (occasionally low-dose opioids may be used for shoulder-tip pain following thoracic surgery)
- Check the level of the epidural block
  - Stop the infusion if arm or respiratory weakness occur
  - A local anaesthetic bolus (or catheter adjustment) may be needed for low/one-sided blocks; inform the anaesthetist/pain team
  - Failed epidurals may need re-siting, if this is a possibility delay giving any LMWH until after the patient has been reviewed
  - Consider CVP-guided administration of fluids with/without inotropic support for hypotension following epidural bolusing

### Further management
- Check epidural insertion sites daily: remove epidurals if there is any concern about infected entry site

### Pitfalls/difficult situations
- A loss of leg motor and sensory function in patients with thoracic or abdominal epidurals may indicate epidural haematoma or abscess; inform the anaesthetist/pain team
- Stop epidural infusions if aggressive resuscitation for hypotension is required

### Further reading
Stone M, Wheatley B (2002). Patient-controlled analgesia. *Br J Anaesth CEPD Rev* **2**, 79–82.
📖 OHCC p. 532, OHEA pp.160, 226, 318–322.

# Trauma and burns

# ☠ Trauma

Critical care emergencies secondary to trauma can be divided into two main categories
- Life-threatening
  - Airway: laryngeal or tracheal injury
  - Breathing: tension pneumothorax, massive haemothorax, cardiac tamponade, flail segment, cardiac contusion
  - Circulation: shock states (hypovolaemic, cardiogenic, septic)
- Limb-threatening
  - Vascular compromise
  - Neurological injury
  - Compartment syndrome

A primary survey (following the ABC format) should be performed and life-threatening injuries treated simultaneously.

Life-threatening injuries may have already been identified and managed in the primary survey in the A&E department and operating theatre prior to the patient's admission to critical care. However, new pathologies can develop, or old ones recur, and so the ICU doctor should always return to the ATLS style of management should a trauma patient become unstable.

Limb-threatening injuries (i.e. compartment syndrome) may not have been identified prior to ICU admission, or may have developed during resuscitative measures.

## Approach

- In all cases it is essential to ensure that those treating the patient are safe to carry out their work
- Consider C-spine and/or other spinal immobilization
- Give 100% oxygen in acute emergencies; in less acute scenarios titrate the oxygen required to keep $SaO_2$ >95%
- Connect any monitoring available: aim to have $SaO_2$, continuous ECG, and non-invasive BP monitoring as a minimum
- Obtain a history and detailed information: the minimum should include an 'AMPLE' history (see p. 2)
- Obtain information from the patient, relatives, or paramedics concerning the mechanism of injury. High-risk injuries include:
  - Pedestrian versus car; car versus car; motor bicycle accident (MBA)
  - Ejection from car; turned over car
  - Fall >1m (or five stairs); fall from a horse
  - Penetrating injuries

### Primary survey

#### Airway

- Look for evidence of airway obstruction: decreased conscious level, foreign body/matter, expanding neck haematoma, laryngeal fracture, stridor
- If obstruction is present perform a jaw thrust and insert an oropharyngeal airway if required (chin lift and head-tilt should be avoided in patients with suspected C-spine injuries)
  - Nasopharyngeal airways may be inserted (avoid if possible in patients with suspected BOS fractures)

- Where obstruction is present consider endotracheal intubation or an emergency needle cricothyroidotomy/tracheostomy (see p. 16)
- Consider endotracheal intubation if the airway is at risk

### Breathing

- Look for evidence of respiratory compromise: hypoxia (reduced $PaO_2$ or $SaO_2$), dyspnoea and/or tachypnoea, absent or abnormal chest movement, loss of chest wall integrity (flail segment), pulmonary aspiration, massive bleeding
- Exclude/treat life-threatening conditions (e.g. tension pneumothorax, massive haemothorax*)
- Consider endotracheal intubation and mechanical ventilation in patients with actual or imminent respiratory distress

### Circulation

- Look for evidence of circulation inadequacy: tachycardia, weak pulse, hypotension, cold peripheries, prolonged capillary refill (>2 seconds: difficult to interpret in associated hypothermia)
- Look for obvious or concealed blood/fluid loss: palpate the abdomen, feel for blood pools (flanks, hollow of neck/back, groin), look for pelvic instability, look for long-bone fractures
- Exclude life-threatening conditions such as cardiac temponade (raised CVP/JVP, pulsus paradoxus, diminished heart sounds, low voltage ECG), tension pneumtothorax[†], haemorrhage, or arrhythmia
  - Assess degree of shock
  - Establish wide-bore IV access (2x 16G cannulae)
- Commence fluid/blood replacement and treatment of hypovolaemic shock: give 500 ml of colloid within 5–10 minutes and reassess

### Disability/neurology

- Rapidly assess the patient's neurological status using GCS or the system: **A**lert, responds to **V**oice, responds to **P**ain, or is **U**nresponsive
- Check for pupil signs and plantar responses
- Check for Battle's sign and scalp, nose, or ear haemorrhage; perform otoscopy now or during secondary survey

### Exposure/general

- Measure the patient's core temperature
  - Rewarming should be commenced if required[‡]
- Establish full exposure of affected area
- Provide analgesia as required

---

* The insertion of a chest drain to treat massive haemothorax may precipitate further catastrophic haemorrhage; obtain IV access first and have IV fluids prepared

† Tension pneumothorax may present as a respiratory or circulatory emergency

‡ Where ROSC has occurred following cardiac arrest, active warming may be inappropriate

Investigations
- BM test should be taken

As soon as IV access is established the following blood tests should be taken:
- Cross-match
- FBC (bedside Hb tests may be available)
- U&Es, LFTs
- Serum glucose
- Consider paracetamol, salicylate, alcohol
- Consider β-HCG

Also consider:
- ABGs
- Bench co-oximetry for carbon monoxide
- ECG
- Where severe abdominal bleeding is suspected consider performing diagnostic peritoneal lavage (DPL) to confirm the presence of blood

Imaging of major trauma should include:
- Lateral C-spine, CXR, pelvis
- Other long bones may be X-rayed as clinically indicated
- AP and 'peg' views of the C-spine may also be considered, but CT of neck may be more appropriate (see p. 189)
- CT of head, chest, neck, or abdomen/pelvis may be required
- Rapid abdominal US scanning may be available to detect intra-abdominal haemorrhage

Differential diagnoses

Medical conditions may coexist with, or cause, trauma, including:
- Alcohol intoxication
- Syncope/seizures from any cause, especially SAH or cardiac arrhythmias
- Diabetic hypoglycaemia

Further management
- Once the patient has been stabilized, the primary survey completed, and initial investigations performed, examination should proceed to a secondary survey (a head-to-toe examination looking for less severe injuries, some of which may still be limb threatening)
- Hypotension associated with intra-abdominal or intra-thoracic haemorrhage may require immediate surgery before a full secondary survey has been completed
- The secondary survey should include full assessment of:
  - Head (see p. 182)
  - Neck
  - Chest and abdomen
  - Pelvis
  - Limbs
- The patient should then be log-rolled and the back, spine, and perineum (including anal sphincter tone) examined

- The patient should be moved off any spinal immobilization boards at the time of log-rolling
- Cardiovascularly unstable patients should be catheterized to monitor urine output

## Specific injuries involving critical care

### Spinal cord injuries

- In major trauma all patients should initially be assumed to have a spinal injury and spinal precautions used, including hard collar, sandbags, head strapping, and log-rolling
- High spinal injuries may result in loss of phrenic or intercostals nerve function, necessitating endotracheal intubation and ventilation
  - Suxamethonium is safe to use within the first 48 hours of a spinal injury; once muscle atrophy has commenced there is a risk of hyperkalaemia
- Spinal shock and autonomic disruption may occur; other causes of hypotension such as occult haemorrhage should be excluded
  - Spinal shock may require vasopressors
- Many centres commence high-dose steroids within the first 8 hours of spinal cord injuries: methylprednisolone IV 30 mg/kg in 15minutes, then 5.4 mg/kg/hr for 23 hours
- Where it has not been possible to rule out spinal cord injury in an unconscious patient admitted to the ICU, carry out the investigations recommended on p. 189
- Considerations for the long-term care of paralysed patients can be found on p. 203

### Pulmonary contusion

- Pulmonary contusions may develop in the first 24 hours after blunt chest injury causing characteristic CXR changes
- Increasing oxygen requirement may indicate the need for endotracheal intubation and mechanical ventilation
- Chest injuries with associated rib, T-spine, or clavicular fractures are more likely to be affected

### Pneumothorax/tension pneumothorax (see p. 78)

### Haemothorax (see p. 80)

- This may occur early, at the time of the injury, or late if intercostal vessels are damaged by fractured ribs

### Rib fractures

- Severe pain may limit the ability of the patient to cough or deep breathe, and insertion of a thoracic epidural may be required for pain relief
  - Atelectasis and pneumonia may occur as a late complication of rib fractures, especially where respiration is limited by pain
- The presence of rib fractures increases the likelihood of pneumothoraces, especially in mechanically ventilated patients
- The presence of multiple rib fractures, especially those involving the upper three or four ribs, is associated with underlying lung or mediastinal injuries

## Flail chest

- Flail chest occurs when a segment of chest wall loses continuity with the rest of the bony structure (usually as a result of two fractures) and effectively 'floats free'
  - In normal respiration the chest can expand and generate a negative pressure; where a flail segment is present it may be sucked in by the negative pressure, rather than air through the airways
- Paradoxical breathing may be obvious (flail segment moving in with respiration)
- Dyspnoea/tachypnoea may be present
- Endotracheal intubation and mechanical ventilation are likely to be required
- As with other rib fractures
  - Good analgesia is required for weaning from ventilation
  - Underlying trauma may be present

## Cardiac contusion

- Cardiac contusion may occur as a result of blunt chest injuries
- ECG changes may include VEs, sinus tachycardia, AF, RBBB, ST segment changes
- ECG monitoring should be continued for 24 hours as severe arrhythmias may develop
- Severe right-sided contusions may result in a raised CVP
- Consider the possibility that myocardial ischaemia *precipitated* the trauma
- Consider checking cardiac enzymes and obtaining a cardiac echo

## Cardiac tamponade (see p. 146)

## Shooting

- 'Low-velocity' injuries (handgun bullets) cause damage along the bullet track; 'high-velocity' injuries (rifle bullets) may cause extensive cavitation areas within the wound
- Entrance/exit wound size does not predict the degree of wound cavity
- Bullet or bone fragments may cause further damage
- The wound tract will be soiled by environmental contaminants
  - Wound exploration, debridement, and excision may be undertaken; delayed primary suture (DPS) is likely to be necessary
- Antibiotic prophylaxis should be given

## Aortic disruption

- Rapid deceleration injuries affecting the chest may cause great vessel disruption, which may initially be contained by haematoma
- Hypotension is normally caused by another bleeding site (as rapid aortic bleeding is rapidly fatal)
- The presence of CXR changes (see p. 403) should prompt CT angiography or TOE

### Intra-abdominal haemorrhage

- Intra-abdominal haemorrhage should be suspected in hypotensive victims of major trauma, especially where there is penetrating abdominal trauma, blunt trauma causing external abdominal bruising, signs of peritoneal irritation*, haematuria, thoracolumbar fractures, pelvic fractures, lower rib fractures
- Investigations may include
  - Laparotomy (or laparoscopy)
  - US of abdomen
  - Diagnostic peritoneal lavage (positive if ≥100 000 RBC/mm³, ≥500 WBC/mm³, bacteria present on Gram stain)
  - CT abdomen

### Pitfalls/difficult situations

- Nerve damage is often difficult to detect in a sedated patient; a high level of suspicion should be maintained depending upon the mechanism of injury (penetrating/crushing trauma) or associated injuries (fractures/dislocations)
- Arterial injury usually presents with a cold pale pulseless limb; treatment may involve simply realigning a fractured limb, or vascular surgery
- Compartment syndrome may be often difficult to detect in sedated patients; a high level of suspicion must be maintained when there are high-risk injuries present (forearm/leg fractures, crush injuries)
- The tetanus immunization status of the patient should be established in case a further booster injection is required
- Trauma may be associated with worse outcomes in the elderly, pregnant, or malnourished, or those with severe comorbidities

### CXR findings associated with traumatic aortic disruption

- Widened mediastinum
- Distorted poorly defined aortic knuckle
- Tracheal deviation (to the right)
- Loss of space between the pulmonary artery and the aorta
- Depression of the left main bronchus
- Oesophageal/nasogastric tube deviation (to the right)
- Paratracheal striping
- Left haemothorax
- Fractures of ribs 1 or 2; scapula fractures
- Pleural or apical caps
- Widened paraspinal interfaces

### Further reading

Deitch EA, Dayal SD (2006). Intensive care unit management of the trauma patient. *Crit Care Med* **34**, 2294–301.
OHCC pp. 500, 508, OHEA pp. 36, 128, 186.

---

* The signs of an acute abdomen may not be present, especially where a patient has been given neuromuscular blockade for endotracheal intubation and mechanical ventilation

## ☠ Severe burns

### Causes

Burns are commonly associated with
• Dry heat contact
• Wet heat contact (scalds)
• Electricity
• Chemical damage

### Presentation and assessment

Burn thickness may be:
• Superficial    first degree
• Intermediate    second degree
• Deep dermal    third degree

Body surface area (BSA) coverage of a burn can be calculated by:
• Palm of the patient's hand ~1% (and any skin are of approximately the same size is also 1%), **or**
• Chest    18%
• Back    18%
• Whole of head    9%
• Whole of arm    9% (each)
• Front of leg    9% (each)
• Back of leg    9% (each)
• Genitalia    1%

BSA is difficult to assess at initial presentation and is best done by a burns team. It should be reassessed at 24 hours.

The location of burns is also important
• Airway involvement (see p. 28: singed nasal hair, hoarse voice, soot in airway)
• Special areas: head and neck, hands and feet, major joints, chest, groin
• Circumferential burns

The mechanism of injury/associated trauma should assessed, especially
• Duration of exposure to injury
• Nature of burn
• Likelihood of airway damage/CO poisoning should be assessed: Did the burn occur in an enclosed space? Were toxins/accelerants present?

### Investigations

• Cross-match
• ABGs and COHb by co-oximetry
• FBC, coagulation studies
• U&Es, LFTs, serum CK
• Toxicology if appropriate
• ECG
• CXR
• C-spine and trauma-series X-rays if appropriate
• Consider head CT scan if neurology abnormal
• Consider sending urine for myoglobin

## Immediate management

- Give 100% $O_2$; support airway, breathing, and circulation as required
- Use spinal precautions if spinal trauma a possibility
- Undertake a primary survey and commence resuscitation
- Obtain an AMPLE history (p. 2)
- Keep patients NBM
- Involve the burns/plastics team early

## Airway (see also p. 66 for inhalational injuries)

- Early endotracheal intubation should be considered where
  - GCS ≤8 or rapidly decreasing
  - Burns are widespread
  - There is facial or airway involvement
- Use an uncut tube to allow for facial swelling
- Suxamethonium is safe to use in the immediate setting (unless there are other contraindications)

## Breathing

- Ventilatory support may be required
- Consider the possibility of associated chest trauma
- Eschar formation across the chest may limit respiration and require surgical intervention
- COHb levels >20% will require 100% $FiO_2$ until COHb <5%

## Circulation

- Insert 2x large (16G) cannulae
- If the patient is hypotensive, consider a bolus of 20 ml/kg IV colloid
- Estimate degree of burn and commence resuscitation using an appropriate formula (see below)
- Insert urinary catheter, arterial line, and CVP

## Other

- Ensure adequate analgesia; titrate morphine boluses IV
- Monitor temperature; large-area burns can result in rapid cooling
  - Losses can be reduced by occlusive watertight dressings and by nursing patients in a warm environment
  - Perform a secondary survey

## Burns fluid resuscitation formulae

### Parklands

Use Hartmann's solution IV
First 24 hours requirement: body weight x BSA x 4 ml)
Give half over 8 hours and half over next 16 hours

### Muir and Barclay

Use IV colloid (human albumin solution 4.5%)
First 4 hours requirement: body weight x BSA x 0.5 ml)
Give this fluid volume six times in the first 36 hours after the injury over the following lengths of time: 4, 4, 4, 6, 6, and 12 hours

**In addition to either of the above, patients require 1–1.5 ml/kg/hour of maintenance crystalloid (or NG feed)**

**Further management**

- Complete a tertiary survey in trauma cases once the patient is stable
- Hypotension due to vasodilatation is common during ICU stay despite patients being well filled
  - Where possible, vasopressors should be avoided as they will compromise skin healing; this should be balanced against the risk of hypotension
  - Consider monitoring cardiac output
  - Dopamine or dobutamine may be the preferred first-line inotropes
  - Aim for a core–peripheral temperature gradient of <2°C
- Respiratory support
  - ARDS is common; a lung protective ventilation protocol should be adopted
  - Airway involvement will produce severe oedema; the airway should be assessed prior to extubation (see p. 29)
  - Broncho-alveolar lavages with $NaHCO_3$ 1.4% may be considered if there is soot in the bronchi
- RRT is likely to be required
- Haemolysis can occur with full-thickness burns; blood transfusions may be required, aiming for Hb 8–10 g/dl
- Feeding requirements in severely burned patients are increased
  - Gastric stasis is common; consider NJ feeding or TPN if NG feeding fails
  - Commence stress ulcer prophylaxis
- Monitor for developing sepsis (burns are initially sterile but rapidly become colonized)
  - Typical organisms include *Staphylococcus aureus*, streptococci, *Pseudomonas*, *Acinetobacter*
  - SIRS is likely to be present already; sepsis should be suspected if organ failure (especially cardiovascular compromise or renal failure) worsens or WCC increases
  - Suggested empirical antibiotic therapy in the event of deterioration might include piptazobactam IV 4.5 g 8-hourly and vancomycin IV 500 mg 6-hourly (this should be discussed with a microbiologist as soon as practicable)
- Temperature control may become difficult, especially if full body dressing are required; if hyperpyrexia occurs consider:
  - Antipyretics
  - Neuromuscular blockade
  - Extra-corporeal cooling (e.g. RRT)
  - Taking down dressings
- Regular monitoring and correction of electrolytes is required
- Surgery may be required for debridement, grafting, or synthetic skin cover
  - Patients are often cardiovascularly unstable afterwards
  - Blood loss may be profound
  - Antibiotic cover may be required
- Dressing changes may be extremely painful; consider providing analgesia and sedation with ketamine IV 1–2 mg/kg (alternatively consider remifentanil infusion)

## Indications for admission

### To a burns unit
- >10% BSA burn or >5% full-thickness burn
- Burn to hands, feet, genitalia, perineum, joint
- Burns to face
- Electrical/chemical burns
- Circumferential burns (limbs or chest)
- Extremes of age

### To a burns ICU
- Burns affecting >30% body surface area (BSA)
- Burns affecting upper chest, neck, or face (affecting airway)
- Burns affecting the airway
- Smoke inhalation
- COHb >20%
- Secondary complications (e.g. sepsis, renal failure, major trauma)

## Pitfalls/difficult situations

- Do not assume that a patient has been adequately assessed or resuscitated prior to ICU admission, especially following inter-hospital transfer
- If in doubt, intubate; delay may make a difficult intubation impossible
- Do not use suxamethonium >48 hours or <1 year after a major burn; severe hyperkalaemia may develop
- Some prolonged contact burns are associated with overdose and/or compartment syndrome
- Consider cyanide toxicity as a cause of unexplained metabolic acidosis (see p. 451)
- Burns >60% have a high mortality, especially if associated with inhalation injury

## Further reading

Hettiaratchy S, Papini R (2004). Initial management of a major burn: I-overview *BMJ* **328**, 1555–7.
Clarke J (1999). Burns. *Br Med Bull* **55**, 885–94.
📖 OHCC p. 510, OHEA pp. 130, 334.

# ☢ Electrocution

Electrocution disrupts the normal electrical function of cells (e.g. ventricular fibrillation, skeletal muscle tetany), or causes internal and external burns

## Causes

- The current involved is the major determinant of tissue damage
  - AC current can produce tetany; DC shocks tend to 'throw' the victim clear
- Microshock can occur when low-current electricity flows directly to the myocardium via an indwelling catheter or pacing lines (<1 mA may cause VF)

## Presentation and assessment

Signs and symptoms may include the following:

- General: burns are commonly seen (surface damage may be superficial compared with internal injuries)
  - Direct, arc, and flame burns may be seen (from adjacent source)
  - Where the electrical path involves a limb the increased current density may cause greater tissue damage
- Cardiac: asystole—VF/VT may occur with high currents (or micro-shock)
  - Myocardial injury or burns may occur, causing ischaemia
- Respiratory: respiratory muscle tetany may cause respiratory arrest
- Neurological: paraplegia, quadriplegia and/or autonomic instability may occur which generally resolve over a period of hours
- Other: feathering/fern patterns and 'spider' entry/exit wounds may be seen on the skin in lightning injuries
  - Muscoloskeletal injuries (including long-bone fractures) may be caused by tetany
  - There may be associated trauma (including C-spine) injuries

## Investigations

- ABGs
- U&Es
- Serum CK
- Cardiac enzymes (to detect myocardial injury)
- ECG: check for atrial arrhythmia, transient ST segment changes
- Urine myoglobin
- Long-bone X-rays (if fractures suspected)

## Differential diagnoses

- Seizures
- Spontaneous dysrhythmias

### Immediate management

- Ensure that there is no ongoing risk of electrocution to staff or victim
- Commence BLS/ALS as appropriate and treat dysrhythmias
  - Prolonged resuscitation efforts are appropriate
- Use C-spine immobilization if there is associated trauma
- Give 100% $O_2$; support airway, breathing, and circulation as required
- Use continuous ECG monitoring
- Remove any burning/smouldering clothing
- Commence burns resuscitation

### Further management

- Electrical burns may cause airway swelling; consider early endotracheal intubation even if patient has adequate ventilation
- Fractures should be immobilized
- Muscle tetany, or compartment syndromes secondary to muscle damage, fractures, or burns, may result in myoglbinuria and rhabdomyolysis
  - Fasciotomy may be required

### Pitfalls/difficult situations

- Estimating BSA (and therefore fluid resuscitation requirements) can be difficult as there may be severe deep tissue injury with only limited superficial involvement

### Further reading

Circulation 2005;112;154-155; Part 10.9: Electric Shock and Lightning Strike.

International Liaison Committee on Resuscitation (1997). Special resuscitation situations: an advisory statement. *Circulation* **95**, 2196–210.

Jain S, Bandi V (1999). Electrical and lightning injuries. *Crit Care Clin* **15**, 319–31.

Cooper, M.A. (1995). Emergent care of lightning and electrical injuries. *Semin Neurol* **15**, 268–78.

📖 OHCC p. 524.

# ☼ Near-drowning

Drowning is typically defined as death from asphyxia within 24 hours of a submersion episode. Survival for longer than this is near-drowning.

## Causes

- 'Wet drowning' occurs when the submersion victim attempts to breathe underwater and aspirates significant quantities of water
- 'Dry drowning' occurs when laryngospasm prevents aspiration
- There is minimal clinical difference between saltwater and freshwater near-drowning
- Aspiration of >20 ml/kg water is required to produce significant electrolyte abnormalities.
- Primary CNS injury is caused by hypoxaemia at the time of the near-drowning episode; secondary injury may occur as a result of ongoing pulmonary damage, reperfusion injury, or multi-organ dysfunction

## Presentation and assessment

Severity may vary considerably: patients may be asymptomatic, or signs and symptoms may include:

- General: hypothermia
- Neurological: anxiety, delirium, coma (secondary to hypoxaemia or cerebral oedema)
- Cardiovascular: severe hypotension may occur secondary to:
  - Hypovolaemia (fluid shifts)
  - Myocardial dysfunction (secondary to hypoxaemia, hypothermia, acidosis, electrolyte abnormalities)
- Respiratory: cough, tachypnoea, dyspnoea, wheeze
  - ALI/ARDS may develop (development may be delayed)
- Other: multiple organ dysfunction syndrome (MODS) may occur

## Investigations

- ABGs
- FBC, coagulation screen (including fibrinogen, D-dimers, and FDPs)
- U&Es, LFTs
- Serum glucose, calcium, magnesium, phosphate
- Blood alcohol level
- ECG
- CXR
- ECHO (if significant CVS instability)
- Consider CT head (if cerebral oedema or infarction suspected)
- Consider drug screen

## Differential diagnoses

- Hypothermia
- Epilepsy

## Immediate management

- Give 100% $O_2$; support airway, breathing, and circulation as required
- Endotracheal intubation may be required for respiratory support or airway protection
- Respiratory support should be provided to maintain oxygen saturations >95% (NIV or IPPV may be required)
- Fluid resuscitation with/without inotropes may be required to maintain a reasonable perfusion pressure (MAP ≥65 mmHg)
  - A CVC may be required to guide fluid resuscitation and allow vasoactive support if required
- Continuous ECG monitoring in view of risk of dysrhythmias
- Rewarm as appropriate to the degree of hypothermia (p. 260)
- Nurse in at least a 15°–30° head-up position to minimize cerebral oedema
- Consider inserting an NGT(or OGT if head or facial trauma are present) in order to drain ingested water or debris

## Further management

- Bronchoscopy may be required in order to remove foreign bodies or water debris
- Consider urinary catheterization to monitor urine output
- Consider inserting an arterial line for cardiovascular monitoring and repeated blood gas analyses
- Treat any associated diseases or complications
  - Traumatic injuries
  - Seizure (see p. 166)
  - Cardiac disease, dysrhythmias, and syncope
  - Exhaustion and hypothermia
  - Hypoglycaemia
  - Alcohol or drug use

## Pitfalls/difficult situations

- Even where an apparently full recovery has rapidly occurred, patients should be kept in hospital for monitoring as delayed respiratory compromise may occur
- C-spine injuries may be present in near-drowning victims (C-spine protection should remain in place until injury is excluded)
- In cases of paediatric near-drowning consider the possibility of non-accidental injury

## Further reading

Harries M (2003). Near drowning *BMJ*, **327**,1336–8.
OHCC p. 526, OHEA p.120.

# Obstetric critical care

# ⓘ Critical illness in pregnancy

Critical illness may complicate, or occur shortly after, pregnancy. Severe pregnancy-related illnesses may also require critical care intervention and management; these include pre-eclampsia and eclampsia, the HELLP syndrome, major haemorrhage, and amniotic fluid embolism. The same general principles apply as for any critical illness; life-threatening problems are identified and treated first.

Fetal well-being relies upon successful maternal resuscitation. Treating the maternal critical illness takes precedence. Occasionally it may be necessary to deliver the fetus so as to optimize maternal resuscitation and fetal survival (mostly in the third trimester). In cardiac arrests emergency Caesarean section should take place alongside CPR.

## Assessment (physiological changes of pregnancy)

The physiological changes which occur in pregnancy must be considered when assessing and treating pregnant women

- **Cardiovascular**
  - Plasma volume increases steadily up to 34 weeks gestation; in late pregnancy a haematocrit of 30–35% is not uncommon
  - Significant blood loss may occur without apparent maternal compromise (fetal distress may still occur)
  - Maternal heart rate may be increased by 25% in late pregnancy with a resultant increase in cardiac output of up to 1.5 L/min
  - Supine positioning reduces venous return and cardiac output in the second half of pregnancy because of significant aorto-caval compression
  - Blood pressure typically falls by 5–15 mmHg during the second trimester, returning to normal levels in the third trimester
- **Respiratory**
  - Inspiratory capacity increases, functional residual capacity (FRC) decreases, and overall respiratory reserve reduces as pregnancy advances
  - Minute volume increases with increased tidal volume, leading to hypocapnia ($PaCO_2$ ~4kPa) and a compensated respiratory alkalosis
  - Oxygen consumption increases during pregnancy which, combined with the decrease in FRC, leads to rapid desaturation in the event of significant airway/breathing difficulties
- **Renal**
  - Glomerular filtration rate and renal plasma flow increase during pregnancy; serum urea and creatinine levels decrease (by up to 50% of normal)
  - Glycosuria is common
- **Gastrointestinal tract**
  - Gastric emptying is delayed leading to increased risk of aspiration
- **Drug handling**
  - Maternal drug handling may be altered by changes occurring in pregnancy (e.g. serum albumin levels fall to levels of 20–30 g/L)
  - Teratogenic/harmful effects of drugs to the fetus must be considered at different stages of the pregnancy

## Immediate management

A multidisciplinary approach should be adopted with input from senior critical care/anaesthetic, obstetric, and midwifery disciplines
- Give $O_2$ and support airway, breathing, and circulation as required
- If endotracheal intubation is required, a rapid sequence intubation will be required to minimize the risk of aspiration
  - If endotracheal intubation is becoming increasing likely consider giving prophylactic ranitidine 150 mg PO (or equivalent), if possible also give sodium citrate 30 ml PO just prior to intubation
  - The incidence of difficult intubation increases in late pregnancy, especially in patients with pre-eclampsia; immediate availability of intubation adjuncts and familiarization with difficult airway protocols is required (see p. 23–4)
  - Rapid desaturation at induction is likely (see above)
- Mechanical ventilation may be difficult in heavily pregnant women; PEEP will be required to avoid further loss of FRC
- Aggressive fluid resuscitation and/or inotropes may be required
  - In a pregnant patient a right-sided wedge, or even lateral positioning, will decrease the effects of aorto-caval compression (even in the early stages of pregnancy)
  - Manual displacement of the uterus may be useful in an emergency
- In cases of critical illness where pre-term delivery is likely to occur consider giving early steroids (two doses of betamethasone 12 mg 24 hours apart) to improve fetal lung function post delivery

## Further management (following emergency delivery)

- It may be possible to facilitate the baby visiting the mother whilst she is in a critical care environment; this should be encouraged
- Breast-feeding is more likely to succeed if established early; where appropriate it should be encouraged within critical care
- Drugs which are expressed in breast-milk should be avoided if possible
- The incidence of thrombotic events increases in the post-partum period; thromboprophylaxis should be instituted when appropriate
- Routine post-partum examinations by obstetricians or midwives should still be conducted in patients in critical care settings
- Anti-D rhesus immunization should be given to at-risk mothers

## Pitfalls/difficult situations

- Consider the possibility of epidural complications or local anaesthetic toxicity in the differential diagnosis; discuss with the anaesthetist
- The management of patients with severe coexisting disease, partic-ularly congenital cardiac abnormalities, will require specialist advice
- Prophylaxis against potentially severe complications (e.g. anti-epileptic medications) should not be withheld unless absolutely necessary
- If delivery is expected in a critical care patient paediatric support will be required to assess and resuscitate the newborn

## Further reading

📖 OHEA pp. 142, 168, 170.

## :⚙: Severe pre-eclampsia/eclampsia

Pre-eclampsia (or pre-eclamptic toxaemia (PET)) occurs after the twentieth week of pregnancy (and can occur in the post-partum period). Severe proteinuria, neurological symptoms, and severe pregnancy-induced hypertension (PIH), with systolic >170 mmHg or diastolic >110 mmHg (on two occasions) are the typical features of severe pre-eclampsia. Death occurs as a result of CVA, hepatic failure, cardiac failure, or pulmonary complications.

Eclampsia is the occurrence of major seizure activity in the presence of pre-eclampsia (38% occur ante-partum, 18% intra-partum, 44% post-partum). It may occur before the signs of hypertension or proteinuria.

### Causes

Risk factors for pre-eclampsia include:
- A strong family history of PIH or PET
- Previous hypertension
- Diabetes mellitus
- Obesity
- Increasing maternal age
- First pregnancy
- Multiple pregnancies or polyhydramnios

### Presentation and assessment

Pre-eclampsia, even when severe, may be asymptomatic and only discovered by routine blood pressure screening, or when complications such as eclampsia occur. Signs and symptoms, when they occur, consist of:
- Neurological: headache and/or blurred vision (cerebral oedema), hyper-reflexia, seizures
- Respiratory: dyspnoea on exertion, pulmonary oedema, ARDS
- Cardiovascular: hypertension (>170/110 mmHg)
- Gastrointestinal: nausea and vomiting, epigastric discomfort (hepatic engorgement/ischaemia)
- Renal: proteinuria, marked oliguria (often <0.25 ml/kg/hour)
- General: peripheral oedema; facial and laryngeal oedema

### Investigations

- FBC, thrombocytopenia may be seen (platelets <100 × 10⁹/L)
- Coagulation studies, as DIC can occur
- U&Es: may be deranged as ARF can occur
- LFTs: may be deranged; hypoproteinaemia may occur
- Serum urate, raised in PET (>10 × the gestational age in weeks in µmol/L, or >360 µmol/L, or >6 mg/dl)
- Serum glucose
- Urinalysis for proteinuria: urine dipstick ( proteinuria: ≥ + + seen; *severe proteinurea*: ≥ + + + seen), 24 hour collection (proteinuria, ≥0.3 g/24 hours; *severe proteinurea*, >1 g/24 hours)
- Ultrasound of the fetus, to examine for fetal well-being

## Differential diagnoses

- Seizures: epilepsy, encephalitis/meningitis, CVA
- Hypertension: pre-existing hypertension, pain, agitation

## Immediate management

A multidisciplinary approach should be adopted with input from senior critical care/anaesthetic, obstetric, and midwifery disciplines
- Give $O_2$ and support airway, breathing, and circulation as required
- Overall aims include stabilization of blood pressure, prevention of eclamptic seizures, and opportune delivery of the baby

*Hypertension treatment*
- The aim should be to reduce diastolic BP to around 90–100 mmHg; precipitous drops in blood pressure should be avoided
  - First-line treatment should be labetalol 200 mg PO, repeated after 30 min if required; if oral labetalol is ineffective consider labetalol 50 mg IV repeated every 5 min to a maximum of 200 mg, followed by infusion at 5–50 mg/hour
  - Second-line: if labetalol is not tolerated or contraindicated give nifedipine 10 mg PO; it can be repeated after 30 min if required
  - Third-line: consider hydralazine 5–10 mg by slow IV bolus, repeated after 15 mins, followed by an infusion at 5–15 mg/hour

*Treatment and/or prevention of eclamptic seizures*
- Magnesium sulphate IV 4 g over 15–20 min, followed by an infusion of 1–1.5 g/hour for at least 24 hours
  - A further dose of magnesium sulphate 2 g over 15–20 min can be given if further seizures occur
- Close observation for evidence of magnesium toxicity is essential (see p. 232)
- Second-line eclampsia treatments are only rarely required if blood pressure control and magnesium have been used, but include:
  - IV phenytoin or benzodiazepines
  - Induction of anaesthesia with endotracheal intubation and ventilation – The presence of upper airway oedema suggests that difficult intubation will be more likely
- The definitive treatment for severe pre-eclampsia/eclampsia is delivery of the baby
  - The decision to deliver must weigh up the needs of the mother against the maturity of the baby
  - Seizures and other symptoms should be controlled prior to proceeding to delivery/Caesarean section
  - Consider IV steroids for fetal lung development (see p. 415)
- Patients may be transferred to critical care for enhanced monitoring and vital organ support pre- or post-delivery

**Further management**

- The role of central venous pressure monitoring is unclear: it can aid fluid management, but is not always required if urine output/fluid balance is strictly monitored; it is more difficult in the presence of agitation, dyspnoea, oedema, and coagulopathy
- Traditionally, fluid restriction has been practised (to avoid precipitating acute pulmonary/cerebral oedema); a policy of controlled volume expansion with crystalloids/colloids is also adopted by some centres. A target urine output of ≥0.25 ml/kg/hour is acceptable in the absence of other renal insults

**Pitfalls/difficult situations**

- Endotracheal intubation may cause a profound hypertensive surge. Short-acting IV opiates, or IV anti-hypertensives such as labetalol, should be used to blunt this effect
- Up to 10% of women with severe pre-eclampsia, and 25–50% of women with eclampsia are affected by the HELLP syndrome

# HELLP syndrome

HELLP syndrome consists of **H**aemolysis, **E**levated **L**iver enzymes, and **L**ow **P**latelets. It may occur as an entity on its own, or in association with pre-eclampsia. The associated mortality is reported to be as high as 24% of patients.

## Causes

This is a multisystem disease consisting of generalized vasospasm and coagulation defects. No common precipitating factor has been identified.

Haemolysis is due to a microangiopathic haemolytic anaemia; elevated liver enzymes are due to hepatic necrosis (in severe cases, intra-hepatic haemorrhage, subcapsular haematoma, or hepatic rupture may occur); low platelets/thrombocytopenia is due to increased consumption/destruction

## Presentation and assessment

The signs and symptoms overlap with those of PET

- Neurological: headache and/or blurred vision (cerebral oedema), hyper-reflexia, seizures
- Respiratory: dyspnoea on exertion, pulmonary oedema, ARDS
- Cardiovascular: hypertension (>160/110 mmHg)
- Gastrointestinal: right upper quadrant tenderness, nausea and vomiting, epigastric discomfort (hepatic engorgement/ischaemia)
- Renal: proteinuria, marked oliguria (often <0.25 ml/kg/hour)
- General: malaise, bruising/petechiae, peripheral oedema, facial and laryngeal oedema

## Investigations

Investigations are used to confirm the diagnosis and monitor the progression of the disease; they should be taken early and repeated 6-hourly

- FBC: haemolysis will be evidenced by an abnormal film (spherocytes, schistocytes, burr cells); low platelets will be confirmed by a thrombocytopenia of $<100 \times 10^9$/L
- Coagulation studies/fibrinogen (usually normal, unless DIC present)
- U&Es
- LFTs: elevated liver enzymes will be seen (AST >70 U/L); haemolysis will also lead to a high bilirubin and an elevated LDH (>600 U/L)
- Serum haptoglobins: haemolysis will reduce haptoglobins (<0.3 g/L)
- Serum glucose and serum urate
- Urine, dipstick, or 24 hour collection for proteinuria (as for pre-eclampsia)
- Abdominal ultrasound and fetal ultrasound

## Differential diagnoses

- Acute fatty liver of pregnancy, hepatitis, pancreatitis
- Thrombotic thrombocytopenic purpura
- Haemolytic uraemic syndrome

## Immediate management

A multidisciplinary approach should be adopted with input from senior critical care/anaesthetic, obstetric, and midwifery disciplines

- Give $O_2$ and support airway, breathing, and circulation as required
- Correction of thrombocytopenia may be required:
  - Patients with a platelet count >40 × 10$^9$/L are unlikely to bleed
  - Transfusion is generally only required if the platelet count drops to <20 × 10$^9$/L
  - Patients who undergo Caesarean section should be transfused to a platelet count >50 × 10$^9$/L
- Patients with DIC should be given FFP and packed red blood cells.

(see also preceding section on pre-eclampsia management)

- Seizure prophylaxis: magnesium sulphate should be administered to prevent seizures regardless of whether hypertension is present
- Antihypertensives: should be administered according to the protocol for for pre-eclampsia
- Fluids: as for pre-eclampsia
- Betamethasone should be given for fetal lung maturity (see p. 415)
- Delivery: the definitive treatment for severe HELLP syndrome is delivery of the baby; any decision to deliver must weigh up the needs of the mother against the maturity of the baby

## Further management

- High-dose steroids (dexamethasone 10 mg IV 12-hourly) are used in some centres in order to improve the laboratory abnormalities; lengthen time to delivery and facilitate maturity of fetal lungs
  - Steroids are continued until LFT abnormalities are resolving and the platelet count is >100 × 10$^9$/L
- Consider plasmaphoresis after delivery
- Epoprostenol and ketanserin have also been used as treatment

### Pitfalls/difficult situations

- Post-partum haemorrhage will require aggressive early treatment

### Further reading

Hart E, Coley S (2003). The diagnosis and management of pre-eclampsia. *Br J Anaesth CEPD Rev* **3**, 38–42.

📖 OHCC pp. 538, 540, OHEA pp. 154, 158.

# ☢ Amniotic fluid embolism

Amniotic fluid embolism (AFE) can occur if amniotic fluid enters the maternal circulation, triggering an anaphylactoid reaction and/or DIC

## Causes

Risk factors are unclear though older age and increasing parity are likely to be associated.

AFE can occur at any time in late pregnancy, during or after labour/delivery (by vaginal delivery or Caesarean section), and also after termination.

## Presentation and assessment

Typically there is a biphasic presentation.

*Phase 1*

- Respiratory: dyspnoea, tachypnoea, pulmonary oedema, hypoxia, cyanosis
  - Pulmonary hypertension and right heart failure (secondary to pulmonary artery vasospasm/obstruction)
- Cardiovascular: hypotension, cardiovascular collapse, cardiac arrest
- Neurological: tonic–clonic seizures
- Other: fetal bradycardia

Up to half of the survivors of phase 1 may enter phase 2

*Phase 2*

- DIC with massive haemorrhage secondary to the coagulopathy

Occasionally either fatal consumptive coagulopathy or grand mal seizure activity may be the initial presenting features of AFE.

## Investigations

- ABGs
- FBC
- Coagulation studies/fibrinogen
- U&Es
- LFTs
- Serum glucose
- Consider serum tryptase (see Anaphylaxis, p. 112)
- 12-lead ECG
- Cardiac echocardiography
- CT pulmonary angiogram, or VQ scan (VQ scan may be more appropriate if patient has not delivered (lower radiation dose))
- CT head scan may be required
- If a PAFC has been inserted a pulmonary artery blood sample may be examined for fetal cells or amniotic fluid (a finding associated with, but not diagnostic of, AFE); urine may also be examined

**Differential diagnoses**

- Pulmonary embolus, air embolus, or fat embolus
- Anaphylaxis
- Sepsis
- Local anaesthetic toxicity/regional anaesthesia complications
- Pre-eclampsia/eclampsia
- Occult haemorrhage (e.g. placental abruption, uterine rupture)

**Immediate management**

A multidisciplinary approach should be adopted with input from senior critical care/anaesthetic, obstetric, and midwifery disciplines

- Give $O_2$ and support airway, breathing, and circulation as required
- Intubation and mechanical ventilation is often required
  - Non-invasive ventilatory support may be considered in some cases
- Aggressive fluid resuscitation with vasopressor/inotropic support is likely to be required for haemodynamic instability
- Anaphylaxis is often difficult to exclude: treatment with adrenaline, steroids, and antihistamine according to the anaphylaxis protocol (see p. 112) is often required
- Seizures occur as a result of cerebral anoxia and should be treated according to the protocol for status epilepticus (see p. 166) with benzodiazepines as first-line agent, **except**
  - If eclampsia is a likely differential diagnosis consider using magnesium sulphate (see p. 417) as the first line agent (eclampsia is associated with *hypertension*; AFE is associated with *hypotension*, which will be exacerbated by magnesium)
- The fetus should be delivered as soon as is practically possible to prevent further AFE
- If phase 1 is survived then transfer to critical care for close monitoring and vital organ support is likely to be required
- Early invasive monitoring is advised
- The coagulopathy/DIC which occurs in phase 2 should be aggressively corrected
  - Packed red cells, platelets, FFP, and cryoprecipitate are all likely to be required
  - For continued bleeding consider recombinant factor VIIa
- ARDS commonly develops; lung-protective ventilation strategy should be adopted

**Further management**
- Insertion of a PAFC may aid fluid management

**Pitfalls/difficult situations**
- Maternal mortality is between 50% and 75%, and those who survive are often left with significant neurological injury

**Further reading**
📖 OHCC p. 544, OHEA p. 152.

# ☼ Massive obstetric haemorrhage

Massive obstetric haemorrhage is defined as one or more of the following:
- Estimated blood loss ≥2500 ml*
- Transfusion of ≥5 units of blood
- Blood loss precipitating treatment for coagulopathy (e.g. fresh frozen plasma, cryoprecipitate, platelets)

Haemorrhage may be ante-partum (APH), occurring before delivery but after 24 weeks gestation, or post-partum (PPH), occurring during or after delivery.

## Causes
- Ectopic pregnancy
- Placental abruption
- Placenta praevia
- Sepsis: septic abortion or puerperal sepsis
- Uterine atony
- Placenta accrete
- Uterine/cervical/vaginal trauma
- Uterine rupture
- Retained products of conception
- Coagulopathy, especially DIC

## Presentation and assessment
The definition of massive haemorrhage assumes that >20–30% of total blood volume has already been lost. The presentation is similar to haemorrhage from other causes (see p. 114), and includes:
- Neurological: anxiety, thirst, drowsiness or unconsciousness
- Respiratory: dyspnoea, tachypnoea
- Cardiovascular: tachycardia (may be obtunded by regional anaesthesia; bradycardia is generally a late/pre-terminal sign), delayed capillary refill, hypotension
- Renal: oliguria/anuria
- Other: pallor

Bleeding PV or from the Caesarean section wound (or into the post-operative drains) may be seen. Occasionally bleeding is occult (e.g. uterine rupture or placental abruption), and abdominal pain may be present.
- Fetal CTG or blood gases may be abnormal

## Investigations
- ABGs
- FBC
- Coagulation studies/fibrinogen
- U&Es
- LFTs
- Serum calcium
- Where bleeding is associated with suspected concealed pregnancy β-HCG (urine or blood) or abdominal ultrasound may aid the diagnosis

* Blood loss may be very difficult to estimate as it may be mixed with amniotic fluid during delivery.

**Differential diagnoses**
- Amniotic fluid embolus
- Anaphylaxis
- Sepsis
- Local anaesthetic toxicity/regional anaesthesia complications
- Vasovagal response (to uterine stimulation)

**Immediate management**

A multidisciplinary approach should be adopted with input from senior critical care/anaesthetic, obstetric, and midwifery disciplines
- Give $O_2$ and support airway, breathing, and circulation as required
- Intubation and mechanical ventilation are likely to be required, and will facilitate any surgery
- Left lateral positioning to avoid aorto-caval compression is needed
- Aggressive fluid resuscitation is required (warmed fluids if possible)
  - Accurate estimation of blood loss is essential
  - Large-bore IV cannulae will be required for rapid fluid infusion
  - Invasive monitoring, particularly central venous pressure monitoring, will be required
  - Early packed red cell transfusion is likely to be needed, with O-negative blood if required
  - The use of bedside/portable Hb monitoring will guide transfusion
  - Arrange for cell salvage if possible
- Ensure prompt recognition and aggressive treatment of coagulopathies
  - Transfuse FFP, cryoprecipitate, and platelets as required
  - Consider vitamin K
  - Liaise with haematologists
  - Repeatedly check coagulation screen and fibrinogen
  - Consider recombinant factor VIIa for severe uncontrolled coagulopathy
- Post-partum uterine atony may respond to:
  - Manual massage/bimanual compression
  - Oxytocin (5 IU slow bolus, followed by an infusion at 10 IU/hour)
  - Followed by carboprost 250 µg IM or intra-uterine, up to every 15 min over 2 hours
  - Alternatively ergometrine 500 µg IM
- Available surgical treatments depend upon the cause of the bleeding (see also Pitfalls)
  - Traumatic tears may be repaired
  - Retained products of conception/retained placenta may be removed
  - Bleeding from placental site (e.g. placenta praevia) may respond to pressure (e.g. Sengstaken–Blakemore tube)
  - Uterine atony may respond to a brace suture (B Lynch), internal iliac artery ligation, hysterectomy, or interventional radiological treatments if there is access to these
  - Temporary aortic compression may 'buy time'

**Further management**

- Post-operative monitoring should be in a high-dependency environment and should ideally include arterial and central venous pressure monitoring
- Coagulopathy/DIC, clotting factor deficiency, or thrombocytopenia may require treatment with platelets, FFP, or cryoprecipitate
  - Where possible treatment should be guided by haematology
- Other complications of massive haemorrhage may include
  - Hypothermia requiring active warming via a warm air blanket and warmed IV fluids (re-warming will also improve the efficacy of clotting factors)
  - Transfusion-related acute lung injury (TRALI) may require support with non-invasive CPAP or ventilation; or with mechanical ventilation with a lung-protective strategy
  - Acute tubular necrosis: renal support may require volume resuscitation, maintenance of adequate perfusion pressure, or even renal replacement therapy
  - Hyperkalaemia: consider treatment with insulin/dextrose, or salbutamol
  - Hypocalacemia requiring calcium replacement if resistant hypotension is present
  - Massive transfusion may result in citrate toxicity

**Pitfalls/difficult situations**

- Recurrent haemorrhage can prove difficult to control; options include:
  - Returning to theatre for further surgical interventions
  - Further aggressive correction of coagulopathy
  - The use of recombinant factor VIIa
  - Angiographic embolization
- Regional anaesthesia may 'hide' abdominal pain associated with concealed bleeding such as uterine rupture
- The increase in circulating blood volume which occurs in pregnancy may delay the onset of symptoms associated with haemorrhage

**Further reading**

Banks A, Norris A (2005). Massive haemorrhage in pregnancy. *Br J Anaesth CEPD Rev* **5**, 195–8.
OHCC p. 542, OHEA p. 148.

# Poisoning and overdose

# :Ö: Emergency management

Poisonings or overdose (OD) may be intentional or unintentional. It can occur via ingestion, injection, or inhalation, or rarely by transdermal or other routes. It may be obvious from the history and presentation, or it may require a high index of suspicion to identify. In practice the emergency management of poisoning involves:

- Initial resuscitation
- Identification, where possible, of likely agent
- Specific treatments or antidotes
- General supportive measures

## Causes

Common poisoning agents

- Pharmaceutical products including paracetamol (and paracetamol-containing products), aspirin (and other analgesics or NSAIDs), opiates/opioids, benzodiazepines and 'Z-drugs' (e.g. zopiclone), antidepressants (including SSRIs and tricyclics), and barbiturates
- Recreational drugs including alcohol (the most common drug to be co-ingested either with recreational drugs or as part of self-poisoning), opiates/opioids, cocaine, amphetamines, ecstasy, gamma-hydroxybutyric acid (GHB), hallucinogenics (e.g. LSD), glues, and volatile chemicals
- Industrial chemicals, household chemicals, and environmental toxins including inhaled poisons (e.g. carbon monoxide and cyanide), organophosphates, paraquat, methanol, ethylene glycol, household products (e.g. batteries, cleaning agents, and detergents)
- Animal, fish, and insect bites/stings

## Presentation and assessment

Presentations associated with poisoning include:

- History of attempted suicide, psychiatric illness, or substance abuse
- Airway or respiratory signs and symptoms
  - Respiratory depression
  - Aspiration or pneumonitis
  - Bronchospasm
  - Oropharyngeal burns
- Cardiovascular
  - Hypotension, hypertension, cardiovascular collapse, cardiac arrest
  - ECG: tricyclics, antipsychotics, and many other drugs cause conduction defects and arrhythmias which may be resistant to treatment
- Neurological
  - Agitation, confusion, or hallucinations
  - Unexplained unconsciousness, especially if associated with compartment syndrome or prolonged contact burns
  - Convulsions
  - Profound weakness or, conversely, muscle rigidity or dystonia
  - Ataxia or nystagmus
- Gastrointestinal: vomiting or diarrhoea; liver failure
- Renal: renal failure, rhabdomyolysis

- Other associations
  - Hypo- or hyperthermia
  - Self-harm injuries
  - Trauma, burns, drowning, and head injuries
  - Electrolyte imbalance, especially sodium, potassium, or glucose
  - Metabolic acidosis, especially with a raised osmolal or anion gap (see p. 212)

Individual signs and symptoms are associated with certain poisons (Tables 14.1–14.4). Certain clusters of symptoms may occur together when poisoning with certain agents or groups of agents has occurred; these are commonly referred to as 'toxidromes' (Table 14.5).

## Investigations

The need for investigations will be dictated by the severity of the patient's condition and the most likely causative agent(s), but may include:

- ABGs
- FBC, coagulation studies
- Blood methaemoglobin concentration (normal is <1.5%)
- RBC cholinesterase activity (in organophosphate poisoning)
- U&Es, LFTs, serum calcium (in ethylene glycol poisoning), and phosphate (in paracetamol-induced renal failure)
- Serum CK
- Serum glucose
- Expired air (or blood) alcohol levels
- Paracetamol and salicylate levels—check timings
- Specific drug serum levels may also be indicated for other substances including valproic acid, methanol, phenytoin, theophylline, iron, lithium, carbamazepine, digoxin, ethylene glycol, and carboxyhaemoglobin
- Urine for myoglobin
- Consider taking blood, urine, and gastric aspirate samples for toxicology, or for storage in case later analysis is required
- 12-lead ECG
- CXR may be indicated if aspiration is suspected and prior to hyperbaric oxygen therapy
- AXR may be useful if ingestion of radio-opaque substances is suspected: chloral hydrate, heavy metals, iron, enteric-coated or sustained release preparations, 'body packing'
- Consider head CT scan or LP to exclude other causes of unconsciousness
- Other X-rays or scans may be required for any associated injuries

## Differential diagnoses

- Conditions causing altered consciousness, altered behaviour, or respiratory depression including head injuries, meningitis/encephalitis, hypogylcaemia and post-ictal state
- Conditions causing cardiovascular collapse including anaphylaxis
- Conditions causing muscle weakness (e.g. Guillain Barré and botulism)
- Conditions causing non-specific symptoms such as vomiting or hypothermia including infections or sepsis, neurological injury/subarachnoid haemorrhage and radiation sickness

**Table 14.1** Cardiorespiratory changes

| Signs and symptoms | Potential poisons |
| --- | --- |
| Respiratory depression Hypoventilation | Alcohols. barbiturates, benzodiazepines, botulinum toxin, neuromuscular blocking agents, opioids, sedatives, strychnine, tranquillizers, tricyclic antidepressants |
| Tachypnoea | Ethylene glycol, isoniazid, methanol, pentachloro-phenol, salicylates |
| Pulmonary oedema | Cocaine, chlorophenoxy herbicides, ethylene glycol, hydrocarbons, irritant gases, organic solvents, opioids, paraquat, phosgene, salicylates |
| Pneumothorax | Cocaine |
| Bradycardia | β-Blockers, calcium-channel antagonists, carbamates, cholinergics, clonidine, digoxin, lithium, metoclopramide, opioids, organopho-sphates, phenylpropanolamine, physostigmine, propoxyphene, quinidine |
| Tachycardia | Amphetamines, anticholinergics, antihistamines, caffeine, carbon monoxide, cocaine, cyanide, hydralazine, hydrogen levothyroxine , sulphide/phencyclidine, phenothiazines, sympathomimetics, theophylline, tricyclic antidepressants |
| Dysrhythmias | β-Blockers, chloroquine, cyanide, digoxin, phenothiazines, quinidine, theophylline, tricyclic antidepressants |
| Hypotension | β-Blockers, calcium-channel antagonists, ethanol, opioids, sedatives, tranquillizers |
| Hypertension | Anticholinergics, sympathomimetics |

**Table 14.2** Temperature, skin, and oral changes

| Signs and symptoms | Potential poisons |
| --- | --- |
| Hyperthermia | Anticholinergics, amphetamines, antihistamines, cocaine, dinitrophenols, hydroxybenzonitriles, LSD, MAOIs, phencyclidine, phenothiazines, pentochloro-phenols, procainamide, quinidine, salicylates, tricyclic antidepressants |
| Hypothermia | Barbiturates, carbon monoxide, colchicine, ethanol, lithium, opioids, phenothiazines, sedatives, tricyclic antidepressants |
| Excess salivation | Cholinesterase inhibitors, strychnine |
| Dry mouth | Anticholinergics, opioids, tricyclic antidepressants, phenothiazines |
| Sweating | Cholinergics, hypoglycaemics, sympathomimetics |
| Dry skin | Anticholinergics |
| Hair loss | Thallium |
| Acne | Bromide, organochlorine |

**Table 14.3** Neurological and eye changes

| Signs and symptoms | Potential poisons |
| --- | --- |
| Coma, decreased consciousness | Alcohols, benzodiazepines, barbiturates, bethanechol, carbamates, clonidine, GHB, hypoglycaemic agents, lithium, nicotine, opioids, organophosphates, physostigmine, pilocarpine, salicylates, tranquilizers, tricyclic antidepressants |
| Convulsions | Amphetamines, anticholinergics, antihistamines, antipsychotics, caffeine, camphor, carbamates, carbon monoxide, chlorinated hydrocarbons, cocaine, ethylene glycol, isoniazid, lead, lidocaine, lindane, lithium, methanol, nicotine, organophosphates, orphenadrine, phencyclidine, propranolol, salicylates, strychnine, theophylline, tricyclic antidepressants |
| Paraesthesia | Thallium |
| Ataxia/nystagmus | Antihistamines, bromides, barbiturates, carbamazepine, carbon monoxide, diphenylhydantoin, ethanol, phenytoin, piperazine, sedatives, thallium |
| Miosis | Barbiturates, carbamates, cholinergics, clonidine, ethanol, isopropyl alcohol, organophosphates, opioids, phencyclidine, phenothiazines, physostigmine, pilocarpine |
| Mydriasis | Amphetamines, anticholinergics, antihistamines, cocaine, dopamine, glutethimide, LSD, MAOIs, phencylidine, tricyclic antidepressants |
| Blindness | Quinine, methanol |

**Table 14.4** Gastrointestinal and renal changes

| Signs and symptoms | Potential poisons |
| --- | --- |
| Vomiting | Aspirin, iron, fluoride, theophylline |
| GI bleed | Anticoagulants, corrosive compounds, NSAIDs, salicylates |
| Liver failure | Carbon tetrachloride, parcetamol |
| Diarrhoea | Arsenic, cholinesterase inhibitors |
| Constipation | Lead, opioids, thallium |
| Urinary retention | Atropine, opioids, tricyclc antidepressants |
| Incontinence | Carbamates, organophosphates |
| Crystals in urine | Ethylene glycol, primidone |
| Renal failure | *Amanita* toxin, aminoglycosides, cadmium, carbon tetrachloride, ethylene glycol, oxalates, paracetamol, polymycin, mercury, methanol |

**Table 14.5** Toxidromes and combinations of symptoms and the likely associated poisons

| Toxidromes | Constellation of signs and symptoms | Possible toxins |
|---|---|---|
| Anticholinergic activity | Agitation, delirium, diminished consciousness, mydriasis hyperthermia, dry skin and mucosal membranes, flushing, tachycardia, bowel stasis, urinary retention | Anticholinergic alkaloids (e.g. in plants such as Belladonna), antihistamines, anti parkinsonian drugs, atropine, baclofen, cyclopentolate, phenothiazines, propantheline, scopolamine, tricyclic antidepressants |
| Cholinergic activity (muscarinic and/or nicotinic effects) | Miosis or mydriasis, blurred vision, sweating, excess salivation, lacrimation or bronchial secretions, wheezing or dyspnoea, tachycardia or bradycardia, hypertension, vomiting and diarrhoea, abdominal cramps, urinary and faecal incontinence, muscle weakness, fasciculations, | Acetylcholinesterase inhibitors: carbamates, neostigmine, organophosphates (pesticides or agents such as sarin), physostigmine, pyridostigmine Acetylcholine agonists: carbachol, choline, metacholine, pilocarpine |
| Sympathetic hyperactivity α and β adrenergic activity | Agitation, mydriasis, sweating, flushing, pyrexia, tachycardia, hypertension | Amphetamines, cocaine, ecstasy, ephedrine, PCP, phencyclidine, pseudoephedrine |
| If predominantly β-adrenergic | Tremor, tachycardia, hypotension | Caffeine, salbutamol, terbutaline, theophylline |
| If predominantly α-adrenergic | Bradycardia, hypertension | Phenylephrine, phenylpropanolamine |
| Extrapyramidal | Cog-wheel rigidity, tremor, trismus, hyper-reflexia, dyskinesis, dystonia, posturing, opisthotonos, choreoathetosis | Haloperidol, olanzapine, phenothiazines, risperidone |

| | | |
|---|---|---|
| Hallucinogenic | Agitation, psychosis, hallucinations, mydriasis, hyperthermia | Amphetamines, cannabinoids, cocaine, lsd |
| Narcotic | Decreased consciousness, miosis, bradypnoea, bradycardia, hypotension, hypothermia, bowel stasis | Clonidine, dextromethorphan, opiates, pentazocine, propoxyphene |
| Sedative | Confusion, slurred speech, decreased consciousness, normal or reduced respiratory rate, normotension, normocardia | Anticonvulsants, antipsychotics, barbiturates, benzodiazepines, ethanol, GHB, meprobamate |
| Volatile inhalation | Euphoria, confusion, slurred speech, headache, restlessness, ataxia, seizures, respiratory depression, dysrhythmias | Acetone, chlorinated hydrocarbons, fluorocarbons, hydrocarbons (petrol, butane,propaner), nitrites (isobutyl, amyl, butyl), toluene |
| Serotonin | Agitation, confusion, mydriasis, flushing, sweating, tremor, hyper-reflexia, clonus, myoclonus, trismus, hyperthermia, tachypnoea, tachycardia, hypertension | Amphetamine, ecstasy, MAOIs, serotonin re-uptake inhibitors |
| Chemical pneumonitis | Cough, dyspnoea, wheeze, respiratory distress, cyanosis, fever. Can occur without aspiration or loss of consciousness | Essential oils, petroleum distillates, turpentine, white spirit |
| Methaemoglobinaemia | Headache, diminished consciousness, dyspnoea, tachypnoea, severe hypoxia, tachycardia, chocolate-coloured blood | Alanine dyes, benzocaine, chlorates, chloroquine, dapsone, nitrates and nitrites, nitrobenzene, nitrophenol, phenacetin, phenazopyridine, primaquine, sodium nitroprusside |

## Immediate management

**Rapid simultaneous assessment of the patient, and of the likely agent(s) involved, may aid management**

*Identification of poison(s):*
- Details of which agent(s), how much, and how long ago should be actively sought. The following may help:
  - History from patient, family, other witnesses, or paramedics
  - History of repeat prescriptions from GP
  - Examination of patient for signs associated with certain drugs
  - Examination of pill bottles or tablets; a pill identification system such as the computer-aided tablet and capsule identification program (TICTAC) may be required

## Resuscitation
- Give $O_2$; support airway, breathing, and circulation as required

*Airway support*
- Endotracheal intubation may be required in the following circumstances
  - Diminished consciousness (GCS ≤9, or rapidly deteriorating)
  - Hypoxia
  - The patient is at risk of aspiration
  - The patient is agitated, or combative, and not mentally competent
  - Any corrosive substances have been ingested

*Breathing support*
- Ensure ventilation is adequate; use mechanical ventilation if necessary
  - Respiratory stimulants are unhelpful
  - In conditions where there is extreme acidosis it may be appropriate to hyperventilate the patient for a short period

*Circulatory support*
- Fluid loading may be required to treat hypotension
  - Tachypnoea, sweating, and unconsciousness can lead to fluid depletion
  - Hypotension may be the result of arrhythmias requiring treatment
  - Inotropes are occasionally required, but may interact with overdoses of cardiovascular drugs; where there is doubt discuss their use with an expert in poisonings
- Hypertension can occur with some drugs, particularly amphetamines and cocaine; hypotensive agents may be required
- Treat any cardiac arrhythmias and conduction defects which may compromise the circulation(see pp. 136 and 140)
  - Correction of hypoxia, acidosis (both metabolic and respiratory), and electrolytes will be required
  - Where tricyclic antidepressants are involved consider giving a bolus of 50–100 ml sodium bicarbonate 8.4% IV

- Certain drugs may prolong the QT interval resulting in torsade de pointes; consider giving magnesium sulphate 8 mmol (2 g) in 100 ml 5% dextrose IV over 2–5 minutes followed by an infusion of 2–4 mmol/hour (0.5–1 g/hour) (10 mmol) and potassium supplementation (40 mmol in 100 ml 5% dextrose over 1–4 hours via a central line aiming for a plasma concentration of 4.5–5.0 mmol/L)
- Profound bradycardia may be caused by certain agents, and may be unresponsive to drug therapy; consider
  - Early transvenous or transcutaneous pacing
  - In β-blocker overdose: treatment with glucagon 1 mg IV/IM
  - In calcium antagonist overdose: treatment with calcium chloride 10 ml 10% IV
  - In digoxin overdose: treatment with Fab fragments may help

*Neurological support*
- Convulsions are mostly brief and non-sustained; where status epilepticus occurs first-line treatment is with a short-acting benzodiazepine such as lorazepam 4 mg IV (see p. 166)
  - Be aware that many patients will have taken benzodiazepines as part of their overdose 'cocktail'
- Dystonic reactions can occur and may require treatment with procyclidine 5–10 mg IV

## Prevention of absorption

*Activated charcoal*
- Consider giving activated charcoal 50–100 g PO for enteral poisonings presenting within 1–2 hours (later administration may be useful in delayed-release preparations)
- In patients with diminished consciousness charcoal can be safely delivered via a nasogastric tube if the airway is protected by a cuffed endotracheal tube and the nasogastric tube position has been positively confirmed
- Can be used in repeated 4-hourly doses for certain drugs, including barbiturates, carbamazepine, dapsone, quinine, and theophylline
- Ineffective against alcohols, solvents, metal salts (e.g. iron and lithium), petroleum distillates, DDT, and malathion
- Do not give alongside an oral antidote

*Gastric lavage*
- Gastric lavage is only useful if performed within 1 hour of ingestion and works best on drugs not absorbed by charcoal (e.g. iron)
- In patients with diminished consciousness the airway must be protected by a cuffed endotracheal tube
- Not to be used if corrosive substances or hydrocarbons (e.g. petrol) have been ingested due to risk of gut perforation or pneumonitis
- Sudden deterioration may occur due to a bolus of gastric contents being forced past pylorus and so rapidly absorbed

*Forced emesis*
- Forced emesis with agents such as ipecacuanha is no longer recommended; it is not very effective, increases likelihood of aspiration, can cause regurgitation of corrosive substances to mouth and oesophagus, and limits the effectiveness of activated charcoal

**Further management**
- Consider contacting a specialist poisons unit to discuss complex cases

*Agitation*
- Look for and treat causes of agitation, e.g. full bladder or hypoxia
- Sedation may be required in agitated patients, but may provoke a drop in consciousness requiring intubation and it is often worth considering elective endotracheal intubation; sedation may also worsen any hypotension
- Antipsychotics are sometimes used to treat agitation, but may lower the seizure threshold

*Coma*
- If either opioids or benzodiazepines are suspected of contributing to a decreased level of consciousness, consider giving either naloxone (0.6–1.2 mg IV) or flumazenil (0.5 mg IV) as a diagnostic challenge to confirm the diagnosis. Be aware that flumazenil may lower the seizure threshold, and can provoke dysrhythmias (avoid in suspected tricyclic overdose)

*Hypothermia*
- Hypothermia is classically associated with barbiturate poisoning, but can occur with other drugs, and is common following prolonged unconsciousness
- Hypothermia may be profound and rewarming may be required (see p. 260); there may be an associated bradycardia (see p. 136)

*Hyperthermia*
- Hyperthermia is associated with stimulants and neuroleptic and antimuscarinic drugs; cooling and specific anti-hyperthermic therapy may be required (see p. 252)

*Other*
- Catheterization and urine output measurements may be required
- Regular blood sugar measurements may be required in order to monitor/treat any hypoglycaemia
- Invasive monitoring and continuous ECG monitoring are required for many poisonings and overdoses

*Antidotes and specific treatments*
- Antidotes or treatments may be available for certain drugs and chemicals (see Table 14.6)

*Active removal of drugs and poisons*
- Haemodialysis may be useful for ethanol, methanol, ethylene glycol, salicylates, theophylline, lithium

- Haemoperfusion may be useful for phenobarbitone, theophylline, carbamazepine (charcoal haemoperfusion columns can be obtained from manufacturers or poisons centres)
- Forced diuresis may be used for basic or acidic water-soluble drugs that are renally excreted
  - Diuresis is encouraged with mannitol or furosemide
  - Urine is alkalinized with bicarbonate or acidified with ammonium hydroxide
  - Urinary alkalinization may be considered for aspirin/salicylates, phenobarbital and phenoxyacetate herbicides
  - Urinary acidification may be considered for amphetamines, quinine, and phencyclidine
  - Electrolytes (including magnesium) should be monitored
  - Care must be taken to avoid fluid overload or dehydration
- Whole bowel irrigation using polyethylene glycol to promote bowel transit and liquefy stool has only limited evidence of effectiveness, but has been used in the following circumstances:
  - For sustained-release drug preparations, and drugs not absorbed by charcoal (e.g. iron and lithium)
  - For 'body-packers' (drug couriers who have ingested condoms filled with drugs)

**Table 14.6** Specific antidotes and treatments

| Drug or chemical | Antidote(s) |
| --- | --- |
| Anticholinergics | Physostigmine |
| β-Blockers | Glucagon |
| Benzodiazepines | Flumazenil |
| Calcium-channel blockers | Calcium chloride/gluconate |
| Cyanide | Sodium nitrate with sodium thiosulphate<br>Dicobalt edentate<br>Hydroxycobalamin |
| Digoxin | Fab fragments |
| Ethylene glycol/methanol | Ethanol or fomepizole |
| Heavy metal poisoning | Sodium calcium edentate<br>Penicillamine<br>Dimercaprol<br>DMSA/DMPS |
| Insulin/hypoglycaemics | Glucose, glucagon |
| Iron | Desferrioxamine |
| Isoniazid | Pyridoxine |
| Methaemoglobinaemia | Methylene blue |
| Opiates/opioids | Naloxone |
| Organophosphates/nerve agents | Atropine or pralidoxime |
| Paracetamol | Acetylcysteine or methionine |
| Snake bites | Anti-venom |
| Warfarin | Vitamin K and/or FFP |

### Pitfalls/difficult situations

- Accidental or deliberate self-poisoning is commonly associated with other injuries, including trauma
- The use of multiple agents is common in self-poisoning, and signs and symptoms are often a mixture of those caused by various drugs
- The combination of stimulant and sedatives (particularly GHB) taken together can result in profound fluctuations in consciousness
- Where there is any doubt as to the aetiology of decreased consciousness a CT scan is indicated, especially where the only poisoning agent is alcohol
  - Alcohol is commonly associated with both head trauma and intracranial bleeding
- Paracetamol and salicylate are extremely common ingredients in overdose 'cocktails'; it is customary to check plasma levels for these agents in all cases of self-poisoning, even when there is no evidence for their ingestion
- Prior to blood levels being available, or where no blood tests exist, treatment can be based upon the calculated maximum dose (e.g. if all the available pill bottles were full at the time of ingestion)
- Blood levels of toxins taken too soon after ingestion may be falsely low
- Identification of tablets, plants, or snakes brought in to hospital is often wrong; expert advice may be required via either direct contact or programs such as TICTAC
- Self-poisoning requires appropriate evaluation of any future suicide risk; ideally this should be arranged prior to ICU discharge

### Legal pitfalls

- Deaths from poisoning should be reported to the coroner
- Most patients will cooperate with treatment although some, particularly those who have attempted suicide, may refuse it
  - Patients who are mentally competent have the right to refuse any, and all, treatment … even if they risk death in doing so
  - Mental competency requires the ability to understand, retain, believe, and evaluate information
- Life-saving treatments may be administered to patients against their will only if they are not mentally competent
- When in doubt ask for senior advice or psychiatric advice early
- Carefully document any refusal of treatment, or any treatment against a patient's wishes

## Further reading/sources of information

Mokhlesi B, Leiken JB, Murray P, Corbridge TC (2003). Adult toxicology in critical care. Part I: general approach to the intoxicated patient. *Chest* **123**, 577–92.

Riordan M, Rylance G, Berry K (2002). Poisoning in children 1: General management. *Arch Dis Child* **87**, 392–6.

*British National Formulary*. Emergency treatment of poisoning chapter.

TOXBASE. Web-based database of the National Poisons Information Service available to registered users (i.e. A&E departments). Available online at: http://www.spib.axl.co.uk/

Poisons Information Centres. Tel: 0870 600 6266.

TICTAC tablet identification system. Available online at: http://tictac.vhn.net/home/

Mental Capacity Act 2005. Stationery Office, London. Available online at: http://www.opsi.gov.uk/acts/acts2005/20050009.htm

📖 OHCC p. 452.

# Analgesics

## ① Paracetamol poisoning

Paracetamol, a hepatotoxic analgesic found in many over-the-counter medications, is commonly associated with deliberate overdoses.

### Causes

Paracetamol poisoning occurs when healthy individuals take moderate to large overdoses. Certain patients have depleted stores of glutathione and are susceptible to hepatotoxicity at much lower doses

- Malnourished: anorexia, alcoholism, HIV
- Taking enzyme-inducing drugs: carbamazepine, phenobarbital, phenytoin, primidone, rifampicin, St John's Wort

### Presentation and assessment

- Initial presentation is mostly asymptomatic unless other agents are also involved, although nausea and vomiting may occur
- Delayed presentation (12 hours–4 days) can be accompanied by RUQ pain with liver and/or renal failure

### Investigations

- ABGs, if compromised
- FBC and coagulation studies
- U&Es, LFTs
- Serum glucose
- Salicylate and paracetamol levels

Immediate management (see also p. 434)

- Give $O_2$; support airway, breathing, and circulation as required
Other treatment relies on restoring hepatic glutathione
- Treatment is guided by plasma levels taken >4 hours after ingestion; levels earlier than this can be misleading; high-risk patients require treatment at lower plasma levels(see above and Table 14.6)
- Give IV N-acetylcysteine (diluted in 5% dextrose):
  - 150 mk/kg IV over 15 minutes, then
  - 50 mg/kg IV over 4 hours, then
  - 100 mg/kg IV over 16 hours
- N-acetylcysteine is best started <10 hours after ingestion, but can still be given up to 36 hours
  - If the history is suggestive of an overdose requiring treatment then N-acetylcysteine can be commenced whilst awaiting levels

Alternatively methionine can be given if the poisoning is <12 hours and there is no vomiting

Further management (see also p. 436)

- Monitor for hepatotoxicity using serial PT/INR and bilirubin measurements. LFT changes often occur late. Renal failure may also occur
- Signs of impending hepatic or hepatorenal failure include INR >3, oliguria, increased creatinine, hypoglycaemia, acidosis and encephalopathy. They should prompt discussion with a specialist liver centre

## Pitfalls/difficult situations

- Paracetamol co-drugs
  - Cold and decongestant combinations may contain paracetamol and vasoactive preparations such as pseudoephedrine; this may result in moderate transient hypertension in overdose
  - Co-codamol and similar preparations contain codeine, and treatment for opioid side effects may be required
  - Co-proxamol contains dextropropoxythene which has long-acting opioid effects and also produces a cardiotoxic metabolite; cardiovascular compromise and arrhythmias may occur. The administration of magnesium sulphate and/or sodium bicarbonate may be useful

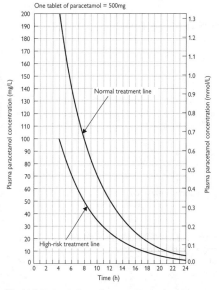

**Fig 14.1** Patients whose plasma paracetamol concentrations are above the normal treament line should be treated with acetylcysteine by IV infusion (or, if acetylcysteine cannot be used, with methionine PO, provided that the overdose has been taken within 10–12 hours and the patient is not vomiting).

Patients on enzyme-inducing drugs (e.g. carbamazepine, phenobarbital, phenytoin, primidone, rifampicin, alcohol, and St John's Wort) or who are malnourished (e.g. in anorexia, in alcoholism, or those who are HIV positive) should be treated if their plasma paracetamol concentration is above the high-risk treament line.

The prognostic accuracy after 15 hours is uncertain but a plasma paracetamol concentration above the relevant treatment line should be regarded as carrying a serious risk of liver damage.

## Further reading

📖 OHCC p. 456

## ☺: Aspirin/salicylate poisoning

Life-threatening salicylate overdoses can result in complex clinical pictures which are difficult to manage.

### Causes
- Aspirin ingestion
- Salicylic acid ingestion
- Oil of wintergreen

### Presentation and assessment
Initial respiratory alkalosis, from respiratory stimulation, gives way to a metabolic acidosis which is an indicator of poor prognosis. Other system derangements can also occur:
- Respiratory:
  - Hyperventilation
  - Pulmonary oedema (non-cardiogenic)
- Cardiovascular
  - Tachycardia
  - Dehydration
  - Vasodilatation
  - Cardiovascular collapse
- Neurological
  - Agitation
  - Deafness/tinnitus
  - Cerebral oedema/encephalopathy
  - Convulsions
  - Coma
  - Tetany
- Metabolic
  - Hypokalaemia
  - Hypoglycaemia (predominantly in children)
- Other
  - Hyperpyrexia
  - Renal failure
  - Petechiae or gastric erosions from platelet dysfunction (although major haemorrhage is rarely a problem)
  - Profound sweating
  - Nausea and vomiting

### Investigations
- ABGs: serial measurements will allow the monitoring of progression of illness
- FBC
- U&Es (serial measurements), LFTs
- Serum glucose
- Salicylate and paracetamol levels
  - Plasma concentrations <700 mg/L (5.1 mmol/L) are associated with less severe symptoms
- CXR may be indicated if there is respiratory compromise

*Differential diagnoses*
- Subdural haematoma
- Dehydration
- Hyperthermia

Immediate management (see also p. 434)

- Give $O_2$; support airway, breathing, and circulation as required
- Give activated charcoal if appropriate (see p. 435), some centres use multiple doses to enhance elimination, though its role is debatable
- Aggressive IV fluid replacement will be required
- Treatment is guided by plasma salicylate levels
  - Delayed absorption may occur, so a repeat level after 4 hours is advised
  - Levels >12 hours after ingestion may be misleadingly low
  - Acidaemia, or severe symptoms, also indicate high levels
- Levels >500 mg/L (3.6 mmol/L) should prompt consideration of urinary alkalinization by giving 200–300 ml IV boluses of 8.4% sodium bicarbonate (sodium bicarbonate may also be considered for correction of metabolic acidaemia)
- Levels >700 mg/L (5.1 mmol/L) are an indication for haemodialysis
- Potassium levels checked and replaced concurrently with urinary alkalinization
- Serial blood glucose measurement (and correction) is required

Further management (see also p. 436)
- Serial blood tests are required as above
- A salicylate level <25 mg/L should be aimed for

Pitfalls/difficult situations
- Treat if blood levels are low but symptoms are severe; also treat if asymptomatic but with high blood levels
- Children and infants are much more sensitive to salicylate poisoning and have a lower trigger level for treatment (see current edition of BNF)
- In pregnant patients consider elective Caesarean section

⑦ **NSAIDs**

Most NSAIDs are relatively benign in overdose. GI pain, nausea, and vomiting are common. Convulsions can occur, especially with mefenamic acid. GI bleeds, renal failure, coma, and arrhythmias can occur but are rare. There is no specific treatment. FBC and U&E monitoring may be advisable after large overdoses.

Further reading
📖 OHCC p. 454.

# Antidepressants

### :Ö: Tricyclic antidepressants

Tricyclic antidepressants (TCAs) are commonly involved in self-poisoning. Alongside their anticholinergic effects they have neurological and cardio-toxic effects (caused by sodium-channel blockade).

#### Causes

There are many tricyclics, modified tricyclics, and related compounds. The more common ones include amitriptyline, clomipramine, dosulepin, imipramine, lofepramine, trimipramine, mianserin, and trazadone. Dosulepin is probably the most cardiotoxic.

#### Presentation and assessment

Signs and symptoms of overdose may include:

- Anticholinergic effects: dry skin, tachycardia, dilated pupils, blurred vision, urinary retention
- Neurological: decreased consciousness, convulsions, hyper-reflexia
- Respiratory: bradypnoea, respiratory acidosis
- Cardiovascular: hypotension, tachycardia or bradycardia may develop
  - ECG: minor ECG changes are common (PR and QT prolongation), QRS > 120 msec is associated with increased incidence of dysrhythmias
- Other: metabolic acidosis and hypokalaemia may develop

#### Investigations

- Plasma levels do not aid management
- ABGs: serial measurements will allow the monitoring of progression of illness
- FBC
- U&Es, LFTs
- Serum CK
- Serum glucose
- Expired air or blood alcohol levels
- Paracetamol and salicylate levels
- 12-lead ECG
- Consider head CT scan to exclude other causes of unconsciousness

#### Differential diagnoses

The combination of neurological and cardiac signs and symptoms is found in other illnesses including:

- Intracranial haemorrhage/subarachnoid haemorrhage
- Meningitis/encephalitis
- Sepsis

**Immediate management** (see also p. 434)

- Give O$_2$; support airway, breathing, and circulation as required
- ECG monitoring is essential
- Give activated charcoal if appropriate (see p. 435),
  - Gastric lavage is not recommended as it may cause a bolus effect by pushing medication through the pylorus
- Acidosis worsens cardiotoxicity
  - If decreased consciousness, bradypnoea, and respiratory acidosis are present, endotracheal intubation and ventilation are indicated
  - Temporarily increasing minute volume to create a respiratory alkalosis may 'buy time'
  - Metabolic acidosis should be treated with 50 ml 8.4% sodium bicarbonate IV, especially in the presence of a widened QRS
- Fluid replacement should be with 0.9% saline or isotonic sodium-containing fluids
- Hypotension may occasionally require inotropes
  - Resistant hypotension may respond to IV glucagon
- Seizures are best treated with benzodiazepines; phenytoin may worsen cardiotoxicity
- Dysrhythmias are best treated with IV sodium bicarbonate in the first instance
  - Lidocaine or esmolol may be the best second-line choices as other anti-arrhythmics may have marked negative-inotropic or cardiotoxic effects

**Further management** (see p. 436)

**Pitfalls/difficult situations**

- Seizures often precede dysrhythmias
- Prolonged resuscitation for cardiac arrests associated with tricyclic overdose is associated with better than expected outcomes

### ☼ SSRIs

SSRIs are safer in overdose. They have fewer anticholinergic effects, and although convulsions and arrythmias can occur, they are uncommon. ECG monitoring for symptomatic cases is advisable.

Combinations of SSRIs or the inclusion of an MAOI can occasionally result in serotonin toxicity (p. 258).

**Further reading**
📖 OHCC p. 460

## :○: MAOIs

Monoamine oxidase inhibitors (MAOIs) include phenelzine, isocar-boxazid, tranylcypromine, and moclobemide. They are less commonly prescribed than other antidepressants.

### Causes

- Overdose of MAOIs can result in noradrenergic and serotinergic effects which can be severe.
- Combinations of SSRIs or the inclusion of an MAOI can occasionally result in serotonin toxicity (see p. 258).
- A hypertensive reaction can be triggered in patients on MAOIs by the ingestion of amine-rich foods such as certain cheeses and red wine (the 'cheese reaction').
- MAOIs are known to interact with certain anaesthetic agents (see Pitfalls).

### Presentation and assessment

Signs and symptoms typically occur 12–24 hours after ingestion, and include:

- Neurological: agitation, dyskinesia, decreased consciousness, seizures
- Autonomic instability: hypotension or hypertension, tachycardia
  - Hypertension may be severe and symptomatic (with encephalopathy or intracerebral haemorrhage)
- Serotinergic toxicity: flushing, sweating, hyperthermia, tremor, hyper-reflexia, clonus, myoclonus, trismus, tachypnoea
- Rhabdomyolysis, DIC, acute renal failure, haemolysis, and metabolic acidosis are all recognized complications

### Investigations

- ABGs: serial measurements will allow the monitoring of progression of illness
- FBC, coagulation studies
- U&Es, LFTs
- Serum CK
- Serum glucose
- Expired air or blood alcohol levels
- Paracetamol and salicylate levels
- 12-lead ECG

### Differential diagnoses

- Thyroid storm
- Malignant hyperthermia/neuroleptic malignant syndrome

Immediate management (see also p. 434)

- Give $O_2$; support airway, breathing, and circulation as required
- ECG monitoring is essential
- Give activated charcoal if appropriate (see p. 436)
- Hypertension often responds to gentle sedation with benzodiazepines (see p. 152 as a guide to management of hypertension)
  - If hypertension is resistant, α-blocking drugs may be started (phentolamine, phenoxybenzamine, doxazosin)
  - Consider IV hydralazine or GTN if further antihypertensives are required
  - Do not use β-blockers as they will result in unopposed α stimulation
- Hyperthermia can be treated with general cooling measures, including cooled IV fluids
  - If hyperthermia is resistant to simple cooling, consider giving IV dantrolene (1–10 mg/kg) and/or sedation, endotracheal intubation, and neuromuscular blockade

Further management

- Symptoms may persist for 1–2 days
- Complications should be monitored and treated
  - Serial U&Es and CK measurements may be required to monitor for rhabdomyolysis and renal failure
  - Serial FBC and coagulation studies may be required to monitor for DIC

Pitfalls/difficult situations

- MAOIs are known to interact with:
  - Certain opioids, particularly pethidine, to cause serotinergic symptoms; morphine would appear to be the drug of choice
  - Indirect acting sympathomimetics such as ephedrine and metaraminol may precipitate hypertensive crises
  - Drugs with indirect acting sympathomimetic effects (pancuronium, ketamine, cocaine) may also precipitate hypertensive crises
- Where inotropic support is required, direct-acting drugs such as adrenaline, noradrenaline, and phenylephrine may be preferred
- The effect of older MAOIs may persist for up to 3 weeks

# Sedatives

## ☼ Benzodiazepines

Benzodiazepines are often taken along with other drugs in overdoses. Occasionally their presence may actually counteract the deleterious effects of other drugs (e.g. convulsions).

### Presentation and assessment

Benzodiazepines are relatively benign on their own. They may cause sedative symptoms, including respiratory depression, mild bradycardia, and decreased consciousness, but these rarely require active treatment.

### Investigations (see p. 420)

Isolation of urinary metabolites may be possible for some benzodiazepines, and may be worth considering if a criminal investigation may take place (see Pitfalls).

### Differential diagnoses

- Conditions causing altered consciousness, altered behaviour, or respiratory depression including head injuries, meningitis/encephalitis, hypoglycaemia and post-ictal state

### Immediate management (see also p. 434)

- Give $O_2$; support airway, breathing, and circulation as required
- Give activated charcoal if appropriate (see p. 435)
- Consider giving flumazenil 500 µg IV, repeated up to 3 mg
  - Flumazenil may trigger agitation or convulsions; do not give to patients who are post-ictal or who have had head injuries
  - Flumazenil can also trigger arrhythmias and heart block; avoid if tricyclic overdose is suspected
  - Flumazenil is short acting and so symptoms may return; an infusion (0.5–1mg/hour) may be appropriate

### Further management (see p. 436)

### Pitfalls/difficult situations

- Benzodiazepines have been used as 'date rape' drugs; a low threshold of suspicion may be required

## ☼ Barbiturates

### Presentation and assessment

Barbiturate poisoning presents with a similar clinical picture to that seen with benzodiazepines except that certain symptoms may be more severe
- Decreased consciousness/coma
- Respiratory depression/apnoea
- Hypotension/cardiovascular collapse

Other associated signs and symptoms include:
- Hypothermia
- Pulmonary oedema (an occasional finding)

**Immediate management** (see also p. 434)

- Give O$_2$; support airway, breathing, and circulation as required
- Give activated charcoal if appropriate (see p. 435)
- Treatment is generally supportive
- Hypotension may be profound, requiring aggressive fluid resuscitation and/or inotropes

## ☼ GHB

Gamma-hydroxybutyric acid (GHB) is generally a recreational drug but, like benzodiazepines, it has been used to 'spike' drinks as a 'date rape' drug.

It produces a 'high', but it is also sedative and is often taken with stimulants such as amphetamines. Individual responses are unpredictable but coma with bradycardia and hypotension are common. Rapid swings in GCS can occur, as can rapid recovery from profound coma to self-extubation.

Metabolic acidosis can occur, as can hypernatraemia, hyperglycaemia, and hypokalaemia. Investigations should include ABGs, U&Es, and glucose. A head CT scan may be required

Temporary airway support is often all that is required. GHB is metabolized rapidly.

## Further reading

Kam PC, Yoong FF (1998). Gamma-hydroxybutyric acid: an emerging recreational drug. *Anaesthesia* **53**, 1195–8.
📖 OHCC p. 458.

# Inhaled poisons

### ☼ Carbon monoxide

Carbon monoxide is a colourless, tasteless, and odourless gas. Poisoning may be intentional but is also often accidental.

#### Causes

It must always be considered in house-fire victims or those trapped in an enclosed space with a fire. It can also be an occult diagnosis (e.g. due to faulty boilers) and should be considered as a cause of unexplained unconsciousness, headache, confusion, or breathlessness.

#### Presentation and assessment

Carboxyhaemaglobin poisoning is strongly associated with severe burns and inhalational injuries (see pp. 28 and 66). Other signs and symptoms are non-specific and a high index of suspicion is required.

- Cherry red skin is only present sometimes; cyanosis is more common

The severity of poisoning depends upon the clinical findings
- Minor neurological changes: headache, ataxia, nystagmus, hyper-reflexia, drowsiness
- Major neurological: cerebral oedema, convulsions, coma
- Cardiac: arrhythmias, myocardial infarct, cardiovascular collapse, ECG evidence of ischaemia
- Other: pulmonary oedema, metabolic acidosis, rhabdomyolysis, or renal failure

Routine clinical findings may become less reliable indicators of illness
- $PaO_2$ is often normal
- $SaO_2$ may be artificially high

#### Investigations (see also p. 429)
- COHb: the diagnosis can be confirmed using bench co-oximetry to measure levels of carboxyhaemoglobin; they are only a rough guide to the severity of poisoning
- ABGs
- FBC
- U&Es, LFTs
- Serum CK, urine for myoglobin
- Cardiac enzymes
- 12-lead ECG
- CXR
- Consider head CT scan to exclude other causes of unconsciousness

---

**Carboxyhaemoglobin levels**[*]

- 3–5%      normal
- 6–10 %    normal for smokers
- >25%      late neurological complications likely
- >60%      highly likely to die

[*] Carboxyhaemoglobin levels do not always equate to severity of poisoning

---

### Differential diagnoses
- Simple viral infections
- Any cause of metabolic acidosis, especially cyanide poisoning
- Meningitis/encephalitis

**Immediate management** (see also p. 434)

- Support airway, breathing, and circulation as required
- Assess and treat burns as appropriate (see p. 435)
- High-concentration $O_2$ is required regardless of $PaO_2$
  - Treatment should be continued for at least 6 hours, longer if COHb remains >5–10%
  - Alkalosis should be avoided if possible
- Hyperbaric oxygen may be of benefit but is difficult to deliver
  - Many patients are too unstable to transfer
  - In cases where COHb >25% the possibility of late-onset neurological complications may be lessened by hyperbaric oxygen
  - Other indications include COHb >40%, episode of unconsciousness, neurological disturbance, ECG changes, and pregnancy
  - Cerebral oedema may require treatment with mannitol

**Further management** (see also p. 436)
- Consider taking a urine sample for a pregnancy test

### :☺: Cyanide

Cyanide poisoning is associated with smoke inhalation injuries and with industrial accidents. As with carbon monoxide, a high index of suspicion is required. Signs and symptoms may include headache, convulsions, coma, tachypnoea, cardiac ischaemia, arrhythmias, pulmonary oedema metabolic acidosis, and cardiac arrest.

### Investigations (see also p. 429)
- FBC, coagulation studies, U&Es, LFTs, ABGs, and ECG are all required.
- Blood should be taken for cyanide levels, but treatment should not be delayed

**Immediate management** (see also p. 434)

- Patients should be decontaminated prior to examination/treatment
- Support airway, breathing, and circulation as required
- High-concentration $O_2$ is required
  - Inhaled amyl nitrite may provide a rapid temporary treatment
  - Consider IV sodium nitrite (10 ml of 3% over 3 minutes) followed by sodium thiosulphate (25 ml of 50% over 10 minutes)
  - Dicobalt edetate is toxic and reserved for confirmed severe cases

### Further reading
📖 OHCC p. 466.

# Industrial chemicals

## :Ö: Organophosphates and carbamates

Industrial exposure and deliberate self-poisonings with organophosphates and carbamates are common, particularly in the developing world.

Chemical nerve agents (e.g. G-agents such as sarin, tabun, and soman, and V-agents such as VX gas) are similar to organophosphates, and require similar treatment.

### Presentation and assessment

These agents can act via ingestion, via inhalation, or transdermally. A classic 'toxidrome' of cholinergic effects may be seen (see Table 14.5) including excess salivation and secretions, miosis, blurred vision, bronchospasm, bronchorrhoea, bradycardia (and other arrhythmias), vomiting, diarrhoea and abdominal cramps, convulsions, and coma. Later findings include muscle weakness, fasciculations, and paralysis.

Carbamate poisoning is generally less severe and of shorter duration.

### Investigations (see p. 429)

- RBC cholinesterase activity can be measured in organophosphate poisoning
- U&Es and ECG are indicated for arrhythmia management
- Serum glucose: hypoglycaemia is common

### Immediate management (see also p. 434)

- Patients should be decontaminated prior to examination/treatment
- Give O₂; support airway, breathing, and circulation as required
  - Mechanical ventilation or other respiratory support may be required if bronchial secretions cause respiratory distress
- Atropine 2 mg IV should be given every 20 minutes until pupils dilate, skin is dry, and tachycardia occurs
- In moderate to severe cases pralidoxime can be given (within 24 hours) 30 mg/kg IV with one to two further doses as required
  - Benzodiazepines may be required to control seizures (p. 166)

### Further management (see also p. 436)

- Paralysis requiring ventilation may occur days after ingestion

## :Ö: Paraquat

The initial features of paraquat poisoning are those of ingestion of a corrosive agent. Cardiovascular collapse, pulmonary oedema, and metabolic acidosis may occur. Urine testing can confirm the diagnosis, and plasma concentrations may give prognostic information. Initial treatment with oral/NG Fuller's earth may be of benefit. High oxygen concentrations may worsen pulmonary toxicity.

Later complications include liver or renal failure, but a progressive alveolitis over a few days is the most common cause of death.

### :Q: Phenoxyacetates

Phenoxyacetate pesticide poisoning is less common than with organophosphates. Signs and symptoms include:

- Neurological: diminished consciousness, seizures
- Neuromuscular: myotonia, myositis, weakness, fasciculation
- Gastrointestinal: mouth and throat burning, nausea, vomiting, diarrhoea
- Other: sweating, hypertension, hyperthermia, rhabdomyolysis

*Investigations* (see p. 429)

- ABGs (metabolic acidosis is common)
- U&Es and serum calcium (hypocalcaemia is common)
- Serum glucose (hypoglycaemia is common)
- Serum CK, urine myoglobin will be required

**Immediate management** (see also p. 434)

- Patients should be decontaminated prior to examination/treatment
- Give O₂; support airway, breathing, and circulation as required
  - Neuromuscular weakness may require mechanical ventilation
- 2,4-dichlorophenoxyacetic acid and mecoprop may be treated with forced alkaline diuresis
- Other phenoxyacetates may be treated by haemodialysis

### :Q: Strychnine

Strychnine poisoning causes intense muscle spasms which may resemble tonic–clonic epilepsy (although the patient should be awake) or tetanus. Respiratory distress requiring endotracheal intubation and mechanical ventilation with neuromuscular blockade may occur. U&Es and CK should be measured as hyperthermia, rhabdomyolysis, and renal failure may occur requiring supportive treatment.

### :Q: Chlorine

Chlorine exposure may cause haemoptysis, dyspnoea, bronchospasm, and pulmonary oedema. Symptoms may occur up to 24 hours after exposure, but are unlikely if ocular symptoms are not present (where the eyes have been exposed).

Laryngeal damage will necessitate early endotracheal intubation (see p. 28). Bronchodilators may help alleviate respiratory distress, but mechanical ventilation is likely to be required in severe cases.

**Further reading**

📖 OHCC pp. 468, 472.

# Alcohols and hydrocarbons

## ☼ Ethanol/alcohol

As well as being found in alcoholic drinks, ethanol is also present in household products (e.g. mouthwashes and aftershaves). It is often co-ingested with other poisons.

### Presentation and assessment

Severe ethanol intoxication, particularly in relatively ethanol-naïve individuals, may cause hypothermia, convulsions, coma, respiratory depression, and hypotension. Metabolic acidosis, hypoglycaemia, and hypokalaemia may also occur.

### Investigations (see p. 429)

- ABGs
- U&Es
- Serum glucose
- Blood alcohol levels (<0.8 g/L, UK driving limit; >5 g/L, severe ethanol toxicity)

### Immediate management (see also p. 434)

- Give $O_2$; support airway, breathing, and circulation as required
- Respiratory depression or loss of airway reflexes may necessitate endotracheal intubation and mechanical ventilation
- Aggressive fluid resuscitation may be required to counteract ethanol-induced vasodilatation
- Correction of hypothermia may be required (see p. 260)
- Correction of glucose and electrolytes may be required
  - If there is doubt concerning the patient's nutritional status give thiamine as Pabrinex® vials 1 and 2 before administration of glucose to avoid precipitating Wernike's syndrome
- Consider haemodialysis if blood alcohol is high or symptoms are severe

### Further management (see also p. 436)

- Consider performing a tertiary survey to look for evidence of occult trauma associated with acute alcohol intoxication

## ☼ Ethylene glycol and methanol

Ethylene glycol and methanol are both found in antifreeze solutions; methanol is also found as a solvent in various household products.

### Presentation and assessment

Ethylene glycol can result in intoxication, confusion, decreased consciousness, coma, convulsions, nystagmus, nausea and vomiting, tachycardia, hypertension, cardiogenic shock, pulmonary oedema, tachypnoea, metabolic acidosis, or renal failure

Methanol can result in intoxication, confusion, headache, decreased consciousness, ataxia, coma, convulsions, visual disturbance, nausea, vomiting, abdominal pain, tachypnoea, metabolic acidosis, or renal failure

*Investigations* (see p. 429)
- ABGS: both methanol and ethylene glycol cause metabolic acidosis with a raised anion gap(>12 mmol/L) and osmolar gap (>10 mOsm)
- Serum U&Es and calcium (hypocalcaemia occurs with ethylene glycol poisoning)
- Serum glucose, as hyperglycaemia occurs with methanol poisoning
- Serum methanol and ethylene glycol levels should be measured
- Serum ethanol levels will be required to guide treatment
- Urine microscopy (oxalate crystals are seen in ethylene glycol poisoning)

Immediate management (see also p. 434)
- Give $O_2$; support airway, breathing, and circulation as required
- Charcoal is ineffective; gastric lavage may be appropriate
- Ethanol should be given
  - Orally (loading dose 1 ml/kg 50%/50 g/~1 cup of spirits)
  - **Or** IV (loading dose 7.5 ml/kg 10% over 30 minutes)
  - A blood alcohol level of 0.8 g/L should be aimed for
- Alternatively IV fomepizole (loading dose 15 mg/kg over 30 minutes, followed by 10 mg/kg 12-hourly) may be used
- Folinic acid 30 mg IV 6-hourly should be given in methanol poisoning
- IV sodium bicarbonate may be required to treat acidosis
- Haemodialysis may be required for the treatment of acidosis or acute renal failure
  - The maintenance doses of ethanol or fomepizole should be increased if dialysis is used

## ☼ Petroleum, white spirit, and other hydrocarbons

These can cause intoxication, agitation, depressed consciousness, and coma. Vomiting is common. Pneumonitis may occur up to 24 hours later, even in the absence of an obvious aspiration event. Dysrhythmias may occur with volatile poisoning.

Consider ABGs and CXR if there are respiratory complications.

Activated charcoal is ineffective. Gastric lavage is not recommended. If laryngeal oedema is present, early intubation should be considered even if the patient is currently asymptomatic. ECG monitoring is advised. Bronchodilators may help in the treatment of hypoxia.

**Further reading**
📖 OHCC p. 470.

# Recreational drugs

## ☼ Opiates/opioids

Opioid poisoning is associated with intentional overdose of prescription medications, or inadvertent overdose of illicit opioids (prescription or otherwise). In both cases they are commonly taken in combination with other drugs such as benzodiazepines.

### Presentation and assessment

Opioid poisoning is classically associated with a 'toxidrome' (see Table 14.5) including decreased consciousness, miosis, bradypnoea, bradycardia, hypotension, hypothermia, and bowel stasis.

Other signs and symptoms may include:
- Track marks and skin infections
- Convulsions
- Pulmonary oedema

### Investigations (see p. 429)
- ABGs are required to monitor acidosis
- CXR may be indicated if pulmonary oedema is present

### Immediate management (see also p. 434)

- Give O₂; support airway, breathing, and circulation as required
- Treatment is mainly supportive consisting of airway/respiratory support
  - Pulmonary oedema may require the addition of PEEP or CPAP
- Hypotension may require aggressive fluid therapy and/or inotropes
- Opiate reversal with IV naloxone (0.4–2 mg) can be attempted
  - Naloxone is shorter acting than most opiates and so repeat doses may be required
  - Consider a naloxone IV infusion (4 µg/ml run at >1 µg/kg/hour, titrated to effect)

### Pitfalls/difficult situations
- Trauma and compartment syndrome are associated with opioids
- Unusual infections such as tetanus and botulism are associated with illicit IV or IM drug usage, as are HIV, HBV, and HCV; appropriate precautions should be taken
- Paracetamol co-drugs contain opioids including dextropropoxyphene which has long-acting opioid effects and has a cardiotoxic metabolite

## ☼ Cocaine

Severe poisoning with cocaine may cause:
- Severe hypertension
- Hyper-reflexia, convulsions, coma, intracranial bleeds, or infarcts
- Myocardial ischaemia, arrythmias, cardiogenic shock, cardiac arrest
- Hyperthermia
- Rhabdomyolysis and renal failure

**Immediate management** (see also p. 434)

- Give $O_2$; support airway, breathing, and circulation as required
- ECG monitoring is essential
- Treat hypertension with benzodiazepines, α-blockers, or IV nitrates
  - β-blockers may worsen hypertension
  - IV or sublingual nitrates should also be used to treat chest pain
- Ischaemic crises should be treated with aspirin
  - Myocardial ischaemia is unlikely to benefit from thrombolysis
- Hyperthermia should be treated by cooling and other treatments, including dantrolene if required (see p. 252)

### ☼ Amphetamines and ecstasy

Amphetamines and methylenedioxymethamphetamine (ecstasy) can cause agitation, convulsions, and coma. Arrhythmias are common, as is hypertension. Patients are often dehydrated, although in some patients excessive water consumption leads to a hypo-osmolar state.

Investigations should include FBC, coagulation studies, U&Es, LFTs, serum CK, serum glucose, and ECG.

Hypertension caused by amphetamines or ecstasy should be treated in the same way as hypertension caused by cocaine.

An idiosyncratic hyperthermic reaction can occur and is associated with muscle rigidity, rhabdomyolysis, metabolic acidosis, renal failure, hepatic failure, convulsions, coma, and DIC. Cooling and other treatment for hyperthermia may be required (see p. 252) along with dantrolene.

### ☼ Ketamine and LSD

Ketamine is sedative in nature, although emergence delirium and agitation may occur requiring treatment with benzodiazepines. Airway support may be required, and in severe poisoning treatment for convulsions and raised ICP may be required.

LSD is mostly relatively benign. Hallucinations may lead to marked agitation or bizarre behaviour. Coma, convulsions, bleeding, and pyrexia sometimes occur. Sedation may be required with benzodiazepines.

### Cannabis

Cannabis is relatively safe except when injected. IV cannabis can cause hypotension, pulmonary oedema, DIC, and renal failure, which may be managed with supportive therapy.

**Further reading**
📖 OHCC pp. 462, 464.

# Miscellaneous poisons

## ☼ Corrosives, acids, alkalis, and bleaches

The main acute risk with these agents is airway or pharyngeal damage. If laryngeal oedema is present, early intubation should be considered even if the patient is currently asymptomatic. Early ENT or thoracic surgical involvement should be considered.

Activated charcoal does not work and gastric lavage should not be attempted. Later complications include GI burns which may require surgical intervention.

## ☼ Bites and stings

Many snake bites are 'dry' (no injected venom), requiring no treatment, and many other bites or stings are of low toxicity. Expert advice is required to identify animals/insects and to direct treatment.

Toxicity is generally either local (tissue necrosis) or systemic (cardiotoxic, neurotoxic, or coagulopathic, either via direct inhibition or consumption of clotting factors).

Initially a compression lymph bandage may be applied (not a tourniquet) to slow the spread of any toxins. Anti-venom may be advised for the treatment of certain snake bites; otherwise treatment is supportive.

Bites, stings, and anti-venom may cause anaphylaxis or anaphylactoid reactions (see p. 112).

## ⑦ Lead

The acute presentation of lead poisoning is an encephalopathy with ataxia, convulsions, and coma, associated with abdominal pain and vomiting. A peripheral motor neuropathy (foot and wrist drop) may occur.

### Investigations (see p. 429)
- Blood lead levels can be estimated
- FBC may reveal anaemia with basophilic stippling and RBC fluorescence
- U&Es may reveal renal dysfunction

---

### Immediate management (see also p. 434)

- Give $O_2$; support airway, breathing, and circulation as required
- Charcoal does not work
- Chelation therapy with IV EDTA or oral DMSA (preferred) should be considered

---

### Further management (see also p. 436)
- An ingested source should be looked for, as should any environmental contaminants

## ☼ Iron

Iron poisoning usually occurs as a result of deliberate or accidental ingestion of large quantities of iron tablets. Iron initially acts as a GI irritant and may cause nausea and vomiting, abdominal pain, and GI bleeding. Decreased consciousness and convulsions may occur if overdose is severe, accompanied by hypotension, pulmonary oedema, and metabolic acidosis.

Further complications may occur up to 48 hours after ingestion and can include liver failure and/or renal failure, with accompanying metabolic acidosis, hypoglycaemia, and cardiovascular collapse.

### Investigations (see p. 429)
- Serum iron levels should be taken 4 hours post ingestion (or just prior to desferrioxamine if given at <4 hours). Later iron levels may be artificially low
- ABGs to monitor for acidosis
- FBC, coagulation screen
- U&Es, LFTs
- Serum glucose
- AXR may be useful to identify tablets

### Immediate management (see also p. 434)
- Give O₂; support airway, breathing, and circulation as required
- Charcoal does not work but gastric lavage is likely to be of benefit (if within 1 hour of ingestion or if AXR reveals intra-gastric tablets)
- Cardiovascular support with fluids/inotropes may be required
- Desferrioxamine (15 mg/kg/hour IV, up to 80 mg/kg/day)may be indicated
  - For patients with severe symptoms (do not delay whilst waiting for iron levels)
  - If serum iron >90 µmol/L (5 mg/L)
  - Desferrioxamine causes hypotension
- Whole bowel irrigation may be indicated for large overdoses

### Further management (see also p. 436)
- Bowel ischaemia may occur, requiring surgical treatment
- Pyloric stenosis causing gastric outlet obstruction is a late complication

## ☀ Lithium

Lithium poisoning may be an acute event, but is more often a complication of chronic therapy where levels are raised by the addition of diuretics, or by renal dysfunction. Lithium poisoning may cause agitation, decreased consciousness, convulsions, hyper-reflexia, myclonus, ataxia, hypotension, arrhythmias and heart block, and renal failure.

*Investigations* (see p. 429)

- Serum lithium concentrations should be measured at 6 hours
  - 0.4–1.2 mmol/L is the therapeutic range
  - >2.5 mmol/L is associated with toxicity
- U&Es, to monitor for renal failure and hypernatraemia
- Serum $Ca^{2+}$, to monitor for hypercalcaemia
- 12-lead ECG, may reveal conduction abnormalities or ST/T wave changes

**Immediate management** (see also p. 434)

- Give $O_2$; support airway, breathing, and circulation as required
- Charcoal does not work, but gastric lavage may be of benefit (if appropriate)
- ECG monitoring is recommended
- Volume replacement with isotonic saline fluids may be required
- Haemodialysis should be considered where any of the following are present
  - Levels >7.5 mmol/L for acute overdoses in patients who are lithium naive
  - Levels >2.5 mmol/L in patients on chronic treatment
  - In acute-on-chronic OD
  - Where symptoms are severe
- Haemofiltration may be used, but is less effective and will take longer to reduce levels

**Further management** (see also p. 436)

### :Q: Local anaesthetic toxicity

Local anaesthetic toxicity within critical care can occur if IV injection/infusion occurs (e.g. a local anaesthetic epidural infusion bag is mistaken for IV fluids), or if the soft tissue dose given exceeds the maximum recommended dose.

---

*Maximum recommended local anaesthetic doses*
- Bupivacaine/levobupivacaine    2 mg/kg
- Ropivacaine    3 mg/kg
- Lidocaine    3 mg/kg
- Lidocaine with adrenaline    6 mg/kg
- Prilocaine    6 mg/kg

---

Signs and symptoms include:
- Orofacial tingling/numbness,
- Tinnitus
- Blurred vision
- Muscle twitching
- Decreased consciousness
- Seizures
- Respiratory arrest
- Circulatory collapse with resistant arrhythmias

**Immediate management** (see also p. 434)
- Stop giving the drug
- Give $O_2$; support airway, breathing, and circulation as required
- Endotracheal intubation and mechanical ventilation may be required
- Treat seizures as appropriate
- Consider treating cardiovascular collapse/arrest with
  - Intralipid 20% IV 1 ml/kg over 1 minute, repeated every 3–5 minutes to a maximum of 3 ml/kg

**Further management** (see also p. 436)

**Further reading**

Picard J, Meek T (2006). Lipid emulsion to treat overdose of local anaesthetic: the gift of the glob *Anaesthesia* **61**, 107–9.

# Miscellaneous conditions

# ☼ Toxic epidermal necrolysis

Toxic epidermal necrolysis (TEN), also known as Lyell's syndrome, is a rare skin disorder characterized by extensive epidermal necrosis. Re-epithelization occurs in 14–21 days, leaving minimal scarring, but severe systemic disturbance can occur during that time.

## Causes

● Drugs are by far the most common cause, especially
  • Anticonvulsants
  • Antibiotics
  • Antiretrovirals
  • NSAIDS

The culprit drug has usually been introduced 2–6 weeks prior to onset of the prodrome.

## Presentation and assessment

● General: there is a prodromal phase of fever and malaise
● Skin: acute coalescing macular exanthema, progressing rapidly to full-thickness epidermal necrosis
  • Prominent skin pain and tenderness
  • Bullae may occur
  • Epidermis sloughs off in large sheets
  • Lateral pressure on erythematous skin may induce epidermal separation (Nikolsky sign: this is not recommended in clinical practice)
  • Mucosal involvement of the eyes, mouth, and perineum may occur
● Respiratory: bronchial tree desquamation can cause hypoxia, pneumonia, and ARDS

## Investigations

● Skin biopsy showing full-thickness epidermal necrosis, sub-epidermal separation, and sparse or absent dermal infiltrate is diagnostic
  • Immunoflurescence is negative
  • A rapid diagnosis may be established by frozen section histology of the blister roof
● ABGs if hypoxic
● FBC
● U&Es, blood glucose, LFTs
● Serum magnesium, phosphate, calcium, and zinc may all be appropriate as large fluid shifts occur
● CXR if there is lung involvement
● Blood culture, sputum culture, and wound swabs (may need to be repeated as surveillance for infection is important)

## Differential diagnoses

● Staphylococcal scalded skin syndrome
● Erythema multiforme major
● DRESS (drug rash with eosinophilia and systemic symptoms) syndrome
● Immunobullous diseases (e.g. paraneoplastic pemphigus)

## Immediate management

- Give $O_2$ as required; support airway, breathing, and circulation
- Withdraw all suspected and non-essential medications
- Arrange dermatological review as soon as the condition is suspected
- Consider endotracheal intubation early if there is hypoxia or respiratory involvement (NIV masks are likely to damage facial skin)
- Provide adequate analgesia; pain is likely to be severe
- Ideally patients with TEN should be nursed in an ITU with burns experience as the care is very similar

## Further management

- Careful protection of dermal surfaces and eroded mucosal surfaces is essential using emollients, burns dressings, and pressure area care
- Core temperature readings are essential, and the patient should be nursed in a warm environment
- The role of immunosuppressants in disease management is unclear
  - IV immunoglobulin (0.4–1 mg/kg/day for 4 days) has been used
  - Ciclosporin may be considered
  - Corticosteroids may worsen prognosis
- Sepsis, especially line-related sepsis, is a major cause of mortality; only essential monitoring lines should be introduced
- Careful fluid and electrolyte balance are required
- Provide DVT/PE and stress ulcer prophylaxis
- Provide nutritional support with enteral feeding where possible; if absorption is limited due to protein losing enteropathy consider TPN
- Regular ophthalmological review will be required as eye involvement is common and results in scarring
  - Use of lubricants and topical antibiotics are usual
  - Complications may develop up to 2–3 weeks later; follow-up is essential

## Pitfalls/difficult situations

- The diagnosis is often not considered until the patient is severely ill, TEN lies on a spectrum with Stevens–Johnson syndrome (SJS)
- These patients require full monitoring; this is often difficult as the skin is sore and eroded, and any entry site is a potential source of infection
- Pyrexia is a feature of TEN and does not always represent infection
- Dermatological review may help make the diagnosis in the early stages
- SJS or TEN is more likely to triggered by anti-tuberculous medication if HIV infection is also present; where anti-tuberculous medication is suspected trigger for SJS/TEN, testing for HIV should be considered
- Despite the severe appearance of the condition, scarring is unusual and recovery can be complete; ophthalmic scarring is the main cause of long-term morbidity

## Further reading

Chave TA, Mortimer NJ, Sladden MJ, Hall AP, Hutchinson PE. (2005). Toxic epidermal necrolysis: current evidence, practical management and future directions. *Br J Dermatol*; 153:241-253

Majumdar S, Mockenhaupt M, Roujeau J-C, *et al.* (2002). Interventions for toxic epidermal necrolysis. *Cochrane Database of Systematic Reviews*, Issue 4, CD001435.

# ☼ Tumour lysis syndrome

Tumour lysis syndrome occurs when rapid tumour cell destruction leads to the release of cellular substances, typically 1–5 days after cancer treatment.

## Causes

- Chemotherapy
- Radiotherapy
- Radiofrequency ablation
- May occur spontaneously with Burkitt's lymphoma and some leukaemias

## Presentation and assessment

The biochemical changes associated with tumour lysis syndrome include:
- Hyperphosphataemia
- Hypocalcaemia
- Hyperkalaemia
- Hyperuricaemia

Signs and symptoms may include:
- General: lethargy, malaise
- Cardiovascular: arrhythmias of hyperkalaemia (see p. 220)
  - ECG changes: tall tented T waves, slurring of ST segments into T waves, small P waves, prolonged PR interval, widened QRS, complete heart block, asystole or VF
- Neuromuscular: muscle cramps, tetany
- Neurological: seizures
- Renal: oliguria, ARF

## Investigations

- ABGs
- FBC
- U&Es, LFTs
- Serum calcium, phosphate, magnesium
- Serum urate
- ECG

## Differential diagnoses

- Sampling error
- Trauma, burns
- Tissue ischaemia (ischaemic bowel)
- Haemolysis
- Pancreatitis
- Rhabdomyolysis

## Immediate management

- Give $O_2$ as required; support airway, breathing, and circulation
- Commence ECG monitoring
- Aggressive fluid resuscitation is required
- Treat hyperkalaemia and hyperphosphataemia (pp. 220 and 228)
    - If ECG changes are present give calcium chloride 3–5 ml 10% solution IV over 3 minutes: cardioprotective effect only; will not lower potassium
- Give sodium bicarbonate to alkalinize urine (and aid serum uric acid excretion); aim for urine pH 7–7.5
- Haemodialysis may be required for severe hyperkalaemia, hyperphophataemia, or ARF
- Consider giving allopurinol 300 mg daily at the start of symptoms

## Further management

- Renal and oncological advice should be obtained early

# ☼ Cord compression

Cord compression (or cauda equina syndrome) is commonly associated with lung, breast and prostate cancer, and lymphoma.

**Presentation and assessment**

Symptoms include progressive weakness and then sensory loss. Areflexia and clonus may develop. Painless urinary retention, or bowel and bladder incontinence may be the only signs.

**Investigations**

• Urgent MRI is required

**Differential diagnoses**

• Epidural haematoma or abscess
• Paraneoplastic neuropathy

**Immediate management**

• Give $O_2$ as required; support airway, breathing, and circulation
• Give dexamethasone IV 8–16 mg
• Urgent decompression is required either surgically or via chemo/radiotherapy

**Pitfalls/difficult situations**

• Nerve damage left for >24 hours is unlikely to be salvageable

**Further reading**
📖 OHCC p. 410.

# :O: Ovarian hyperstimulation syndrome

Ovarian hyperstimulation syndrome (OHSS) is caused by iatrogenic ovarian overstimulation in connection with fertility treatments such as *in vitro* fertilization (IVF). OHSS can occur in up to one-third of treatment cycles, but is generally mild.

## Causes

- Gonadotrophins or clomiphene citrate

More common in:
- Younger women
- Small BMI
- Previous OHSS
- PMH of allergies

## Presentation and assessment

OHSS typically occurs 1–2 days after follicular rupture/aspiration. Only 5% of OHSS cases are moderate to severe, and may include the following features:

- General: pyrexia may be present
- Abdominal: abdominal distension, ascites, nausea and vomiting
  - Intra-abdominal haemorrhage may occur
- Cardiovascular: hypotension, tachycardia
- Respiratory: pulmonary oedema and ARDS may develop; hydrothorax may occur
- Renal: oliguria, metabolic acidosis, hyperkalaemia, and ARF may occur
- Other: DVT/PE may occur; WCC may be raised
  - Hyponatraemia may occur

Infection commonly occurs alongside OHSS.

## Investigations

- ABGs
- FBC, coagulation studies
- U&Es, LFTs
- Serum glucose
- Serum CRP
- Septic screen (blood, sputum, urine cultures)
- CXR
- US of abdomen
- Consider CTPA or VQ scan

## Differential diagnoses

- PE
- Intra-abdominal haemorrhage

## Immediate management

- Give $O_2$ as required; support airway, breathing, and circulation
- The rapid development of abdominal distension and ARDS may necessitate endotracheal intubation and mechanical ventilation
- Hydrothorax may require drainage
- Fluid resuscitation is required and inotropes may be necessary
  - Careful monitoring of fluid balance with urinary catheterization and CVC insertion is required
- IAP should be measured; ascites may require drainage
- Renal replacement therapy may become necessary
- Consider empirical antibiotic treatment with piptazobactam IV 4.5 g 8-hourly and gentamicin IV 5 mg/kg daily (discuss with microbiology specialists as soon as appropriate)
- Consider anticoagulation with unfractionated heparin to prevent thrombotic complications

## Further management

- NGT insertion and enteral feeding should be attempted; TPN may have to be considered
- Surgery should generally be avoided unless haemorrhage or ovarian/ ovarian-cyst torsion occur
- Hyponatraemia should be corrected

## Pitfalls/difficult situations

- The large fluid shifts associated with draining ascites may result in intravascular fluid depletion and hypotension

## Further reading

Budev MM, Arroliga AC, Falcone T (2005). Ovarian hyperstimulation syndrome *Crit Care Med* **33**(Suppl), S301–6.

# ! **The potential organ donor**

Patients can only be considered for organ donation if they are in an unresponsive coma with cerebral dysfunction of known irreversible origin (e.g. traumatic brain injury causing raised ICP), which is confirmed by brainstem death tests.

---

**Criteria for brainstem death**

*Exclusions*

- Is the core temperature <35°C?
- Could any narcotics, hypnotics, tranquillizers, or muscle relaxant drugs still be affecting the patient (e.g. been given within the past 12 hours or 24 hours if renal/hepatic failure present)?
- Is there a metabolic, circulatory, or endocrine cause for the coma?

If the answer to any of the above is **yes** then brainstem death cannot be said to exist (*do not perform tests*)

*Brainstem death tests*

- Do the pupils react to light, either directly or consensually?
- Are corneal reflexes present when a cotton bud is gently pressed to the cornea?
- Is there any eye movement following slow injection of 50 ml iced water over a period of 1 minute into both ears with the head flexed at 30°?*
- Is there any limb, facial, or neck movement in response to bilateral supra-orbital nerve pressure? Is there any limb, facial, or neck response to any other somatic area?
- Is a gag reflex present (contraction of the soft palate when the uvula is stimulated)?
- Is a cough reflex present on tracheal suctioning (with the suction catheter passed via the endotracheal tube as far as the carina)?
- Is there any eye movement during the 'doll's eye' manoeuvre?†
- Is there any respiratory effort during an apnoea test (patient given 100% $O_2$ for 10 minutes, $PaCO_2$ allowed to rise to ≥5 kPa; then the patient is disconnected from the ventilator and $PaCO_2$ allowed to rise to >6.65 kPa)?

If the answer to any of the above is **yes** then brainstem death is **not present**

* Tympanic membranes should be examined by otoscopy first.
† Not required but still used by some practitioners.

---

Two doctors (one a consultant with experience in critical care), registered with GMC for 5 years, are required to perform brainstem death tests. Neither may be connected with transplant team. They can perform the tests independently or together. Two sets of tests are required with a gap between (there is no set time period). Death is confirmed after the second set of tests, *but* time of death is after the first test.

The timing of any discussion with the donor's relatives depends upon the individual circumstances. One suggested approach is to perform the first set of brainstem death tests and discuss the patient with the local transplant coordinator before approaching the relatives to obtain assent (an approach is only made if it is likely that organ donation will be possible). Relatives may wish to witness the second set of tests.

Many contraindications to organ donation are relative; a full discussion with the transplant coordinator is essential. Apart from lack of consent other potential contraindications include blood-borne sepsis, extra CNS malignancy, hepatitis B or C, HIV, CJD, and direct myocardial toxicity. In potential thoracic donors, donor age, smoking status, inotrope requirements, organ damage, and $PaO_2$ <19 kPa on $FiO_2$ of 30% (or $PaO_2$ <33 kPa on $FiO_2$ of 50%) may affect the decision. Renal and liver retrieval decisions may be affected by the presence of IDDM, renal/reno-vascular disease, liver disease, fatty liver, or a history of alcohol abuse.

Complications of brainstem death include: hypotension, diabetes insipidus, DIC, arrhythmias, pulmonary oedema, and metabolic acidosis

## Management

- Be guided by the transplant coordinator and the organ retrieval team
- Continue ICU management, including:
  - Physiotherapy, aseptic precautions, antibiotic treatment, nutrition
  - Lung-protective ventilation strategies
- Prevent hypothermia
- Manage cardiovascular status
  - Monitor CVP and aim for CVP or PAOP 10–12 mmHg, cardiac index 2.2–2.5 L/min/m², MAP ≥70 mmHg
  - Treat hypovolaemia, but avoid excessive volume replacement, especially where lung donation is considered
  - Correct anaemia and coagulopathy
- Monitor biochemistry and consider endocrine replacement therapies
  - Aggressively correct hypernatraemia and hypokalaemia
  - Give insulin to keep blood glucose within 4–6 mmol/L
  - Consider vasopressin 1 unit, then 0.5–2 units/hour IV to treat DI[*]
  - Consider steroids: methylprednisolone 15 mg/kg bolus[*]
  - Consider $T_3$ bolus of 4 µg IV, then 3 µg/hour[*]
- Discuss IV lines with the retrieval team/anaesthetist: femoral lines and left upper body lines may need to be changed prior to surgery
- Cross-match blood (4 units) and take other blood samples as advised

\* Not all centres use these protocols; be guided by the transplant coordinator/retrieval team

## Further reading

Edgar P, Bullock R, Bonner S (2004). Management of the potential heart-beating donor *Cont Educ Anaesth Crit Care Pain* **4**, 86–90.

Intensive Care Society (1999). Donation of organs for transplantation the management of the potential donor: a manual for the establishment of local guidelines. Available online at www.ics.ac.uk

📖 OHCC p548, 552.

# ⑦ **Referral to the coroner**

It is not uncommon to be required to discuss the deaths of critically ill patients with a member of the coroner's office. The coroner, or Procurator-fiscal in Scotland, is independent of government. Where a death is unexpected or unexplained, or where it fulfills any of the criteria listed below, it should be discussed with the coroner.

In many cases the coroner will simply ask for confirmation that the death was due to natural causes and that there is a doctor able to issue a death certificate, for example where potentially life-saving surgery has been attempted in an otherwise dying individual.

In other circumstances the coroner may require a post-mortem examination in order to ascertain the cause of death. Should the death not be due to natural causes, the coroner may hold an inquest in order to determine the identity of the deceased, when, where, and how the death occurred, and the cause of death.

---

### Deaths requiring referral to the coroner

- Any death where the cause is unknown or unclear
- Where surgery, anaesthesia, or other medical treatment may have contributed to death, or where an operation was performed after an injury
- Death associated with poisoning, either deliberate or accidental
- Death associated with acute or chronic alcoholism
- Death associated with therapeutic or recreational drug usage
- Any death which may be related to industrial disease
- Death which may be related to an accident
- Death connected to a crime or suspected crime (including deaths where violence or deliberate neglect on the part of another person might be responsible)
- Any death in custody
- Any death where the deceased was receiving a disability pension
- Any death where the deceased was not seen professionally by a doctor during his/her last illness, within 14 days of death, or after death
- Death of a foster child
- Stillbirths where there was a possibility of the child being born alive

---

### Pitfalls/difficult situations

- Organ donation may still be possible in brain-dead individuals who require referral to the coroner; it is worth seeking permission from the coroner first before approaching the family
- There are no time limits as to when a death may be attributable to a violent or medical cause

- There are slightly different rules regarding what should be reported to the Procurator-fiscal in Scotland. They are very similar to those listed above, but are more specific in certain areas:
  - Possible or suspected suicide
  - Accidents: any death arising from the use of a vehicle including an aircraft, a ship, or a train; any death by drowning; any death by burning or scalding or as a result of a fire or explosion
  - Certain deaths of children: any death of a newborn child whose body is found; any death from apparent sudden infant death syndrome (cot death); any death of a child from suffocation including overlaying; any death of a foster child
  - Occupational: any death at work, whether or not as a result of an accident; any death related to occupation, e.g. industrial disease or poisoning
  - Any death following an abortion or attempted abortion
  - Any death as a result of a medical mishap, and any death where a complaint is received which suggests that medical treatment or the absence of treatment may have contributed to the death
  - Any death due to notifiable infectious disease or food poisoning
  - Any death of a person of residence unknown, who died other than in a house

## Further reading

Fertleman M (1997) Education Michael Fertleman A doctor's life after a patient's death: guide to coroners and certificates. *Student BMJ* **5**, 12–13.

Crown Office (1998). *Death and the Procurator-fiscal.* Available online at: http://www.show.scot.nhs.uk/publications/me/death%20and%20pf.htm

# ⑦ Transfers and retrievals

**Types of transfer/retrieval**

- Intra-hospital transfer (e.g. to ICU or to CT scan)
- Inter-hospital transfer (e.g. because the patient requires a specialist investigation or intervention, there is a lack of critical care beds in the referring hospital, or to repatriate the patient)
- Primary retrieval (e.g. from the roadside)[*]
- Secondary retrieval (an inter-hospital transfer using a specialist team from another healthcare facility to retrieve the patient)

**Decision to transfer**

- Is the transfer necessary?
- Does the patient require further stabilization prior to transfer?
  - Will further stabilization delay urgently required treatments (e.g. surgical decompression of intracranial haematomas)?[*]
- Is everything that might be needed to treat any reasonably predictable complication available to accompany the patient?
- Are the correct staff, monitoring equipment, and transfer apparatus available?

**Stabilization and preparation prior to transfer**

- Most procedures are difficult to undertake *en route*; if there is a probability of deterioration then anticipate and prepare for it
- Reasses the patient's history, treatment and examination findings
- Use a checklist wherever possible

**Airway**

- Consider endotracheal intubation if airway may deteriorate (especially in facial burns or trauma, or where GCS may drop to <8)
- Confirm the ETT position and ensure it is secured firmly in place
- Consider whether C-spine precautions are required for transfer
- Some centres replace ETT cuff air with saline prior to air transport

**Breathing**

- If oxygenation/ventilation is poor consider elective intubation and mechanical ventilation prior to transfer
  - NIV is difficult to deliver during transport; IPPV is likely to be more appropriate
- Establish the patient on the transport ventilator *prior to transfer* and check ABGs
  - Transport ventilators often only produce basic levels of respiratory support
- Check for any chest problem; review CXR for evidence of pneumothoraces (difficult to treat in transit, and may expand during air transfer)
  - Consider prophylactic chest drains in cases of chest trauma
  - Consider replacing fluid-locked chest drains with Heimlich valves

---

[*] With the exception of primary retrievals, and transfers for urgently required treatments, there will be sufficient time to fully stabilize the patient. A 'scoop and run' policy should only be adopted where there are insufficient resources available to resuscitate A, B, and C.

### Circulation
- Avoid transferring hypotensive patients where possible
- Ensure a minimum of two secure working large-bore (16G cannulae)
- Control haemorrhage and fluid resuscitate
- Establish on inotropes/vasopressors prior to transfer if required
  - Avoid using high-concentration inotrope solutions where possible (>16 mg adrenaline/noradrenaline in 50 ml) as low-volume siphoning from syringe drivers may occur with repeated transfers
- An invasive arterial line is preferable for BP monitoring
  - NIBP monitoring is possible during road and air transport, but is less reliable and uses more battery power
- Consider CVP for volume monitoring or if multiple drug infusions
- If a PAFC is *in situ* and the waveform cannot be monitored in transit, consider withdrawing it to the RA to avoid inadvertent 'wedging'
- Where dysrhythmias are a problem consider placing adhesive defibrillator pads on the patient prior to 'wrapping'
- Check last measured Hb and $K^+$ results
- Stabilize long-bone/pelvic fractures

### Neurological
- Re-check GCS and neurological status
- Commence any required/recommended treatment for raised ICP
- Establish mechanically ventilated patients on sedative infusions

### Other
- Check available equipment for transfer
  - Assemble and check critical pieces, e.g. self-inflating bags
- 'Mummy-wrap' the patient with blankets (strap in all lines/tubes)
- Ensure pressure-point care and eye protection
- Remove/stop any unnecessary equipment or infusions
- If using air travel consider inserting an NGT and splitting plaster casts
- Consider the mode of transfer (ground versus air)
  - For patients with high oxygen requirements, recent altitude sickness, recent diving injury, pneumothorax, pneumoperitoneum, or pneumocranium: do they really need to fly? Can the aircraft be pressurized to ground level equivalent?
- Discuss morbidly obese patients with ambulance control: specialist bariatric equipment may be required

### Communication and documentation
- All notes, X-rays, CT scans, and blood results should be taken
- A patient summary sheet should be prepared where possible
- Ensure that all parties involved are aware of the transfer: the receiving hospital/unit, the patient/relatives, ambulance control, the accompanying staff
  - Confirm the destination and obtain directions if appropriate
  - Consider a police escort for 'life or death' transfers

**Avoid using your transfer oxygen/batteries until the last minute**

## Transfer practices

- 'Intensive care' monitoring and management should be continued throughout the transfer process
- Two staff should accompany the patient, one of whom should be trained in advanced airway techniques for any patient who is, or may require to be, intubated; both staff should be familiar with transfer equipment
- Wear appropriate clothing
- Phone the receiving unit immediately prior to transfer
- Before leaving, review the patient's condition for a final time and check all the drugs and equipment needed are going with the patient
- Take an emergency phone and the telephone numbers of the transferring and receiving units

### Monitoring

Minimum standard monitoring should include

- Continuous presence of appropriately trained staff
- ECG
- Non-invasive blood pressure
- Arterial oxygen saturation ($SaO_2$)
- End-tidal carbon dioxide ($ETCO_2$) in ventilated patients
- Temperature (preferably core and peripheral)
- Ventilator pressure, disconnect and $FiO_2$ failure alarms

### Management

- Allocate any task-specific roles early (i.e. who is responsible for monitoring specialist equipment such as ICP monitoring)
- Airway
  - Disconnect the ventilator tubing from the ETT every time the patient is transferred from one bed to another (to avoid accidental extubation)
  - The person in charge of the head and airway controls the occurrence of any patient transfers
- Breathing
  - Paralyse and sedate mechanically ventilated patients
  - Do not clamp chest drains
  - Where pneumothoraces occur in mechanically ventilated patients during air/road transfers consider performing a mid-axillary line blunt-dissection thoracocentesis without inserting a chest drain (air should be released, the lung should be palpable confirming re-expansion; a sterile chest drain may be inserted upon arrival)
  - Switch to ambulance/aircraft $O_2$ supply as soon as appropriate
- Circulation
  - Where possible keep infusor pumps at the same level as the patient (some pumps siphon)
  - Vibration in aircraft (particularly rotary wing) may interfere with gravity IV infusions; consider using pressure infusors
  - Defibrillation in aircraft: most modern aircraft are defibrillation-safe; check first!

- Movement
  - Do a visual sweep prior to moving the patient from any location to ensure lines, NGTs, urinary catheters are not going to catch
  - Always ensure that the team are prepared and know exactly how (i.e. log-roll, slowly, etc) and *which way* the patient is going to be moved
  - The 'count' should be 'ready, steady, slide/roll'
  - Secure the patient to any transfer trolley (cot-sides up, safety belts attached) prior to moving trolley; ensure trolley is secured to ambulance/aircraft prior to movement
- The transport vehicle
  - **Never approach/enter an aircraft without permission from the pilot or load-master; follow their instructions at all times**
  - **NEVER approach the rear of a rotary wing aircraft with a tail rotor**
  - Once inside a vehicle secure all equipment
  - Staff should be securely seated during travel
  - Where possible the head and one side of the patient should be accessible.
  - Consider providing ear-defenders, or other protection, to the patient during air transfers
  - Consider providing anti-emetics to the patient (and staff)
  - 'Hot' unloads are rarely necessary; full engine shutdown should normally be allowed to happen before departure from rotary wing aircraft. Where a 'hot' unload is required make sure everyone knows their roles and responsibilities prior to landing (and that ground crew are aware)
- Environment
  - Keep the ambulance/aircraft warm
  - Keep all monitoring within view
  - Retain easy access to IV access
- Documentation: remember to take all relevant patient documents; document the patient's condition during the transfer
  - Perform a detailed handover of the patient to the receiving team

---

**Transfer equipment**

- Ensure you are familiar with available equipment
- When retrieving patients assume that no equipment will be available; take your own
- Use dedicated trolleys for inter-hospital transfers where available
- Airway: Guedel and nasopharyngeal airways (assorted sizes); laryngeal masks (assorted sizes); endotracheal tubes (assorted sizes); laryngoscopes (spare bulbs and battery); intubating stylet; lubricating gel; Magill's forceps; tape for securing tracheal tube; sterile scissors; stethoscope; Yankauer sucker; suction catheters (assorted sizes); nasogastric tubes (assorted sizes); drainage bag

- Ventilation: self-inflating bag and mask with oxygen reservoir and tubing; high-flow breathing circuit; spare valves for portable ventilator; chest drains (assorted sizes); Heimlich flutter valves
- Ventilators: check prior to use; calculate oxygen requirements for trip—an E-sized cylinder will last ~30–60 minutes (discuss with ambulance crew the oxygen they have available); ensure that 2–3 hours of 'back-up' oxygen is available
- Circulation: syringes (assorted sizes); needles (assorted sizes); alcohol wipes; IV cannulae (assorted sizes); arterial cannulae (assorted sizes); central venous cannulae; IV fluids; infusion sets/extensions; three-way taps; dressings/tape; pressure infusors
- Drugs: emergency drugs for cardiac arrest and intubation/reintubation should be available; spare infusions should be prepared for any inotropes, sedatives, or muscle relaxants; predictable emergency drugs should also be available (e.g. anti-seizure medication); spare IV fluid should be available
- Infusion pumps should be checked and spares taken where transfer will be long, or an infusion is critical, in case of battery failure; a defibrillator may be required (ambulance crews may be able to provide this)
- Specialist: consider the need for blood, minor instrument/cutdown set, tracheostomy set
- Clothing: specialist protective clothing should be available for inter-hospital transfers or retrievals; individual's roles should be clearly identifiable
- Where transfer may be weight limited (e.g. in rotary wing aircraft) discuss any requirements with the crew

## Pitfalls/difficult situations

- Most problems during transfer result from inadequate stabilization prior to departure or failure to continue optimal treatment and monitoring during transfer

## Further reading

Intensive Care Society (2002). *Guidelines for the Transport of the Critically Ill Adult*. Intensive Care Society, London.
📖 OHEA p. 418.

# Common emergency procedures

# ⓘ **Rapid-sequence intubation**

Rapid-sequence endotracheal intubation (RSI) is the preferred method for endotracheal intubation where the patient is at risk of aspiration (e.g. full stomach, delayed gastric emptying). Even if you are not competent to perform the procedure you may be called upon to prepare the equipment or assist.

## Indications for intubation

*To protect the airway*
- From risk of aspiration: blood/vomit
- From risk of obstruction
- Because sedation/anaesthesia is required to allow assessment or treatment, particularly in agitated or combative patients

*To permit mechanical ventilation*
- Apnoea or bradypnoea
- Hypoxaemia or inadequate respiratory effort
- Hypercarbia or requirement for hyperventilation
- Cardiovascular instability: to optimize oxygen supply/demand

## Contraindications
- When attempted as an absolute emergency (i.e. impending or actual cardiac arrest), there are no contraindications to attempting endotracheal intubation
- In all other situations (i.e. urgent or semi-elective endotracheal intubation) the operator must be experienced in the technique, and the likelihood of the patient being difficult to intubate must be assessed (p. 22) and appropriate preparations made
- Suxamethonium should not be used in patients with a known allergy to suxamethonium, a history of MH, hyperkalaemia, recent burns (>2 days <1 year), or paralysis

## Equipment
- An assistant (preferably more) is required to monitor the patient, administer drugs, pass equipment to the operator, and apply cricoid pressure
- A facemask and a means of ventilating (i.e. self-inflating bag)
- Cuffed endotracheal tube (as a rough guide, size 8 for females and size 9 for males)
  - Spare ETTs should be available in the sizes above and below the preferred values
  - Some centres pre-cut ETTs to a length of 27–28cm—do not cut ETTs in patients where orofacial swelling is likely (e.g. burns)
- Lubricant gel (to facilitate passage of ETT through vocal cords)
- 10 ml syringe (for inflating ETT cuff)
- Laryngoscope (plus spare) with Mackintosh blades size 3 and 4
- Bougie

- Tape or tie (to secure ETT post-intubation)
- Stethoscope
- Yankauer sucker and suction apparatus
- End-tidal $CO_2$ monitoring
- Equipment for failed intubation (e.g. LMA)
- Intubation drugs
- Resuscitation drugs (atropine and adrenaline)
- Consider having an NGT available

## Anatomical landmarks

- The cricoid cartilage can be identified immediately inferior to the thyroid cartilage; it feels like a wedding ring below the surface of the skin

## Technique

- Check equipment (suction, laryngoscope bulb, ETT cuff)
- Establish IV access
- Aspirate NGT if one is in place
- Ensure the patient is positioned with their head on a pillow (often removed during CPR) so that the head is raised just above the shoulders
- Attach all monitoring

**Head positioning is not possible where trauma is suspected. In such cases an assistant is required to apply manual inline stabilization to the head. The anterior aspect of the hard collar can then be undone or removed prior to attempting tracheal intubation. Where possible, a bougie should be used for trauma intubations in order to minimize the degree of neck movement required**

- Pre-oxygenate with 100% $O_2$ for 3–5 minutes if possible using a facemask and ventilating circuit (gently assist patient's respiration if required, e.g. previously on NIV); remove false teeth
- Have suction on and within reach
- Administer induction agents over 20–30 seconds: any of
  - Thiopental IV 2–4 mg/kg
  - Propofol IV 1–5 mg/kg
  - Etomidate IV 0.1–0.4 mg/kg
  - Ketamine IV 1–3 mg/kg
  - Thiopental and propofol commonly cause hypotension requiring fluid and/or inotropic support. In cardiovascularly unstable patients consider using ketamine (may cause hypertension, tachycardia, or raised ICP) or etomidate (cardiovascularly stable, but causes adrenal suppression; consider giving hydrocortisone 50 mg 8-hourly for 24 hours)
- Apply cricoid pressure (do not release until ETT is in position, $ETCO_2$ is present and the cuff is inflated[*])

- Immediately administer suxamethonium IV 1–2 mg/kg (where suxamethonium is contraindicated use rocuronium IV 0.6–1 mg/kg)
  - Suxamethonium should cause fasciculation within 15–30 seconds (not always observed)
- After 30 seconds (or when fasciculations cease, or 60 seconds if using rocuronium), holding the laryngoscope in your left hand (close to the angle between the handle and blade), insert the blade into the right-hand side of the patient's mouth.
  - Bring the laryngoscope back to the midline, pushing the tongue aside beneath it; advance forwards until the tip of the laryngoscope is in the valecula space, and then lift vertically until the vocal cords are seen
- Pass a size 8–9 ETT through the cords
- Inflate the ETT cuff and attempt ventilation
- Confirm correct position of the ETT within the trachea by:
  - Presence of ETCO$_2$†
  - Obvious chest movement
  - Presence of misting/clearing of the ETT/catheter mount
  - Bilateral chest sounds on auscultation (listen to the chest in the mid-axillary line)
  - Absence of 'bubbling' sounds over the stomach on auscultation
- Secure the ETT in position using tape or tie; make a note of the ETT length at the teeth/gums
- If intubation is successful and the patient stable, consider inserting an NGT or OGT
- Commence a sedative infusion
- Consider a bolus dose of non-depolarizing muscle relaxant to allow for easier setting-up of the ventilator (unless rocuronium already used)
- Confirm the distal position of the ETT on CXR (above the carina)
- Check ABGs

* Cricoid pressure may have to be released in the event of a failed intubation, see p. 23.
† $CO_2$ will not be present if there is no cardiac output, i.e. cardiac arrest.

## Special considerations/complications

- Oesophageal intubation may be difficult to spot. Consider if:
  - Poor chest expansion
  - 'Distant' breath sounds
  - Abdominal distension
  - Progressive cyanosis

**If in doubt remove ETT and re-intubate.**

- If unable to intubate adjust the head and neck position and have one more attempt. If still unable to intubate follow the failed intubation protocol (p. 23)

**Maintain oxygenation at all costs**

- Endobronchial intubation: commonly right-sided causing unilateral chest expansion and breath sounds. withdraw the ETT to 21–23 cm listening for bilateral chest sounds; check position with a CXR

# ① LMA insertion

## Indications

- Within critical care the indications for insertion of an LMA are:
  - To obtain an airway in an emergency: as a bridge to endotracheal intubation (e.g. poor facemask seal during resuscitation)
  - To obtain an airway as a last resort (e.g. failed intubation)

## Contraindications

- In an emergency situation there are no contraindications, but LMAs do not provide a definitive airway and the intention should always be to proceed to endotracheal intubation or tracheostomy as soon as appropriate

## Equipment

- LMAs (sizes 3, 4, and 5)
  - Size 3 for a small female, size 5 for a large male
- Lubricant
- Tape or ties
- 20 or 50 ml syringe
- Yankauer sucker and suction apparatus
- Stethoscope

## Technique

- Check equipment (no blockage within the tubing; LMA cuff is intact when inflated)
- Deflate cuff and apply lubricant to the smooth surface of the cuff/mask
- Position the patient's head on a pillow if possible
- If available ask an assistant to pull the lower jaw downwards
- Insert the cuff/mask end of the LMA into the mouth so that its smooth surface is against the patient's palate
- Using your first two fingers, against the point where the 'mask' and tube connect, the LMA should be advanced until it has moved behind the tongue and in front of the tracheal opening
- Gently inflate the mask with air (size 3, 20 ml; size 4, 30 ml; size 5, 40 ml); the protruding tube end of the LMA usually rises 1–2 cm
- Attach means of ventilation (e.g. a self-inflating bag) and attempt gentle ventilation
  - Check that air entry is present by the presence of $ETCO_2$, obvious chest movement, presence of misting/clearing of the ETT/catheter mount, chest sounds present on auscultation
  - A small air leak is acceptable
- Consider inserting an oropharyngeal airway as a 'bite block'

## Special considerations/complications

- The LMA may curl back on itself during placement, causing it to be malpositioned (attempt to ensure that the smooth surface of the LMA does not curl back as it moves from the soft palate to the posterior pharyngeal wall)
- LMAs provide only minimal protection against aspiration
- The seal produced by an LMA may not be good enough to provide adequate levels of PEEP
- Sore throat is common

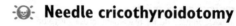

# Needle cricothyroidotomy

### Indications

- To obtain an airway and oxygenate the patient in the event of an obstructed upper airway
- The last resort following a failed intubation where oxygenation is impossible by other means

### Contraindications

- When done as an emergency procedure there are no contraindications

### Equipment

- 14G IV cannula
- 5 ml syringe with 2–3 ml sterile water, attached to the cannula
- Oxygen 'bubble' tubing
  - A hole should be cut in the side of the tubing, or a three-way tap attached

Various prefabricated kits are available which are mostly cannula-over-needle in design

### Anatomical landmarks

- The cricothyroid membrane: immediately below the thyroid cartilage in the midline, above the cricoid ring

### Technique

- Identify the cricothyroid membrane (if the cricothyroid membrane cannot be identified aim for the midline below the thyroid cartilage)
- Stabilize the neck tissues
- Advance the cannula caudally (at an angle of ~45°) into the trachea (aspirate for air as the needle advances)
  - Once air is aspirated fix the stylet and advance the cannula off it; there should be no resistance.
- Attach the oxygen tubing and set the $O_2$ flow rate to 15 L/min
  - 'Jet ventilate' by occluding the hole in the oxygen tube: 1 second on, 4 seconds off
- Proceed to a definitive airway as soon as possible (arrange for anaesthetic assistance with/without ENT cover

## Complications

- Needle cricothyroidotomies are a temporary means of maintaining oxygenation. The intention should be to proceed to endotracheal intubation or tracheostomy as soon as possible
- An escape route for insufflated air is required; if the upper airway is completely obstructed barotrauma will occur
  - Turn down the oxygen flow rate
  - Further needle cricothyroidotomies may be inserted to allow gas to escape
  - Even without airway obstruction the high pressures involved may cause barotrauma
- The cannula is easily kinked or misplaced; paratracheal gas insufflation may result
- $CO_2$ will accumulate

### Surgical cricothyroidotomy

Should a needle cricothyroidotomy prove inadequate and there is no other means of securing an alternative airway, a larger surgical crico-thyroidotomy may be attempted using the same landmarks as before
- Make a 2 cm transverse incision through the skin and cricothyroid membrane
- Dilate the tract with artery forceps (or the handle of the scalpel)
- Insert an endotracheal or tracheostomy tube (the smallest size immediately available, typically size 6.5)
- Inflate the cuff and ventilate as normal (confirming position within the trachea as per normal endotracheal intubation)

This technique is technically more demanding, but does provide a definitive airway through which full ventilatory support can be provided

# :☻: Needle thoracocentesis

**Indications**
- Suspected tension pneumothorax

**Contraindications**
- Where the anterior chest wall cannot be accessed consider performing a needle thoracocentesis in the mid-anterior axillary line (at the fifth intercostal space)

**Equipment**
- 14–16G IV cannula

**Anatomical landmarks**
- Anterior chest wall, mid-clavicular line, second intercostal space (at the level of the angle of Louis)

**Technique**
- Insert the cannula just above top edge of third rib (to avoid the neurovascular bundle along the lower edge of the second rib) and remove the stylet/needle
  - In spontaneously breathing patients a hiss of air occurs if a tension pneumothorax is present
  - In mechanically ventilated patients non-tensioning pneumothoraces can also cause a hiss
- If a tension pneumothorax is present its decompression should improve cardiovascular and/or respiratory compromise. If it does not, consider whether a contralateral tension pneumothorax is present
- After performing a needle thoracocentesis an intercostal chest drain should be inserted as soon as practicable

**Complications**
- A needle thoracocentesis performed where no pneumothorax was present will cause a pneumothorax to occur; proceed to intercostal chest drain insertion in all cases
- The cannula may kink allowing the tension pneumothorax to re-accumulate (further decompression may be required)
- Tension pneumothoraces requiring needle decompression can still occur with chest drains in place (e.g. if they are kinked)
- Bleeding/haemothorax
- Lung laceration/broncho-pleural fistula

# ① Intercostal chest drain insertion

## Indications

- Drainage of pneumothorax, haemothorax, pleural effusion or empyema

## Contraindications

- Presence of pleural adhesion (lung stuck to the chest wall)
- Coagulopathy (or thrombocytopenia) is a relative contraindication

## Equipment

- Full sterile preparation
  - Hat, mask, gown, gloves, drapes, and skin-cleansing solution
- Syringe, 25G needle, and lidocaine 2% or 1%
- Scalpel
- Chest drain (sizes 20–32Fr); remove the trocar
- Spencer–Wells forceps (or needle holders)
  - 'Load' the chest drain onto the forceps using the distal side-hole
- Sutures
- Underwater drain, or Heimlich valve assembly
- Sterile dressing and adhesive dressings

### Anatomical landmarks

- Fifth intercostal space, mid-anterior axillary line

## Technique

- Prepare the skin with sterilizing solution
- Infiltrate 4–5 ml lidocaine subcutaneously and down into the muscles over the top edge of the sixth rib
- Perform a 2–3 cm transverse skin incision
- Perform blunt dissection down to pleura over top edge of sixth rib (to avoid the neurovascular bundle along the lower edge of fifth rib)
- Pierce the pleura with a fingertip and perform a finger sweep
- The chest drain should be guided into the pleural space using the attached Spencer–Wells forceps
- Detach and withdraw the forceps and then advance the drain by 10–15 cm (depending upon patient's body habitus)
- Hold in place and attach the underwater drain or Heimlich valve assembly (in mechanically ventilated patients the chest drain may be anchored with sutures first)
- Insert anchoring sutures at either end of the skin incision, and tie them off leaving long 'tails'; wrap the tails around the chest drain, throwing ties every two to three turns and ensuring that the suture is tight enough to indent the drain (avoid purse-string sutures)
- Place sterile dressings either side of the drain and fix in place with adhesive dressings
- Obtain a post-insertion CXR

## Complications

- Bleeding/haemothorax
- Lung laceration
- Surgical emphysema
- Failure of the lung to re-expand (if mechanically ventilated consider increasing the level of PEEP)
- Damage to intra-abdominal organs if placed to caudally!

# ① Arterial line insertion

### Indications

- Where beat-to-beat monitoring of blood pressure is desirable (e.g. during the titration of inotropes in cardiovascularly unstable patients)
- Where regular blood sampling is required (particularly arterial blood gas sampling)
- To allow pulse wave contour analysis to calculate cardiac output and systemic vascular resistance

### Contraindications

- Where blood supply to the associated limb is already compromised
- Coagulopathy (or thrombocytopenia) is a relative contraindication
- Where there is localized infection at the site of insertion

### Equipment

- Full sterile preparation
  - Hat, mask, gown, gloves, drapes, and skin-cleansing solution
- Syringe, 25G needle, and lidocaine 2% or 1%
- Arterial line of choice (commonly 20G)
- Transducer set (run through and zeroed)
- Suture
- Sterile dressing

### Anatomical landmarks

- The radial artery is palpable at the wrist; other palpable arteries include
  - Dorsalis pedis on the dorsum of the foot
  - Brachial or femoral arteries (longer arterial lines are available if required for femoral cannulation)
  - Posterior tibial artery at the ankle
  - Ulnar artery is often best avoided as cannulation of the radial artery is likely to have recently been attempted
- Doppler ultrasound may help identify arteries

### Technique

- Prepare the skin with cleansing solution
- Identify the artery by palpation
- Infiltrate puncture site with lidocaine
- Insert the needle/arterial line at an angle of 45°–60° to the skin, pointing proximally, until a flashback is seen
  - If a Seldinger kit is being used the guidewire is advanced; no resistance should be felt
  - If the line is a cannula kit, advance the cannula off the needle; again no resistance should be felt

- For difficult arteries the 'transfixion technique' may be more reliable. Following initial flashback the needle/cannula is advanced through the artery and then slowly withdrawn until blood flows; then the guidewire/cannula is advanced
- Attach the transducer set, suture the line in place, and cover with a sterile dressing

## Complications

- Inability to palpate the artery may occur, particularly in shutdown patients. Consider using the femoral or brachial arteries, or giving a small bolus of ephedrine (3–6 mg IV) or metaraminol (0.5–1.0 mg IV) to cause a transient rise in BP
- If ischaemia occurs distal to the arterial line, remove it
- Carefully label the arterial line to avoid inadvertent injections
- Bleeding/haematoma
- Infection: skin or CRBSI

# ! **Central venous catheter insertion**

**Indications**

- To measure CVP and guide fluid resuscitation
- To administer fluids, drugs (especially inotropes/vasopressors or potassium), or TPN
- Where extra IV access is required
- For CVVH
- Frequent blood sampling
- For specialist interventions: PAFC, temporary transvenous pacing

**Contraindications**

- Uncorrected coagulopathy or thrombocytopenia
- Damaged or infected skin at the point of insertion
- Being unable to lie supine (or head down) is a relative contraindication

**Equipment**

- Full sterile preparation
  - Hat, mask, gown, gloves, drapes, and skin-cleansing solution
- Syringe, needle, and lidocaine 2% or 1%
- Central venous catheter set (or dialysis catheter, PAFC sheath, etc.), which commonly contains
  - Needle and Seldinger wire
  - 5 ml syringe
  - Scalpel
- 20–30 ml sterile saline 0.9%
- 20ml syringe and blood culture bottles (if required)
- Transducer (run through and zeroed)
- Suture
- Sterile dressings
- Ultrasound machine (with sterile sheath and gel)

**Anatomical landmarks**

- Femoral vein (medial to the femoral artery, distal to the inguinal ligament) is the safest major vein to cannulate in an emergency (especially if coagulation status is not known) as inadvertent arterial puncture can be easily controlled
- Internal jugular: lateral to the carotid artery at the level of the thyroid cartilage (high approach) or at the point where the lateral and medial heads of the sternocleidomastoid meet (low approach)
- External jugular: identified by pressing across the base of the lateral side of the neck and occluding the flow of blood, allowing the vein to fill
- Subclavian: may be approached at any point along the middle third of the clavicle by directing the needle under the clavicle, and then towards the suprasternal notch. It is not recommended in emergency situations, unless the operator is skilled in its use, because US guidance is of little use, and there are associated risks of haemorrhage and pneumothorax

## Technique

- Check coagulation studies
- Prepare the CVC by flushing all the lumens through with saline
- Prepare the skin with cleansing solution and drape the patient
- Infiltrate puncture site with lidocaine
- Place the patient in a head-down position for internal jugular or subclavian approaches, head-up for femoral
- Identify the vein using ultrasound where possible (veins are compressible, non-pulsatile, and dilate during Valsalva manoeuvres)
- Half fill the 5 ml syringe with saline and attach the needle
- When ultrasound is used the needle should be perpendicular to the skin. Use short jabbing movements to help identify the needle tip on the ultrasound image
- When ultrasound is not used (not recommended), the relevant anatomy should be established. It is suggested for the internal jugular and femoral routes that, once the artery has been identified, the palpating fingers are only rested gently on the skin during venous puncture so as not to compress the vein
- A continuous gentle negative pressure should be maintained on the syringe until flashback is obtained (this often occurs as the needle is withdrawn because the vein is compressed on insertion)
- Once a flashback occurs the syringe should be disconnected with the needle stabilized. If there is doubt as to whether the needle is in a vein or artery a blood gas sample may be obtained and compared with $SpO_2$
- The Seldinger guidewire should be advanced (20–25 cm at the needle hub is all that is required in most patients); no resistance should be felt
- The needle is then withdrawn and the skin entry point incised with the scalpel
- The dilator should then be inserted (to between half and two-thirds its length) and removed—often easiest using a 'screwing' motion
- The central line is then threaded over the guidewire to the appropriate depth (12–14 cm for RIJ, REJ, or RSC lines; 16–20 cm for left-sided lines; inserted fully to the hub for femoral lines). Control of the guidewire should be maintained at all times to prevent accidental loss of the wire into the vein.
- The guidewire is then removed and the CVC sutured in place. Both the hub *and* adjustable clamp (if used) should be sutured.
- Check that blood can be aspirated from all lumens, and flush them with saline (in septic patients take this opportunity to take sterile blood cultures prior to flushing the line)
- Obtain a CXR for IJ, EJ, or SC lines to confirm correct position (the tip should be in the SVC just above/at the level of the carina) and to exclude pneumothorax and haemothorax

## Complications

- Arterial puncture
- Dysrhythmias
- Pneumothorax
- Haemothorax
- Cardiac tamponade
- Infection: skin or CRBSI

# ☠ IV cutdown

### Indications

- Where emergency IV access is required for fluid resuscitation and no other IV access is obtainable
  - Consider also alternatives such as central venous or intra-osseous access (or ETT access for drugs during cardiac arrest)

### Contraindications

- If the saphenous vein at the ankle is not accessible consider using the median cubital vein at the antecubital fossa

### Equipment

- Syringe, 25G needle, and lidocaine 2% or 1%
- Scalpel
- Artery clips (or similar)
- Surgical ties
- IV cannula (15–18G, stylet removed)
- IV fluid and giving set
- Suture

### Anatomical landmarks

- The great saphenous vein at the ankle
  - 2 cm anterior and 2 cm superior to the medial malleolus

### Technique

- Clean the area with antiseptic solution
- Infiltrate incision site with lidocaine
- Make a 2–3 cm transverse incision
- Use blunt dissection (using artery clips) to identify the vein and lift away a 2–3 cm portion of the vein from the tissues underlying it
- Pass two ties behind the vein, one caudal and one cephalad; tie off the caudal end and keep the cephalad tie as a sling
- Make a small incision in the vein and dilate it using the artery forceps
- Introduce the plastic cannula into the vein and use the sling/tie to secure it in place
- Attach the giving set to the cannula and infuse fluid
- Close the incision with interrupted sutures
- Remove the cannula as soon as the patient is stable and alternative IV access is available

### Complications

- The vein may be difficult to identify; the artery or nerve may be damaged
- Bleeding/haematoma
- Infection: skin, phlebitis, CRBSI

# ☠ External pacing

## Indications

- Complete heart block with associated hypotension
- Ventricular standstill
  - In both cases chemical means should be tried in the first instance if possible (e.g. a bolus of atropine and/or a low-dose adrenaline infusion)

## Contraindications

- The skin must be dry; it must be safe to approach the patient
- Remove GTN patches
- Avoid placement near an implanted pacemaker

## Equipment

- A defibrillator with transcutaneous pacing function
- Adhesive pads to attach to the patient

## Anatomical landmarks

- Pads should be placed over the sternum and apex. Alternatives include
  - Anterior–posterior: to the left of the sternum and just to the left of the midline on the back
  - Side to side: overlying the fourth and fifth intercostal spaces, both sides, in the mid-axillary line

## Technique

- Ensure pads are attached to clean dry skin if possible
- Choose *fixed* mode (consider *demand*, if available, once stable)
- Set the rate for 50–70/min
- Increase the *output* (start at 70 mA) until *capture* occurs: pacing spikes are seen and QRS complexes are triggered by them
- Once capture occurs set the output at 5–10 mA above the threshold
- If no capture occurs at 120 mA, consider resiting the electrodes
- Ensure there is a pulse present with QRS complexes; otherwise treat for PEA
- Muscle twitching is normal; provide sedation or analgesia if there is associated pain

## Complications

- Transcutaneous pacing is a temporary measure only; proceed to transvenous pacing as soon as appropriate
- Minor burning may occur; review the skin areas afterwards and treat as appropriate

# ☠ **Pericardiocentesis**

### Indications

- Cardiac tamponade
  - Pericardiocentesis may also be required for the drainage of large effusions, or in order to obtain diagnostic samples. In these situations it should be performed by an experienced operator under echocardiographic guidance

### Contraindications

- Where this is done during imminent or actual cardiac arrest there are no contraindications

## Equipment

- A 15 cm 16–18G cannula
  - In an emergency a 20G spinal needle (with stylet removed) or a 16–18G IV cannula may suffice
- A 20 ml syringe and a three-way-tap

## Anatomical landmarks

- The left xiphochondral angle

### Technique

- Monitor patient's ECG continuously
- Prepare the sub-xiphoid area with antiseptic solution if time allows
- Insert the cannula at an angle of 30°–45° to the skin, near the left xiphochondral angle, aiming towards the tip of the left scapula
- Advance slowly, aspirating gently at all times
- When fluid/blood is aspirated stop advancing the cannula; advance the catheter over the needle and remove the needle
- Attach the three-way tap and aspirate as much blood/fluid as possible
- Aspirating as little as 100 ml of blood is likely to make a dramatic difference to cardiac output, even in chronic massive effusions
- Secure the cannula in place as blood may re-accumulate
- Arrange formal drainage or surgery as soon as possible

## Complications

- ECG changes may be seen (QRS widening, ST–T wave changes, or ventricular ectopics) if the cannula is advanced too far; withdraw the needle and redirect more posteriorly
- Always perform under echocardiographic guidance unless there is imminent/actual cardiac arrest

# ! Fibreoptic bronchoscopy

### Indications

- Confirmation of ETT or tracheostomy position
- To obtain microbiological samples via suction or BAL
- To localize and control haemoptysis
- To remove secretions, blood clots, or foreign bodies
- To examine for strictures, tumours, or tracheobronchial trauma (including burns or smoke inhalation damage)

### Contraindications

- Relative contraindications include
  - Moderate/severe hypoxaemia or hypercapnia
  - Coagulopathy, SVC obstruction, or other risk of bleeding
  - Near-complete tracheal obstruction
  - Myocardial ischaemia, dysrhythmias, or hypotension

### Equipment

- An assistant to monitor the patient and provide sedation if required
- Gown, gloves, and mask
- A fibreoptic bronchoscope with suction/biopsy channel (already sterilized)
- Light source
- Suction source and suction tubing (attach this to the bronchoscope)
- Angle-piece adapter
- Sputum traps, syringes, 0.9% saline for lavages
- Lubricant

### Anatomical landmarks

- A knowledge of the tracheo-bronchial tree is required

### Technique

- Pre-oxygenate patient by increasing $FiO_2$ to 100%
- Ensure that the patient's ETT is a size 8 or greater
- Consider deepening sedation and/or adding neuromuscular blockade
- Scrub and dress in gown and gloves; technique should be as sterile as possible
- Attach the angle-piece adapter to the ETT and pass the lubricated bronchoscope through it
- Identify the carina and systematically explore the tracheo-bronchial tree, starting on the 'good' side where possible
- Where secretions are present insert the suction trap and collect specimens
- If a BAL is required identify the appropriate site and inject 20–30 ml sterile water which is then suctioned back up into a sputum trap
    - Avoid performing BALs on more than one side (ideally just one lobe)
    - Use ≤100 ml water in total
    - Send BAL samples for microscopy and Gram's stain, culture (consider viral and fungal culture, and immunofluorescence for Legionella or PCC where appropriate)
- Clean and sterilise the bronchoscope after use

### Complications

- Tracheobronchial trauma/bleeding
- Pneumothorax (consider requesting a CXR)

# ① Intra-abdominal pressure measurement

### Indications

- The detection of IAH and ACS in patients with:
  - Blunt abdominal trauma (ACS can develop in up to 15% of patients)
  - Abdominal surgery with primary closure
  - Severe burns with eschar formation
  - Prone positioning
  - Bowel obstruction
  - Haemoperitoneum, pneumoperitoneum
  - Ascites or visceral oedema, infection, liver failure, pancreatitis, massive fluid resuscitation
  - Peritonitis, intra-abdominal abscesses
  - Tumour, haematoma, surgical packs
  - Pelvic fracture

### Contraindications

- The catheter must be patent; clot retention/bladder irrigation is a relative contraindication (discuss with a urologist; irrigation may be temporarily suspended)

### Equipment

- The patient should already have a urinary catheter in place
- A manometry column should be attached to the catheter
  - Alternatively the catheter outflow may be clamped and a transducer set attached to it (using a needle to go through the urine sampling port)
- Sterile water
- 20 ml syringe

### Anatomical landmarks

- The mid-axillary line is the recommended zero-point though some units use the symphysis pubis

### Technique

- The patient should be supine
- 20–25 ml of sterile water should be instilled into the bladder via the catheter
- After 30–60 seconds the pressure should be measured (at end-expiration)

### Complications

- Artificially high readings may be measured; re-check IAP before considering treatment to ensure that any increase is sustained

# ⓘ **Lumbar puncture**

### Indications

- Suspected meningitis
- SAH
- Peripheral neuropathy (e.g. GBS)

### Contraindications

- Raised ICP (perform CT head scan beforehand)
- Uncorrected coagulopathy or thrombocytopenia
- Damaged or infected skin at the point of insertion

### Equipment

- Full sterile preparation
  - Hat, mask, gown, gloves, drapes, and skin-cleansing solution
- Syringe, 25G needle, and lidocaine 2% or 1%
- Introducing needle
- 20–24G atraumatic spinal needle (e.g. Whittacre)
- A CSF manometry set with a three-way tap *or* an arterial/CVP transducer giving set (zeroed to the level of the spine and kept completely sterile)
  - Manometry sets will take a long time to fill with very small gauge needles
- Three sterile universal containers and a glucose measurement bottle

### Anatomical landmarks

- L3/4 interspace: the gap between the spinous processes of L3 and L4, approximately level with the iliac crests

### Technique

- Position the patient on their side, with their chin on their chest and their knees drawn up (the 'fetal' position)
- Identify the L3/4 interspace (if the patient is able to speak, and spinous processes are hard to palpate, ask them to confirm when you are touching the midline)
- Indent the skin (i.e. using the hub of a needle) at the appropriate point
- Scrub, gown (mask, hat, etc.), drape the area, and prepare the skin
- Infiltrate lidocaine around the previously indented area
- Insert the introducer needle into the indented area, staying perpendicular to the skin
- Advance the spinal needle through the introducer until a 'give' is felt as it passes through the dura. Stop. Withdraw and redirect if the patient complains of 'shooting' pains at any point
- Remove the stylet and observe for CSF

- If the subarachnoid space is not found, withdraw the spinal needle into the introducer needle, redirect the introducer needle, and advance again
- If using a manometer, attach it (with the three-way tap in the appropriate position) and let fluid collect to measure the opening pressure. Then use the fluid within the manometer and collect further fluid for samples (see below)
- If using the transducer technique collect the samples first to avoid contamination
- Samples: collect 1–1.5 ml in each of the three universal containers (and also in the glucose bottle) and send for
  - Microscopy and culture, protein, glucose, PCR (and consider cytology, AFBs, cryptococcal antigen, India ink stain, fungal culture, and oligoclonal bands)
- If using the transducer technique, connect to the transducer and allow the trace time to approach the mean (30–60 seconds)
- Remove the needle and dress the wound
- Send a blood glucose sample as well

## Complications

- The most common complication is failure to identify the subarachnoid space; repositioning the patient to increase the lumbar kyphosis often helps
- Post-dural puncture headache is common with larger needles and multiple attempts. If it occurs discuss treatment options with an anaesthetist
- Nerve damage (rare): stop and withdraw if shooting pain occurs
- Infection (as meningitis or as an epidural abscess) or bleeding may occur, but are uncommon
- Coning may occur if raised ICP is present (i.e. not identified beforehand)

# ⓘ Sengstaken–Blakemore tube insertion

### Indications
- Severe upper GI haemorrhage due to varices when other methods (e.g. endoscopic sclerotherapy) cannot be used

### Contraindications
- Oesophageal perforation
- Previous oesophageal surgery

### Equipment
- A Sengstaken–Blakemore tube, or equivalent
  - SSB tubes have three ports (oesophageal and intragastric balloons and gastric aspirate ports)
  - Minnesota tubes have four ports (as above with extra oesophageal aspirate port)
  - Linton–Nachlas tube (has a larger intragastric balloon)
  - Check all balloons prior to use
- 50 ml syringe
- Lubrication
- Mouth guard
- Lidocaine spray 4%
- Marker pen
- Non-toothed clamps (Kelly clamps)

### Anatomical landmarks
- The intragastric balloon should be below the diaphragm on X-ray

### Technique
- Most patients will be intubated and mechanically ventilated to allow insertion of the SSB tube
  - In awake patients, if available and time allows, spray the back of the mouth with 4% lidocaine
  - The patient should be supine or in the left lateral position
- Insert the tube via the mouth using the mouth guard
  - In anaesthetized patients use laryngoscopy to aid oesophageal insertion
- Pass the tube until the gastric balloon is in the stomach; then gently inject 50–100 ml of air into the intragastric port listening with a stethoscope over the stomach to check for sounds of insufflation (also use pressure monitoring to confirm that pressure does not exceed 15 mmHg)
- Inject further air to a total of 200–300 ml (stop if there is patient discomfort) and clamp the port

- Gently apply traction on the tube to bring the gastric balloon up to the fundus
- Check the tube position with a thoraco-abdominal X-ray
- Inflate the oesophageal balloon to a pressure of 20–30 mmHg and clamp
- Return the patient to a 30°–40° head-up position
- Mark the position of the tube at the teeth using a marker pen
- Apply 250 g of traction to the tube
- SSB tubes can stay in place for 1–3 days
- Deflate the oesophageal balloon for 10 minutes every 2–4 hours to decrease the likelihood of oesophageal ischaemia

## Complications
- Re-bleeding
- Oesophageal ischaemia

# ① **Prone positioning**

### Indications

- To improve oxygenation in ALI or ARDS
- To improve the mobilization of secretions and decrease basal atelectasis

### Contraindications

- Facial injuries or burns where loss of airway may occur
- Unstable spinal or pelvic fractures
- Raised IAP; recent abdominal trauma or surgery
- Pregnancy
- Seizures; head injuries with raised ICP
- Raised IOP
- Relative contraindications include
  - Morbid obesity
  - Cardiovascular instability or hypotension
  - Recent tracheostomy
  - Agitation or pain

### Equipment

- Liquid paraffin and gel pads for eye protection
- Five staff (ideally one airway trained)
- Four extra pillows

### Technique

- Check ABGs prior to changing position
- Remove all non-essential monitoring (keep pulse oximetry attached)
- Aspirate NGT and perform tracheal suctioning
- Apply eye protection (as above)
- Ensure analgesia is adequate; increased sedation and neuromuscular blockade may be required
- Check the airway (ensure the ETT is secure and check position at teeth/gums)
- Position two staff at either side of the patient and one at the head ('head' controls the timing of all movement)
- Disconnect ventilator tubing from the patient prior to all moves
- Place the patient's arms by their side (palms in) and place a pillow between the patient's legs
- 'Mummy-wrap' the patient in the sheets they are lying on and slide them to the edge of the bed
- Place pillows beside the patient at the level of the upper chest, the pelvis, and the ankles
- Roll the patient over onto the pillows and ensure that the abdomen 'hangs' free; bring one arm forward and turn the head towards one side, adopting the 'swimmer's position'

- Reconnect the ventilator tubing, all monitoring, and lines
- Position the whole bed 30°–45° head up
- Check all pressure or stress areas (toes, knees, genitalia, elbows, wrists, breasts, neck, chin, lips, nose, eyes, ears); make sure pressure points are hanging free or are very well padded; make sure joints are in physiological acceptable positions

## Complications

- Loss of airway: re-intubation in the prone position is difficult. Should it occur rapidly return the patient to the supine position; if this is impossible an LMA may be inserted as a temporary measure
- Hypotension may occur immediately after turning
- Skin joint or nerve damage may occur
- Dependent facial oedema may occur

# Index